D1498777

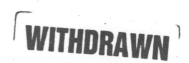

NORTHEAST COMMUNITY COLLEGE LIBRARY

WITHDRAWN

Exotic Animal Medicine

Dedication

As always, to Lisa

For Elsevier:

Commissioning Editor: *Rita Demetriou-Swanwick / Robert Edwards*
Development Editor: *Louisa Welch*
Project Manager: *Christine Johnston*
Designer: *Charles Gray*
Illustration Manager: *Bruce Hogarth*
Illustrator: *Debbie Maizels, Zoobotanica*

Exotic Animal
Medicine
A QUICK REFERENCE GUIDE

Lance Jepson MA, VetMB, CBiol, MIBiol, MRCVS

vet4dragons, Veterinary Referral & Consultancy
Service for Aquatic & Exotic Animals, Haverfordwest, UK

Foreword by
Scott J. Stahl, DVM, DABVP-Avian
Stahl Exotic Animal Veterinary Services, Virginia, USA

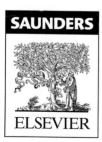

SAUNDERS

ELSEVIER

Edinburgh London New York Oxford Philadelphia St Louis Sydney Toronto 2009

636.089
J549e

SAUNDERS
ELSEVIER

© 2009, Elsevier Limited. All rights reserved.

No part of this publication may be reproduced, stored in a retrieval system, or transmitted in any form or by any means, electronic, mechanical, photocopying, recording or otherwise, without either the prior permission of the publishers or a licence permitting restricted copying in the United Kingdom issued by the Copyright Licensing Agency, 90 Tottenham Court Road, London W1T 4LP. Permissions may be sought directly from Elsevier's Health Sciences Rights Department in Philadelphia , USA: phone: (+1) 215 239 3804, fax: (+1) 215 239 3805, e-mail: healthpermissions@elsevier.com. You may also complete your request on-line via the Elsevier homepage (http://www.elsevier.com), by selecting 'Support and contact' and then 'Copyright and Permission'.

First published 2009
  Reprinted 2010 (twice)

ISBN: 978-0-7020-2873-1

British Library Cataloguing in Publication Data
A catalogue record for this book is available from the British Library

Library of Congress Cataloging in Publication Data
A catalog record for this book is available from the Library of Congress

Knowledge and best practice in this field are constantly changing. As new research and experience broaden our knowledge, changes in practice, treatment and drug therapy may become necessary or appropriate. Readers are advised to check the most current information provided (i) on procedures featured or (ii) by the manufacturer of each product to be administered, to verify the recommended dose or formula, the method and duration of administration, and contraindications. It is the responsibility of the practitioner, relying on their own experience and knowledge of the patient, to make diagnoses, to determine dosages and the best treatment for each individual patient, and to take all appropriate safety precautions.
  To the fullest extent of the law, neither the publisher nor the author assumes any liability for any injury and/or damage.

The Publisher

 ELSEVIER your source for books, journals and multimedia in the health sciences
www.elsevierhealth.com

Working together to grow
libraries in developing countries
www.elsevier.com | www.bookaid.org | www.sabre.org

ELSEVIER   BOOK AID International   Sabre Foundation

The Publisher's policy is to use paper manufactured from sustainable forests

Printed in China

Contents

Acknowledgements

· ·

Exotic pets are more popular than ever. In some cases they provide companionship, in others they are a fascination and a hobby, and in still others, a cause. I am privileged to be a veterinary surgeon who works solely with exotic species. A great many people have influenced and inspired my professional life in both its course and its content. Many of these are colleagues, students or clients who have become more friends than 'customers'. To single them out would be to put one above the other and I cannot do that, but thank you all.

Foreword

It has been almost 10 years now since I first met Lance Jepson. We were both instructors for a British Small Animal Veterinary Association course in Exotic Animal Medicine in Tewkesbury, Gloucestershire. After a long day of teaching, with each of us 'tag team' lecturing to the delegates, we met in the pub that night for some libation. Even though we had spent the entire day on the subject we were both so excited about the growth and potential within the field of exotic animal medicine, we continued to talk into the wee hours of the night. As we parted, we agreed to continue to focus our clinical work on 'exclusively' exotic pets and we each hoped to one day publish a clinically-relevant book to share our enthusiasm with colleagues.

Lance has done just that with this book *Exotic Animal Medicine: A Quick Reference Guide*. Writing such a book is truly a monumental task. What the author has provided here is a practical clinician's guide to approaching the exotic pet. The book is user friendly, works nicely as a quick reference, but also provides a review of pertinent clinical information with detailed rule-out lists.

Perhaps the most valuable part of this book is that Lance provides specific information, including diagnostic approaches, clinical techniques, anesthetic protocols and treatment regimens that have worked for him over many years in clinical practice. These days in an atmosphere of 'data overload' with so many internet sources, journals, magazines and other reference books, it is becoming more difficult for veterinarians to wade through materials to find a source of useful clinically-applicable material. Veterinarians, especially practitioners just getting started in the field of exotic animal medicine, will find this book invaluable.

As promised in the pub that night, Lance has devoted his career to working with these non-traditional pets and with this book has found a way to provide something valuable to his colleagues!

Scott J. Stahl, DVM, DABVP-Avian
Stahl Exotic Animal Veterinary Services
Fairfax, Virginia, USA
www.seavs.com

Introduction

How to use this book

During their training, veterinarians are taught to apply the same core set of clinical skills and thought processes to the health problems and management of several different domestic species. Often due to time constraints and outmoded perceptions, exotic pets fall off the radar. The practising veterinarian often, therefore, feels at a disadvantage when presented with the more unusual species, yet those same core skills, backed by relevant information, can be applied as easily to a bearded dragon as they can to a bearded collie.

Exotic Animal Medicine: A Quick Reference Guide is designed to aid the veterinary clinician to professionally and quickly deal with a wide array of exotic pets and their problems. It allows the veterinarian to create a diagnostic and treatment plan in a short space of time for a wide range of exotic pets, some of which he or she may not be familiar with.

The approach is hoped to be a practical one, combining both clinical signs and/or an organ system perspective. Thus, a parrot may present with a loss of flight (clinical sign) or have a liver disorder diagnosed on blood sampling (organ system). Where relevant, there is cross-referencing between the different sections.

Lists of differential diagnoses

These provide the clinician with a rapid overview of the likely conditions to be encountered in a given animal group. Where no examples are listed but the heading is still included, these should still be considered even though no examples have been reported in the literature. As an example, neoplasia should occur on most lists of differential diagnoses.

Findings on clinical examination

These list the commonest signs seen within the given group of disorders. Not every clinical sign will be seen in every case, and because of this some may appear contradictory. They are given as an aid to diagnosis. Some diseases may present as a syndrome of typical signs and where this occurs an indication of that disease is given in brackets at the end of the description. I have tried to make these complete and accurate wherever possible, but the huge range of individual and species responses to a multitude of diseases and challenges mean that variations outside those listed are possible.

Investigations

A list of the basic types of investigative procedures is offered to stimulate ideas on how to approach a given case. In some cases, useful general tips are given; in others, normal values (or expected abnormalities) that may be difficult to find in the literature are given where it may aid a diagnosis. In some cases, specific tests for certain diseases, e.g. PCRs, are listed to aid the clinician with the tests that are potentially available (although this may vary from country to country). A basic list of investigations is as follows and, where appropriate, is included in each section to act as a reminder:

- Radiography
- Routine haematology and biochemistry
- Culture and sensitivity
- Endoscopy
- Biopsy/necropsy
- Ultrasonography

It is hoped that by the consideration and undertaking of appropriate tests, diagnoses can be achieved, even if these fall outside the potential differential lists. Other more advanced, potential investigative techniques such as MRI and CT scans are not to be ruled out or discounted – where practical, their use can make a significant contribution to the diagnostic procedure, but it is assumed that most practising clinicians will not have ready access to these facilities.

Management

In most cases, the clinician is referred to the section on *Nursing Care* at the beginning of each chapter. In some conditions, specific recommendations are given.

Treatment/specific therapy

For each condition, suggested treatment options are given. Not every drug variation is listed, as there are some excellent resources, such as *The Veterinary Formulary* (Pharmaceutical Press), that amply cover this and to which the clinician may already have access. The majority of the drugs mentioned are not licensed for use in the species described and, where applicable, consent should be gained from the owner before their use. Due consideration should be given to mandatory drug selection procedures where such systems exist, for example the cascade system in the UK.

Ferrets

Ferrets (*Mustela putorius furo*) are thought to be a domesticated form of the European polecat (*M. putorius*) and, not surprisingly, have a history extending back alongside the domestic rabbit. Originally kept as working animals, selective breeding for colour varieties and temperament has resulted in a significant rise in their being kept as pets and show animals.

Table 1.1 The ferret: Key facts

Average life span (years)		5–8+
Weight (kg)	Male	1.0–2.0 kg
	Female	0.5–1.0 kg
Body temperature (°C)		37.8–40
Respiratory rate (per min)		33–36
Heart rate (beats/min)		180–250
Gestation (days)		41–42
Age at weaning (weeks)		6–8
Sexual maturity		4–8 months (in the first spring following birth – typically March)

Consultation and handling

Ferrets vary markedly in their temperament; working ferrets are perhaps slightly more unpredictable, whereas pet ferrets are usually well handled and unlikely to bite unless provoked. When handling a ferret, it can be easily restrained around the neck; a towel can be used – draped over the body before grasping the neck to protect from scratching. For those ferrets determined to bite, scruffing and holding with all four legs off the table will usually relax them to allow a reasonable examination.

Many ferrets intensely enjoy certain commercially available dietary supplements, e.g. Ferretone (8 in 1) to the extent that they will readily tolerate some procedures, e.g. ECG, so long as they are supplied with a steady stream of product to lick.

Always weigh the ferret whenever examined, to monitor weight trends. A healthy ferret above ground walks with a dorsal flexure in its back. Hind-leg paresis can be a non-specific sign of ill-health in the ferret due to weakness of the muscle groups needed to maintain this position.

Odour is a feature of ferret life and is likely to be used for transmitting and receiving information about individuals, such as identification, age, sex and sexual readiness. Most of this smell comes from the sebaceous skin glands, which regress following routine castration or ovario-hysterectomy. The anal sacs can produce a strong-smelling liquid, but this tends only to occur if the ferret is frightened. Therefore the routine anal gland removal ('descenting') of ferrets is largely pointless and could constitute unnecessary surgery.

Blood sampling

Suitable sites for venepuncture are the jugular, cephalic and saphenous veins. Alternatively, the ventral tail artery and veins can be used.

Blood collection from the tail in the ferret

1. The ferret is held on its back with ventral tail shaved.
2. Use a 21 or 23 gauge 25 mm needle.
3. There is a flattened area on the ventral side for the proximal 4–5 cm overlying the ventral concavity of the caudal vertebrae.
4. The artery there is flanked by two veins.
5. The needle is inserted at a shallow angle towards the body around 3–4 cm from the base of the tail.

Note that if blood sampling is done under isoflurane anaesthetic, isoflurane has been linked with a reduction in PCV, haemoglobin level and RBC count. In addition, one may need to centrifuge for 20% longer than in other species and collect $3 \times$ plasma volume required. This may be due to increased erythropoiesis from the spleen.

The typical WBC count is neutrophilic with <30% lymphocytes. Absolute and relative increases in lymphocyte counts may indicate lymphosarcoma.

It is not uncommon for ferrets to have two or more pathologic conditions ongoing at the same time. Combinations include variations on insulinomas, hyperadrenocortism, lymphoma and cardiomyopathy. The clinician should always be aware that the situation may be more complicated that it initially appears and be prepared to investigate several possible clinical problems simultaneously.

Avoid gentamicin, as it has been associated with nephrotoxicity and ototoxicity (deafness) in ferrets.

Nursing care

Thermoregulation

For general principles, see *Thermoregulation* under 'Nursing Care', in Ch. 2, *Rabbits*.

Fluid therapy

The normal maintenance daily water intake for ferrets is 75–100 mL/kg per day. In ferrets, the choice of fluid used is indicated as with other mammals. Fluid replacement calculations are as for other species. All fluids should be warmed to 38°C.

Recommended fluid replacement rates for ferrets

1. Subcutaneous: 30–60 mL.
2. Intraperitoneal: 30–60 mL.
3. Ferrets in shock or suffering from profound losses from vomiting and diarrhoea may need up to 180–240 mL/kg over a 24 h period.
4. Crystalloids: For ferrets the maintenance fluid rate is 75–100 mL/kg per 24 h. Shock rate is up to 100 mL/kg over 1 hour.
5. Colloids. A bolus of 10–15 mL/kg over 30 min can be given up to four times daily.

Blood transfusions

Blood volume is 40–60 mL per ferret. Blood groups have not been demonstrated (Manning & Bell 1990), so there is thought to be no need for cross-matching.

Estimation of blood volume requirement

Based upon an assumption of 70 mL/kg per h maintenance fluid requirement (Orcutt 1998):

$$\text{Anticoagulated blood volume(mL)} = \text{body weight(kg)} \times 70$$

$$\times \frac{\text{PCV desired-PCV recipient}}{\text{PCV of donor in anticoagulant}}$$

Nutritional support

- Ferrets are prone to hypoglycaemia, so nutritional support is imperative. If anorexic for even a comparatively short time, a ferret may be hypoglycaemic, so test with a commercial glucometer on a small sample of blood. Glucose, either i.v. or i.p., can be given to these cases once identified (see *Pancreatic Disorders* for normal blood glucose values).
- Commercially available high-energy dog and cat recovery foods, e.g. Prescription Diet Canine/Feline a/d (Hills Pet Products) are suitable.
- Force-feeding is possible with these supplements at 2–5 mL, 3–4 times daily.

Analgesia

Analgesic doses for ferrets are given in Table 1.2.

Table 1.2 The ferret: Analgesic doses

Analgesic	Dose
Buprenorphine	0.01–0.03 mg/kg s.c., i.m., i.v. every 8–12 h
Butorphanol	0.1–0.5 mg/kg s.c., i.m. or i.v. every 2–4 h
Carprofen	1.0–2.0 mg/kg s.c., i.m. every 12–24 h
Ketoprofen	1.0 mg/kg s.c., i.m. every 12–24 h
Meloxicam	0.1–0.3 mg/kg s.c. or p.o. every 24 h
Morphine	0.5–5.0 mg/kg s.c., i.m. every 2–6 h
Pethidine	5–10 mg/kg s.c., i.m., i.v. every 2–4 h
Nalbuphine	0.5–1.5 mg/kg i.m., i.v. every 2–3 h

Anaesthesia

Ferrets have a very short gut transit time of around 3 h, therefore if starved overnight there is a high risk of hypoglycaemia. Therefore, do not starve preoperatively.

There are many anaesthetic protocols written up in the literature. The author has found the following protocols useful:

Anaesthetic protocol

1. Pre-medication
   a. Acepromazine (ACP) at 0.1–0.3 mg/kg i.m. or s.c.
   b. Diazepam at 2 mg/kg i.m. or s.c.
2. Ferrets are easily induced with 5% isoflurane, head held in a mask.
3. Intubate.

Parenteral anaesthesia

1. Propofol at 2–10 mg/kg i.v.
   or
2. Ketamine at 5 mg/kg; medetomidine at 80 µg/kg; butorphanol at 100 µg/kg, all given simultaneously i.m.
3. Intubate and maintain with isoflurane as necessary.

- Intraoperative care
  - Keep warm (see *Thermoregulation*)
  - Fluids (see *Fluid Therapy*)

- Postoperative care
  - Reverse medetomidine (if used) with atipamezole at 0.4–1.0 mg/kg i.m.
  - Analgesia – as for other small mammals
  - Must be offered food as soon as recovers
  - Keep warm.

Cardiopulmonary resuscitation

1. Intubate and ventilate at 20–30 breaths/min.
2. Reverse medetomidine (if used) with atipamezole at 0.4–1.0 mg/kg i.m.
3. If cardiac arrest, external cardiac massage at around 100 compressions/min.
4. Epinephrine at:
   a. 0.2–0.4 mg/kg diluted in sterile saline intratracheal
   b. 0.2 mg/kg intracardiac, i.v. or i.o.
5. Fluid therapy (see above).
6. If bradycardic, atropine at 0.05 mg/kg i.v. 0.05–0.1 mg/kg intratracheal.

Skin disorders

- Ferrets under a seasonal cycle of hair thinning occurring during the summer months. There are multiple sebaceous glands in the skin that impart both a greasy feel to the coat and the typical musky ferret smell. These glands are more numerous in males, and in some albino males they can produce a dirty, yellow appearance. Routine neutering causes some atrophy of these glands reducing the odour.

Pruritus
- Ectoparasites
  - *Note* that *Sarcoptes scabei* presents in two clinical patterns – generalized and localized to the feet
- Hyperadrenocortism (see *Endocrine Disorders*)
- Pyoderma
  - Staphylococci
  - Streptococci
- *Corynebacterium*
  - *Pasteurella*
  - Actinomyces
  - *E. coli*
- Dermatophytosis.

Alopecia
- Self-mutilation
- Hormonal
- Hyperadrenocortism (see *Endocrine Disorders*, Fig. 1.1)
- Ovarian pedicle neoplasia (Patterson et al 2003)
- Alopecia at tail base (hyperoestrogenism – see *Reproductive System Disorders*)
- Seasonal alopecia

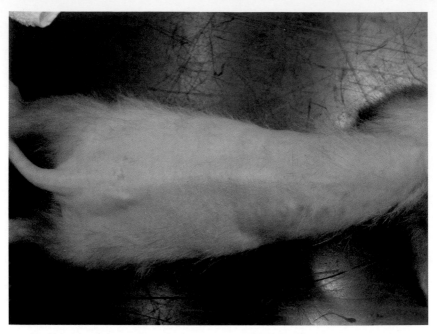

Fig. 1.1. Bilateral symmetrical alopecia in a female ferret with hyperadrenocortism.

- Pregnancy toxaemia/ketosis (see *Reproductive System Disorders*)
- Dermatophytosis
- Mucormycosis (*Absidia corymbifera*)
- Biotin deficiency (feeding raw eggs).

Scaling and crusting

- Canine distemper virus (CDV) (see *Systemic Disorders*)
- Pyoderma
- Dermatophytosis.

Erosions and ulceration

- Excoriation from self-inflicted trauma if pruritic
- Bite wound
- *Blastomyces dermatitidis*
- *Cryptococcus bacillisporus.*

Nodules and non-healing wounds

- Abscess
- Haematoma
- Granuloma
- Swollen mammary glands
    - Painful, discoloured (acute mastitis, neoplasia) (see *Reproductive System Disorders*)

- Non-painful, normal colour (chronic mastitis, neoplasia) (see *Reproductive System Disorders*)
- Swollen, discharging swellings around neck (actinomycosis).

Changes in pigmentation

- Dry, dull coat (poor diet)
- Canine distemper virus (CDV) (see *Systemic Disorders*)
- Swollen painful mammary glands. May turn black (gangrenous) (acute mastitis) (see *Reproductive System Disorders*)
- Ectoparasites
  - Fleas (*Ctenocephalides spp*)
  - Ear mites *Otodectes cyanotis*
  - Ticks
  - *Sarcoptes scabei*
  - Myiasis
  - *Cuterebra spp*
  - *Hypoderma bovis.*

Neoplasia

- Mast cell tumour
- Sebaceous gland adenoma
- Haemangioma
- Squamous cell carcinoma
- Benign cystic adenoma
- Preputial adenocarcinoma
- Dermatofibroma
- Carcinoma
- Fibroma
- Fibrosarcoma
- Histiocytoma
- Sarcoma
- Lymphoma (rarely presents as a skin lesion).

Findings on clinical examination

- Thick brown, waxy exudate from ears (ear mites)
- Pruritus and inflammation limited to feet (*Sarcoptes scabei*)
- Hyperkeratosis of the footpads and erythematous cutaneous rashes in the inguinal area and under the chin. Oculo-nasal discharge (CDV)
- Swellings with discharging sinuses in the cervical area (bite wounds, actinomycosis).

Investigations

1. Microscopy: examine fur pluck, acetate strips or skin scrapes to affected area and examine for ectoparasites
2. Examine material from ear canals for *Otodectes cynotis*
3. Bacteriology and mycology: hair pluck or swab lesions for routine culture and sensitivity
4. Fine-needle aspirate followed by staining with rapid Romanowski stains

5. Biopsy obvious lesions
6. Ultraviolet (Wood's) lamp – positive for *Microsporium canis* only (not all strains fluoresce)
7. Radiography
8. Routine haematology and biochemistry
9. Culture and sensitivity
10. Endoscopy
11. Biopsy
12. Ultrasonography.

Treatment/specific therapy

- Fleas
  - Commercial flea treatments at cat dose rates
  - Lufenuron at 10 mg/kg s.c. or 30 mg/kg p.o. in food
  - Topical spot on preparations of 10% (w/v) imidacloprid (Advantage, Bayer) at 10 mg/kg and 10% (w/v) imidacloprid/50% (w/v) permethrin (Advantix, Bayer) at 10 mg/kg have proven efficacious at flea control on the mink (Larsen et al 2005) and should be safe on the ferret. Environmental flea control will be required
- Sarcoptic mange
  - Ivermectin at 0.2–0.4 mg/kg s.c. every 7–14 days to resolution
  - Selamectin at dose for ear mites (see *Ear mites* below)
  - Moxidectin at dose for ear mites (see *Ear mites* below)
- Ear mites
  - Topical antiparasitic ear preparations, although the small size of the ear canal may prevent effective treatment
  - Selamectin spot-on at 6 mg/kg as a topical spot-on preparation; has proven safe at 45 mg /adult ferret (Stronghold Cat, Pfizer) (Miller et al 2006)
  - 10% imidacloprid/1% moxidectin (Advocate, Bayer) at 1 drop per 100 g body-weight (Beck 2007)
  - Cross infection with dogs and cats in the same household may occur
- Myiasis
  - Removal of larvae
  - Clean and debride wounds
  - Systemic parasiticide, e.g. ivermectin, selectin, imidacloprid
  - Covering antibiosis
  - Supportive therapy if necessary
- Pyoderma, bacterial dermatitis and cellulitis
  - Shave any badly infected areas
  - Topical and parenteral antibiotics
  - Cleaning with chlorhexidine solution may be beneficial
- Surgical removal of abscesses
- Bites and lacerations
  - Clean and debride well
  - Covering broad-spectrum antibiosis
- Actinomycosis
  - Debride and clean lesion
  - Appropriate antibiosis

- Dermatophytosis, *Blastomyces* and mucormycosis
  - Miconazole/chlorhexidine (Malaseb, Leo) shampoo – bath once daily
  - Griseofulvin at 25 mg/kg p.o. s.i.d. for 21–30 days
  - Itraconazole at 25–33 mg/kg p.o. s.i.d. for 30 days
  - Ketoconazole at 10–30 mg/kg p.o. s.i.d. for 60 days
- Cryptococcus
  - Amphotericin B at 150 mg/kg i.v. 3 times weekly for 2–4 months
- Seasonal alopecia
  - In breeding season (March to August). Will regrow
  - Hair loss occurring in winter and early spring may be an early indicator of hyperadrenocortism (see *Endocrine Disorders*)
- Self-mutilation
  - Lack of suitable hiding places or other stressors
  - Females plucking hair for nesting
- Biotin deficiency
  - Associated with diets >10% raw egg
  - Reduce egg intake and supplement with proprietary vitamin formula
- Neoplasia
  - Aggressive surgical resection
  - Chemotherapy may be attempted. Accessible cutaneous tumours can be treated by injecting cisplatin directly into the tissue mass on a weekly basis as a debulking exercise.

Respiratory tract disorders

Ferrets constantly investigate and monitor their environment by sniffing all available surfaces, hence sneezing is not uncommon.

Viral

- Canine distemper virus (CDV) (see *Systemic Disorders*)
- Influenza virus (orthomyxovirus).

Bacterial

- Bacterial pneumonias
- *Streptococcus zooepidemicus, S. pneumoniae,* group C and G *Streptococci*
- *E. coli*
- *Klebsiella pneumoniae*
- *Pseudomonas aeruginosa*
- *Bordetella bronchiseptica*
- *Listeria monocytogenes*
- Mycobacteriosis: *M. bovis, M. abscessus.*

Fungal

- *Cryptococcus*
- *Blastomyces dermatitidis*
- *Coccidioides immitis*
- Other fungal mycoses, e.g. Aspergillus (rare).

Protozoal

* *Pneumocystis carinii.*

Neoplasia

* Lymphoma/lymphosarcoma (see *Systemic Disorders*)
* Lung metastases.

Other non-infectious problems

* Cardiac disorders
* Hyperoestrogenism (see *Reproductive Disorders*)
* Gastric bloat (see *Gastrointestinal Tract Disorders*).

Findings on clinical examination

* Sneezing
* Coughing
* Dyspnoea and tachypnea
* 'Air hunger'
* Cyanosis
* Respiratory signs varying from a catarrhal rhinitis to pneumonia, plus oculo-nasal discharge, hyperkeratosis and gastrointestinal signs (CDV)
* Pale mucous membranes (anaemia – see *Cardiovascular and Haematologic Disorders*)
* Ocular and/or nasal discharges (CDV, influenza)
* Lethargy, dullness, depression, and pyrexia in addition to upper respiratory signs (influenza).

Investigations

1. Tracheal wash/bronchoalveolar lavage
2. Culture and sensitivity
3. Cytology
4. Pleural tap and cytology
5. Radiography
   a. Mediastinal lymphoma with pleural effusions occurs more commonly in younger ferrets
6. Routine haematology and biochemistry
7. Serology for CDV, *Mycobacterium bovis,* influenza (haemagglutination inhibition tests and ELISAs may be of benefit in detecting influenza A)
8. Endoscopy
9. Biopsy
10. Ultrasonography.

Management

1. Give supportive treatment, e.g. fluids, covering antibiosis.
2. Reduce stress levels. Hospitalize away from dogs and noisy cats; keep in darkened position.
3. Supply oxygen, preferably via an 'oxygen-tent'.

4. Mucolytics may be useful, e.g. bromhexine, N-acetyl-cysteine.
5. Pleural effusion – consider tube thoracostomy.

Treatment/specific therapy

- Canine distemper virus (see *Systemic Disorders*)
- Influenza
  - Ferrets are very susceptible to the human influenza virus as well as the H5N1 strain (Govorkova et al 2005) showing pyrexia, anorexia, weight loss, lethargy diarrhoea and death
  - It can be transmitted from ferret to ferret and, more importantly, from human to ferret
  - It may also be a potential zoonosis
  - Usually transient and self-limiting – most ferrets will recover without treatment, although the H5N1 strain is potentially fatal
  - Supportive care including fluids and nutritional support can be given if necessary
  - Diphenhydramine at 1 mg/kg p.o. b.i.d.
  - Amantadine at 6.0 mg/kg p.o. b.i.d. or by nebulization
  - Covering antibiosis to prevent secondary infections (mucopurulent oculo-nasal discharges)
- Bacterial pneumonia
  - Appropriate antibiosis
  - Otherwise care as described under *Management*
- Mycobacteriosis
  - Potential zoonosis so consider euthanasia
  - *M. abscessus* has been successfully treated with clarithromycin (Lunn et al 2005)
- Fungal mycoses
  - Ketoconazole at 10–30 mg/kg p.o. s.i.d. for 60 days.
  - Amphotericin B
    - 0.25–1.0 mg/kg i.v. s.i.d. or every other day until a total dose of 7–25 mg has been given
    - For *Cryptococcus*, 150 mg/kg i.v. 3 times weekly for 2–4 months
- Itraconazole at 25–33 mg/kg p.o. s.i.d. long term
  - *Pneumocystis carinii*
- Pentamidine isethionate at 3–4 mg/kg on alternate days for a maximum of 10 treatments
- Trimethoprim-sulfamethoxazole at 30 mg/kg p.o., s.c. b.i.d.

Gastrointestinal tract disorders

Permanent dental formula of the ferret

$$I : \frac{3}{3}, C : \frac{1}{1}, PM : \frac{3}{3}, M : \frac{1}{2}$$

The permanent incisors erupt at around 6–8 weeks while the other permanents are usually through by 10 weeks.

Deciduous dental formula of the ferret

$$I : \frac{1}{0}, C : \frac{1}{1}, PM : \frac{0}{0}, M : \frac{3}{3}$$

Disorders of the oral cavity

- Dental disease
  - Periodontal disease, gingivitis and dental tartar not uncommon
  - May be associated with moist or semi-moist foods
  - Fractured canines are commonly found but are rarely painful unless the pulp is exposed
  - If pulp/dentine is red/pink (recently exposed) or tan-coloured and the tooth colour has been retained, these teeth can potentially be saved with an amalgam filling (Johnson-Delaney & Nelson 1992)
  - If dull grey is likely to be devitalized; if black, is necrotic
  - Manage as for dog and cat dental disease
- Salivary mucocoele
  - Facial swellings
  - Aspirate sample for analysis including cytology (differentiate from abscess, neoplasia, haematoma)
  - Surgical resection of the affected gland is best option to prevent recurrence. Zygomatic and buccal glands commonly affected – may require removal of zygomatic arch to aid surgical resection (Mullen 1997)
- Neoplasia
  - Salivary gland adenocarcinoma
  - Investigate as for salivary mucocoele
  - Oral fibrosarcoma
    - Solid mass from oral mucosa that gradually grows over the teeth, eventually interfering with feeding
    - Surgical resection, although often becomes a debulking exercise as complete resection difficult.

Differential diagnoses for gastrointestinal disorders

Viral

- Canine distemper virus (CDV) (see *Systemic Disorders*)
- Rotavirus
- Influenza virus (transient diarrhoea)
- Epizootic catarrhal enteritis (green slime disease) (coronavirus).

Bacterial

- *Lawsonia intracellularis* (proliferative bowel disease, PBD)
- *Helicobacter mustelae*
- Salmonellosis, esp. S. *typhimurium*, S. *newport* and S. *choleraesuis*
- *Campylobacter jejuni*
- *Clostridium perfringens* (possible cause of gastric bloat)
- Mycobacteriosis esp. M. *bovis* and M. *avium*
- Anal gland abscess.

Fungal

- *Cryptococcus neoformans var grubii* (Malik et al 2002).

Protozoal

- *Isospora*
- *Giardia*
- *Cryptosporidium*.

Parasitic

- Toxascaris (uncommon)
- Toxocara (uncommon)
- Ancyclostoma (uncommon)
- Cestodes (uncommon).

Nutritional

Neoplasia

- Lymphoma/lymphosarcoma (see *Systemic Disorders*)
- Polyps
- Adenocarcinoma
- Anal gland neoplasia.

Other non-infectious problems

- Eosinophilic gastroenteritis (EGE)
- Megaoesophagus
- Foreign body
- Trichobezoar (hair ball)
- Gastric ulceration (may be iatrogenic, e.g. NSAIDs overdose)
- Gastric bloat
- Rectal prolapse
- Anal sac impaction.

Findings on clinical examination

- Diarrhoea (with or without blood/melaena). For melaena, see also *Urinary Tract Disorders*)
- Green diarrhoea (epizootic catarrhal enteritis, *Hepatic Disorders*)
- Vomiting/gagging
- Dehydration
- Anorexia

- Dysphagia
- Hypersalivation
- Teeth grinding and abdominal pain
- Weight loss
- Gastric distension, dyspnoea, cyanosis
- Haemorrhagic diarrhoea in young ferrets. Occasional rectal prolapse (*Isospora*)
- Faecal tenesmus (especially in ferrets under 1 year of age) (PBD)
- Thickened bowel palpable (PBD, EGE)
- Colitis-like signs – increased amount of mucous and frank blood in the stool (PBD, EGE)
- Vomiting (± blood from erosions or ulcers), black tarry diarrhoea (small intestine), watery diarrhoea with frank blood (large intestine) and weight loss (EGE)
- Enlarged mesenteric lymph nodes may be palpable (EGE)
- Palpable foreign body
- Gastrointestinal signs are rare with CDV, but it should be considered if accompanied by oculo-nasal discharge, hyperkeratosis and respiratory signs.

Investigations

1. Faecal examination
   a. *Isospora* oocysts
   b. MZN staining for *Cryptosporidium*
   c. Nematode eggs
2. Radiography
   a. Megaoesophagus (contrast study with barium at 10 mL/kg p.o.)
   b. Foreign body
3. Routine haematology and biochemistry
   a. Eosinophilia – 10–35% (normal range 3–5%) (EGE – eosinophilia not always present) (parasitism)
   b. Anaemia (severe gastric ulceration – see also *Cardiovascular and Haematologic Disorders*)
   c. Hypoalbuminaemia (severe intestinal disease including PBD, EGE and *Helicobacter*)
4. Serology for CDV, *Helicobacter mustelae*
5. PCR for *Lawsonia*
6. Culture and sensitivity
7. Endoscopy
   a. Gastric ulceration (also biopsy).
8. Biopsy
   a. Lymphoma
   b. *Helicobacter*
9. Ultrasonography
   a. Enlarged mesenteric lymph node (EGE).

Management

1. Fluid therapy (see *Nursing Care*)
2. If vomiting:

a. Do not feed 6–12 h and use antiemetics, e.g. metoclopramide at 0.2–1.0 mg/kg s.c. t.i.d.
b. Monitor blood glucose – consider dextrose/saline fluids.

Treatment/specific therapy

1. Rotavirus
   a. Supportive treatment only
   b. Usually in young ferrets at 2–6 weeks old
2. Influenza virus (see *Respiratory Tract Disorders*)
3. Epizootic catarrhal enteritis
   a. Supportive treatment plus covering antibiotics
4. Bacterial diseases including salmonellosis
   a. See *Management,* above
   b. Appropriate antibiosis
5. Proliferative bowel disease
   a. Chloramphenicol at 50 mg/kg i.m., s.c., p.o., b.i.d.
   b. Metronidazole at 20 mg/kg p.o. b.i.d. for 3 weeks
6. *Helicobacter mustelae*
   a. A common isolate from gastric ulcers, its significance is uncertain
   b. Combination therapy of:
      i. Amoxicillin at 10–20 mg/kg p.o., s.c., b.i.d.
      ii. Metronidazole at 20 mg/kg p.o. b.i.d.
      iii. Bismuth subsalicylate at 0.25–1.0 mL/kg p.o. q.i.d.
7. Mycobacteriosis
   a. Potential zoonosis
   b. Consider euthanasia
8. *Cryptococcus*
   a. Amphotericin B at 150 mg/kg i.v. 3 times weekly for 2–4 months
9. *Isospora*
   a. Sulfadimethoxine at 30 mg/kg b.i.d.
   b. Amprolium at 100 mg/kg p.o. in food or water daily for 7–10 days
10. *Giardia*
    a. Metronidazole at 10–20 mg/kg b.i.d. for 10 days
11. *Cryptosporidium*
    a. Often subclinical
    b. No effective treatment recognized
    c. Potentiated sulphonamides may be of use, as may nitazoxanide at 5 mg/kg s.i.d.
    d. Potential zoonosis so consider euthanasia
12. Nematodes
    a. Fenbendazole at 20 mg/kg p.o. s.i.d. for 5 days or 100 mg/kg as a single dose
    b. Mebendazole at 50 mg/kg p.o. b.i.d. for 2 days
    c. Ivermectin at 0.4–1.0 mg/kg s.c. Repeat after 1 week
13. Cestodes
    a. Praziquantel at 5–10 mg/kg s.c. Repeat after 2 weeks
14. Eosinophilic gastroenteritis
    a. May be an allergic or immune mediated response
    b. Prednisolone at 1.25–2.5 mg/kg p.o. s.i.d., continuing for 3–4 weeks after clinical resolution
    c. Ivermectin at 0.4 mg/kg s.c. once only. Repeat after 2 weeks

15. Megaoesophagus
    a. Feed from a raised platform
    b. Gut motility enhancers, e.g. metoclopramide at 0.2–1.0 mg/kg p.o., s.c. every 6–8 h; cisapride at 0.5 mg/kg p.o. every 8–24 h
    c. If oesophagitis, cimetidine at 5–10 mg/kg p.o., i.v. t.i.d.
16. Gastric ulceration
    a. Investigate possible underlying aetiologies
    b. Cimetidine at above dose
    c. Bismuth subsalicylate at 0.25–1.0 mL/kg p.o. q.i.d.
    d. Sucralfate at 25–30 mg p.o. q.i.d.
    e. For *Helicobacter*, see above
17. Foreign body
    a. Surgical removal
18. Trichobezoars
    a. Likely to require surgical removal
    b. Attempt prevention by regular use of cat laxatives
    c. May be linked to abnormal gut motility arising from underlying gastrointestinal disease, e.g. lymphoma (see *Systemic Disorders*)
19. Gastric bloat
    a. May be related to foreign body or *Clostridium perfringens* overgrowth
    b. Decompress either by passing oesophageal tube, or trocharization
    c. Fluid therapy
    d. Treat as for gastric ulceration
20. Solid neoplasms and polyps
    a. Surgical resection
21. Rectal prolapse
    a. Moisten prolapse, clean up; if necessary apply osmotic solution, e.g. concentrated sugar water to shrink prolapse prior to reinsertion
    b. Replace and insert rectal pursestring suture
    c. Address possible underlying causes
22. Anal sac impaction
    a. Express and treat as for other small animals.

Nutritional disorders

Ferrets have a rapid gut transit time of around 3 h. They should be fed a diet high in protein and fat, and low in fibre.

Ferret nutrition

1. Protein requirement is around 30–40% and the quality must be good – in the region of 85% to 90% digestible. Diets high in plant proteins predispose to urinary calculi (see *Urinary Tract Disorders*).
2. Fat levels should be 15–30%.
3. Carbohydrate levels should be below 40%. The rapid gut transit time and low brush border enzyme levels present in ferrets' result in a poor ability to utilize carbohydrates, and will fail to thrive if the carbohydrate concentration exceeds 40%. Note that the only carbohydrates that ferrets would normally have access to are in the gut contents of their prey.

It can be normal for ferrets to undergo seasonal weight increases, under the influence of photoperiod. This is normal and should not be a cause of concern.

- Hypoglycaemia from starvation (see *Pancreatic Disorders* for management)
- Nutritional osteodystrophy
  - Young kits fed on a low calcium diet (day-old chicks)
  - Deformities of the long bones, soft jaw
  - Supplement with dietary calcium and vitamin D3 supplement
- Hepatic lipidosis
  - Linked to long-term anorexia
  - Aggressive fluid therapy
  - Parenteral nutrition with glucose and vitamins
  - Assisted feeding by syringe (see *Nursing Care*)
  - Calcium gluconate p.o. or propylene glycol p.o. may be of use
  - Dexamethasone at 0.2 mg/kg i.v., s.c. or p.o.

Hepatic disorders

Nutritional

- Hepatic lipidosis
- Copper toxicosis
- Ketosis (see *Reproductive System Disorders*).

Neoplasia

- Lymphoma/lymphosarcoma (see *Systemic Disorders*)
- Metastases, e.g. insulinoma
- Haemangiosarcoma
- Adenocarcinoma
- Hepatocellular adenoma
- Bile duct cyst adenoma
- Biliary carcinoma
- Other non-infectious problems
- Lymphocytic hepatitis
- Cholangiohepatitis.

Findings on clinical examination

- Reduced or loss of appetite
- Vague signs of ill-health
- Abnormal faeces
- Hepatomegaly
- Jaundice (rare)
- Ascites
- Bile-tinged (green) diarrhoea
- Lethargy, hypothermia, hyperthermia, jaundice (copper toxicosis)
- Seizures.

Investigations

1. Radiography
2. Routine haematology and biochemistry
   a. Raised liver enzymes; ALT usually >275 IU/L (normal 78–289 IU/L). ALP may be raised; total bilirubin levels often normal
3. Culture and sensitivity
4. Endoscopy
5. Biopsy
6. Ultrasonography.

Management

1. Fluid therapy (see *Nursing Care*)
2. Lactulose at 150–750 mg/kg p.o. b.i.d. or t.i.d.
3. Milk thistle (*Silybum marianum*) is hepatoprotectant. Dose at 4–15 mg/kg b.i.d. or t.i.d.

Treatment/specific therapy

- Hepatic lipidosis (see *Nutritional Disorders*)
- Copper toxicosis
  - Penicillamine at 10 mg/kg p.o. s.i.d. – offer as divided dose if vomiting occurs
  - Trientine at 10 mg/kg p.o. b.i.d.
  - Supportive therapy
  - Possibly inherited susceptibility
  - Poor prognosis.

Splenic disorders

- Splenomegaly can be a normal finding in ferrets; however it is also found in a range of disorders including, the most significant of which would be:
  - Haemangiosarcoma and haemangioma
  - Cardiac disease (see *Cardiovascular and Haematological Disorders*)
  - Lymphoma/lymphosarcoma (see *Systemic Disorders*)
  - Insulinoma (see *Pancreatic Disorders*)
  - Aleutian disease (see *Systemic Disorders*)
  - Idiopathic splenomegaly.

Treatment

- Address underlying cause
- Splenectomy
  - Hypersplenism
  - Splenic rupture
  - Splenic torsion
  - Neoplasia
  - Splenitis.

Pancreatic disorders

Neoplasia

• Insulinoma (pancreatic beta cell tumour)
• Exocrine pancreatic adenocarcinoma.

Other non-infectious problems

• Diabetes mellitus.

Findings on clinical examination

• Signs of an insulinoma include transient episodes of inactivity where the ferret is unresponsive to external stimuli, hind-limb weakness and eventually seizures, coma and death
• Ataxia and hind-limb paresis
• Lethargy
• Hypersalivation
• 'Glazed-eye' appearance
• Abdominal distension
• Pain
• Abdominal mass palpable.

Investigations

1. Radiography
2. Routine haematology and biochemistry (Table 1.3)
   a. Provisional diagnosis of an insulinoma is based upon a low-fasting blood glucose sample (a 4-h fast will suffice). Insulinomas often also show neutrophilia, leucocytosis and monocytosis plus raised ALT and AST
3. Culture and sensitivity
4. Urinalysis
   a. Glycosuria/ketonuria.

Table 1.3 The ferret: Routine haematology and biochemistry

		Normal range	Insulinoma	Diabetes mellitus
Blood glucose (mmol/L)	Normal resting	5.22–11.49	< 3.89 (commonly 1.12–2.24)	>16.65
	Normal fasting	5.0–6.94		
Normal insulin (pmol/L)		35–250	772.7–12470	
Mean fasting insulin (pmol/L)		58		
Normal insulin/glucose ratio (pmol/mmol)		4.6–44.2		

5. Endoscopy
6. Exploratory surgery and biopsy
7. Ultrasonography.

Management

1. Treatment of hypoglycaemia.

Hypoglycaemia

1. Rub honey or sugared water on to the gingiva, taking care not to get bitten.
2. 0.5–2.0 mL bolus i.v. of 50% dextrose solution given slowly (so as not to overstimulate a possible insulinoma).
3. Fluid therapy (see *Nursing Care*) with 5% dextrose infusion.
4. If ferret fails to respond, can give shock dose of dexamethasone at 4–8 mg/kg i.v., i.m. once only.
5. Diazepam at 1–2 mg i.v. as needed to control if seizures persistent.

Treatment/specific therapy

- Diabetes mellitus
  - Neutral protamine Hagedorn (NPH) insulin at a starting dose of 0.1 IU/ferret b.i.d. s.c. until stabilized. Monitor blood glucose levels
  - Maintain on ultralente insulin s.i.d.
- Insulinoma
  - Surgical resection
    - Fluid therapy with 5% dextrose saline
    - Partial resection or nodulectomy
    - Metastasis is very common
  - Medical management
    - Prednisolone 0.5–2.0 mg/kg p.o. b.i.d., raising until clinical signs subside
    - Diazoxide at 5–10 mg/kg b.i.d. p.o. (may induce vomiting and anorexia)
  - Medical management may give 6–18 months of control of clinical signs, although it will not prevent further growth and spread of the insulinoma
  - Hyperglycaemia following pancreatic surgery will usually resolve within 2 weeks and requires no action
- Pancreatic exocrine adenocarcinoma
  - Readily metastasize. Surgery is a possible option but metastasis highly likely before diagnosis confirmed.

Cardiovascular and haematological disorders

Viral
- Aleutian disease (see *Systemic Disorders*).

Bacterial
- Bacteraemia/septicaemia
- Endocarditis.

Protozoal
- Toxoplasma gondii (myocarditis) (see *Neurological Disorders*).

Parasitic
- Dirofilaria immitis (heartworm).

Neoplasia
- Lymphoma (see *Systemic Disorders*).

Other non-infectious problems
- Cardiomyopathy
- Dilative
- Hypertrophic
- Valvular heart disease
- Hyperoestrogenism (see *Reproductive System Disorders*)
- Gastric ulceration (see *Gastrointestinal Tract Disorders*)
- Congenital disorders.

Findings on clinical examination

- Cyanosis or pallor of the mucous membranes
- Anaemia (hyperoestrogenism, gastric ulceration)
- Slow capillary refill time
- Dyspnoea
- Precordial thrill
- Abnormalities of femoral arterial pulse including weakness, irregularities, pulse deficits
- Dysrhythmia
- Lack of thoracic percussion with auscultation
- Abnormal lung sounds
- Abnormal heart sounds
- Exercise intolerance
- Ascites
- Hepatomegaly, splenomegaly
- Weight loss
- Sudden death.

Investigations

1. Auscultation
2. Blood pressure: systole: 140 ± 35 mmHg; diastole: 110 ± 31 mmHg
3. ECG
   a. Use adhesive ECG contacts designed for children, as metal clips and needles are poorly tolerated in the conscious ferret

    b. Distract the ferret by offering a favoured food or food supplement, e.g. Ferre-tone (8:1)

    c. Normal ferret lead II ECGs:
        1. The P waves are small
        2. The R waves are large
        3. Short QT interval
        4. Elevated ST segment (see Table 1.4)

4. Radiography
    a. Pleural effusions and cardiomegaly are common findings with cardiomyopathy and dirofilariasis
    b. A globoid heart shape often indicative of cardiac disease, usually with increased cardiosternal contact
    c. Anterior mediastinal masses (lymphoma)

Table 1.4 The ferret: Normal lead II ECGs

Parameter	Ketamine-xylazine anaesthesia[a]	Ketamine-diazepam anaesthesia[b]	
		Right lateral recumbency	Sternal recumbency
Heart rate (beats/min)	233 ± 22	250–430	
Frontal plane MEA (°)	+77.22 ± 12	+75–+100	+65–+90
Lead II			
P amplitude (mV)	0.122 ± 0.007	≤0.2	≤0.3
P duration (s)	0.024 ± 0.004	0.01–0.03	
PR interval (s)	0.047 ± 0.003	0.03–0.06	
QRS duration (s)	0.043 ± 0.003	0.02–0.05	
Q wave amplitude (mV)		−0.05–0	
R amplitude (mV)	1.46 ± 0.84	1.0–2.8	1.0–3.1
QT interval (s)	0.12 ± 0.04	0.06–0.16	
S wave amplitude		0	
T amplitude (mV)		−0.4–+0.4	
		Most often >0	>0 or <0
Lead I			
Q(S) wave amplitude (mV)		−0.4–0.0	0
R amplitude (mV)		≤+0.9	≤+1.25
Lead a VF			
R amplitude (mV)		1.0–3.1	

[a]Stamoulis et al 1997.
[b]Bublot et al 2006.

Table 1.5 The ferret: Normal echocardiographic values

Parameter	Mean value
Left ventricle, end-diastolic (mm)	11.0
Left ventricle, end-systolic (mm)	6.4
Left ventricular posterior or free wall (mm)	3.3
Fractional shortening (%)	42
End-point septal separation	

5. Ultrasonography/echocardiography
   a. Normal echocardiographic values for ferrets are shown in Table 1.5 (Stamoulis et al 1997)
   b. Detection of dirofilariasis (Sasai et al 2000)
6. Routine haematology and biochemistry
   a. Microfilaria in peripheral bloodstream (uncommon) (*Dirofilaria*)
   b. Anaemia (hyperoestrogenism, high ectoparasite count, Aleutian disease, gastrointestinal haemorrhage, e.g. gastric ulceration, gastroenteritis)
7. Serology for *Dirofilaria* antigen, toxoplasma
8. Culture and sensitivity
9. Endoscopy
10. Biopsy.

Management

- Reduce stress, e.g. keep in a cool, shaded or darkened area away from potential stressors such as dogs.
- Provide a high oxygen environment.
- For pleural effusion consider tube thoracostomy.

Treatment/specific therapy

- *Dirofilaria immitis*
  - Due to the small size of the ferret, only a few worms may cause serious problems with clinical signs ranging from heart failure to pulmonary edema
  - Treatment is also difficult because the worms may cause thromboembolisms resulting in acute death
  - Treatment protocol
    - Thiacetarsamide at 2.2 mg/kg i.v. b.i.d. for 2 days
    - Start heparin at 100 units/ferret s.c. every 24 h for 21 days
    - After 3 weeks stop heparin and start on aspirin at 22 mg/kg p.o. s.i.d. for 3 months
    - Treat concurrently for cardiac disease if appropriate
    - Alternatively try topical 10% imidacloprid/1.0% moxidectin (Advocate, Bayer) at 0.4 mL per ferret
    - Prevention is with ivermectin at 0.4–1.0 mg/kg s.c. once monthly in areas where heartworm is endemic.

- Cardiomyopathies
  - Dilated (congestive) cardiomyopathy
    - Furosemide at 1–4 mg/kg b.i.d.
    - Enalapril at 0.5 mg/kg p.o. every 48 h. Ferrets appear very sensitive to the hypotensive effects of ACE inhibitors
    - Digoxin at 0.01 mg/kg p.o. s.i.d.
    - Nitroglycerin at 3 mm of 2% ointment applied to skin s.i.d. or b.i.d.
    - Pimobendan at 0.2 mg/kg s.i.d.
  - Hypertrophic cardiomyopathy
    - Atenolol at 0.5–2.0 mg/kg p.o. s.i.d.
    - Diltiazem at 0.5–1.0 mg/kg p.o. b.i.d.
  - Valvular heart disease
    - Treat as for dilated cardiomyopathy
  - Hyperoestrogenism (see *Reproductive System Disorders*).

Systemic disorders

Viral

- Coronavirus
- Canine distemper virus (CDV) (see also *Neurological Disorders*)
- Aleutian disease (parvovirus) (AD)
- Rabies.

Bacterial

- Bacteraemia/septicaemia.

Nutritional

- Copper toxicosis (see *Hepatic Disorders*)
- Ketosis (see *Reproductive System Disorders*).

Neoplasia

- Insulinoma (see *Pancreatic Disorders*)
- Hyperadrenocortism (see *Endocrine Disorders*)
- Lymphoma/lymphosarcoma (see also *Respiratory Tract Disorders* and *Cardiovascular and Haematologic Disorders*)
- Mesothelioma.

Other non-infectious problems

- Hyperoestrogenism (see *Reproductive System Disorders*).

Findings on clinical examination

- Weight loss, dyspnoea, hind-leg weakness, ascites (coronavirus, Aleutian disease, lymphoma)
- Bilateral mucopurulent ocular and/or nasal discharges – the ocular discharge dries to a crust at the eyelid margins sealing the eyes shut (CDV)
- Hyperkeratosis of the footpads and erythematous cutaneous rashes in the inguinal area and under the chin (CDV)

- Chronic upper respiratory infections, dyspnoea, general lethargy, wasting and lymphadenopathy (lymphoma). Peripheral lymphadenopathy is more common in older animals
- Palpable abdominal masses (splenomegaly, mesenteric and/or gastric lymph nodes) (lymphoma)
- Distended abdomen (mesothelioma).

Investigations

1. Radiography
   a. Renomegaly, splenomegaly, lymphadenopathy (coronavirus)
   b. Mediastinal masses, pleural effusions, abdominal masses (lymphoma) (see Table 1.6)
2. Routine haematology and biochemistry
   a. Persistent high white blood cell counts (10×10^9/L or above) with a high lymphocyte count (lymphoma). Consider lymphoma if lymphocytosis ($\geq 3.5 \times 10^9$/L) or 60% lymphocytes. Immature ferrets (<6 m.o.) can have a natural lymphocytosis. In older ferrets with chronic lymphoma there may be a lymphopaenia
   b. Bacterial infections tend to cause a smaller rise in WBC with a relative neutrophilia of >85% with the presence of bands
   c. Hyperglobulinaemia (coronavirus, Aleutian disease). *Note* that not all ferrets with Aleutian disease are hypergammaglobulinaemic (Une et al 2000)
   d. Aleutian disease produces immune complexes that trigger renal disease including glomerular nephritis so renal parameters likely to be high
3. Bone marrow aspirate/lymph node cytology (lymphoma)

Technique for bone marrow aspirate (performed under GA)

1. Prepare at least 4 slides.
2. Draw some EDTA (can mix from EDTA blood tube with sterile saline).
3. Use a 5 or 10 mL syringe with around 1 mL of EDTA solution present.
4. Use an 18 G or 21 G 25 mm needle.
5. Identify the trochanteric fossa.
6. Grind into bone so that needle is parallel to long axis of femur.
7. Perform several aspirates – marrow appears as thick blood.
8. Apply the collected marrow to each of slides.
9. Leave for around 30 s for bone spicules to settle on to slide.
10. With half of the slides, tip and drain away excess including the spicules.
11. For the other half, place a clean slide across at right angles and draw across to create a 'squash' preparation (but without squashing!).
12. Air dry and submit to laboratory.

Table 1.6 The ferret: Grading of lymphoma

Stage 1	Single focus
Stage 2	Two foci on same side of diaphragm
Stage 3	Involving the spleen and lymph node(s)
Stage 4	Multiple sites

4. Abdominal centesis and cytology
5. Serology for CDV, AD, rabies
6. Culture and sensitivity
7. Endoscopy
8. Biopsy/necropsy
   a. Pyogranulomatous enteritis (coronavirus)
   b. Lymphoma (especially mesenteric lymph node, peripheral lymph nodes, spleen, liver and any abnormal organs)
   c. CDV
9. Ultrasonography.

Management

- See *Nursing Care*

Treatment/specific therapy

- Coronavirus
  - Symptomatic treatment only
- Canine distemper virus
  - The incubation period described for CDV in ferrets is from 7–10 days. The usual course of disease, from exposure to death is 12–25 days
  - There is no treatment – consider supportive therapy including covering antibiosis. The mortality rate is close to 100%. Those that do recover are likely to die later from CNS disturbances (see *Neurological Disorders*)
  - Prevent by vaccination. Consult manufacturers first as some CDV vaccines derived from ferret tissue cultures that may increase the risk of vaccine-induced disease. Where possible do not use multivalent vaccines. Where CDV is endemic, an initial vaccination course of 3 injections is recommended at 6–8 weeks of age, 10–12 weeks and 13–14 weeks with annual boosters to follow. If CDV is not endemic a single dose at 12 weeks of age with annual boosters
  - Adverse reactions to vaccination are vomiting and diarrhoea (Moore et al 2005)
  - CDV is readily destroyed by normal cleaning and disinfection routines
- Rabies
  - Significant zoonosis. Euthanize
  - Prevent by vaccination given at 12 weeks of age with an annual booster
- Aleutian disease
  - Many ferrets can be serologically positive for AD but show no clinical signs
  - Supportive therapy
  - Steroids may prove useful in reducing the formation and effect of the immune complexes
- Bacteraemia/septicaemia
  - Appropriate antibiosis
  - Supportive therapy as necessary (see *Nursing Care*)
- Lymphoma/lymphosarcoma
  - Chemotherapy protocols for small animals are regularly altered and updated so if in doubt, consult a veterinary oncologist. The following two protocols (from Brown 1997) have been found to be useful

- Protocol 1 is set out in Table 1.7
- The author finds it useful to give the owner a modified copy of the above protocol adjusted to specific days/dates for administration of the different medications
- Weekly PCV should be performed before administration of next dose of vincristine to assess degree of anaemia; consider halting treatment at values below 20%
- Protocol 2 is set out in Table 1.8
- Palliative treatment for lymphoma
  - Prednisolone at 0.5 mg/kg b.i.d., increasing to control signs. Note that prednisolone treatment alone is likely to make the lymphoma refractory to chemotherapy
  - Vitamin C (ascorbic acid) at 50–100 mg/kg p.o. b.i.d.
  - Regular annual CBC to screen for lymphoma

Table 1.7 The ferret: Chemotherapy protocol 1

Week	Day	Drug	Dose
1	1	Prednisolone	1 mg/kg p.o. b.i.d. Continue throughout treatment
	1	Vincristine	0.12 mg/kg i.v.
	3	Cyclophosphamide	10 mg/kg p.o.
2	8	Vincristine	0.12 mg/kg i.v.
3	15	Vincristine	0.12 mg/kg i.v.
4	22	Vincristine	0.12 mg/kg i.v.
	24	Cyclophosphamide	10 mg/kg p.o.
7	46	Cyclophosphamide	10 mg/kg p.o.
9		Prednisolone	Start reducing dose to end by 4 weeks

Table 1.8 The ferret: Chemotherapy protocol 2

Week	Drug	Dose
1	Vincristine	0.07 mg/kg i.v.
	Asparaginase	400 iu/kg i.p.
	Prednisolone	1 mg/kg p.o. s.i.d. Continue throughout treatment
2	Cyclophosphamide	10 mg/kg p.o.
3	Doxorubicin	1 mg/kg i.v.
4–6	Asparaginase	Discontinue, otherwise as for weeks 1–3
8	Vincristine	0.07 mg/kg i.v.
10	Cyclophosphamide	10 mg/kg p.o.
12	Vincristine	0.07 mg/kg i.v.
14	Methotrexate	0.5 mg/kg i.v.

- Clusters of outbreaks have occurred and in some cases may be due to a retrovirus-like agent (Erdman et al 1995), although attempted detection using FeLV serology, PCR or ELISA all proved negative (Erdman et al 1996)
- Mesothelioma
  - Surgical resection and chemotherapy may be worth attempting but the prognosis is poor.

Musculoskeletal disorders

Viral
- Aleutian disease (see *Systemic Disorders*).

Neoplasia
- Multiple myeloma
- Chondroma
- Chondrosarcoma
- Fibrosarcoma
- Osteoma
- Chordoma.

Other non-infectious problems
- Traumatic fractures
- Any causes of weakness
  - See *Neurologic Disorders*
  - See *Cardiovascular and Haematologic Disorders*
  - See *Systemic Disorders*
  - See *Pancreatic Disorders*.

Findings on clinical examination

- Pain
- Lameness
- Swelling
- Hind-leg paresis/paralysis
- Small rounded mass at tip of tail (chordoma).

Investigations

1. Radiography
2. Osteolysis, pathological fractures (multiple myeloma)
3. Traumatic fractures
4. Routine haematology and biochemistry
5. Culture and sensitivity
6. Endoscopy
7. Biopsy
8. Ultrasonography.

Treatment/specific therapy

- Multiple myeloma
  - No treatment recorded
- Traumatic fractures
  - Repair using standard small animal techniques
- Neoplasia
  - Surgical resection, amputation, chemotherapy or radiation therapy as for other small animals
  - Note that chordomas may metastasize (Munday et al 2004).

Neurological disorders

Viral

- Canine distemper virus (CDV) (see *Systemic Disorders*)
- Rabies.

Bacterial

- Bacterial meningitis or other CNS infection
- Otitis media/interna.

Fungal

- Cryptococcus meningitis
- Blastomycosis.

Protozoal

- Toxoplasmosis.

Nutritional

- Hypoglycaemia
- Ketosis (see *Reproductive System Disorders*).

Neoplasia

- Schwannoma
- Insulinoma (hypoglycaemia) (see *Pancreatic Disorders*)
- Lymphoma (see *Systemic Disorders*)
- T-cell lymphoma (Hanley et al 2004).

Other non-infectious problems

- Toxins
- Spinal lesions, e.g. intervertebral disc prolapse (Lu et al 2004), fractures
- Eosinophilic granulomatous infiltrate (as part of eosinophilic gastroenteritis – see *Gastrointestinal Tract Disorders*).

Findings on clinical examination

- Apparent weakness
- Posterior paralysis/paresis
- Anxiety, lethargy, constipation, bladder atony, posterior paresis, aggression (rabies)
- Seizures (uncommon except with chronic neurotrophic form of CDV)
- Salivation, muscle tremors, seizures and coma (CDV)
- Otitis externa (see also 'Ear mites' in *Skin Disorders*).

Investigations

1. Full neurological examination
2. Radiography
   a. Myelography – access as for CSF tap (see below)
   b. 0.25–0.5 mL/kg iohexol
3. Routine haematology and biochemistry
4. Serology for toxoplasmosis
5. Culture and sensitivity.

Cerebrospinal fluid tap in the ferret

1. Collect as would do from dog or cat.
2. Sites for CSF tap are the atlanto-occipital joint and lumbar (L5-L6) region.
3. Use a 21 or 22 gauge needle.

---

6. Endoscopy
7. Biopsy
8. Ultrasonography.

Management

- Important to differentiate from other causes of weakness (insulinoma, lymphoma, etc.).

Treatment/specific therapy

- Rabies (see *Systemic Disorders*)
- Bacterial CNS infection
  - Appropriate antibiosis
  - Supportive care
- Fungal infections
  - Ketoconazole at 10–30 mg/kg p.o. s.i.d. for 60 days
  - Amphotericin B
    - 0.25–1.0 mg/kg i.v. s.i.d. or every other day until a total dose of 7–25 mg has been given
    - For *Cryptococcus*, 150 mg/kg i.v. 3 times weekly for 2–4 months

- Itraconazole at 25–33 mg/kg p.o. s.i.d. long term
- Toxoplasmosis
  - Clindamycin at 12.5 mg/kg p.o. b.i.d. for at least 2 weeks
  - Combination therapy consisting of:
    - Co-trimoxazole at 30 mg/kg b.i.d. p.o.
  - Pyrimethamine at 0.5 mg/kg b.i.d. p.o.
  - Folic acid at 3.0–5.0 s.i.d.
- Hypoglycaemia
  - For management of hypoglycaemic episodes, see *Pancreatic Disorders*
- Orthopaedic conditions
  - Treat as for other small animals.

Ophthalmic disorders

The ferret eye is similar to the canine eye except that the pupil is horizontal rather than vertical.

Viral

- Canine distemper virus (CDV) (see *Systemic Disorders*)
- Influenza A (see *Respiratory Tract Disorders*).

Protozoal

- Toxoplasmosis (see *Neurological Disorders*).

Nutritional

- Hypovitaminosis A.

Neoplasia

- Carcinoma of the ocular globe
- Other non-infectious problems
- Salivary mucocoele (see *Gastrointestinal Tract Disorders*)
- Hereditary cataracts
- Idiopathic cataracts
- Retinal degeneration (may be hereditary).

Findings on clinical examination

- Corneal ulceration
- Conjunctivitis (influenza, CDV, hypovitaminosis A)
- Nasal discharge
- Uveitis
- Corneal oedema, hypopyon, and synechiae
- Cataracts
- Exophthalmus
- Megaglobus/glaucoma
- Night blindness (hypovitaminosis A, retinal degeneration)
- Periocular swelling (salivary mucocoele)
- Cataracts (hereditary, hypovitaminosis A, idiopathic)

- Bilateral mucopurulent ocular and/or nasal discharges – the ocular discharge dries to a crust at the eyelid margins sealing the eyes shut. Hyperkeratosis of the foot-pads and skin rashes (CDV).

Investigations

1. Ophthalmic examination
   a. Schirmer tear test 5.31 ± 1.32 mm/min (Montiani-Ferreira et al 2006)
   b. Central corneal thickness 0.337 ± 0.020 mm
2. Topical fluorescein to assess extent of ulceration
3. Tonometry
   a. Intraocular pressure 14.5 ± 3.27 mmHg
4. Skull radiography
5. Routine haematology and biochemistry
6. Serology for CDV, toxoplasmosis
7. Culture and sensitivity
8. Biopsy
9. Ultrasonography.

Treatment/specific therapy

- Corneal ulceration
  - Topical and systemic antibiosis
  - Once infection cleared, treat as for other small animals, e.g. scarification to encourage healing, conjunctival grafts, etc.
- Uveitis
  - Topical ophthalmic steroid or NSAID preparations
  - Topical ophthalmic antibiotic preparations plus systemic antibiosis if appropriate
  - Enucleation if severe
- Cataracts
  - Treat for any uveitis as above.
  - Cataract removal either surgically or by phacoemulsification
- Neoplasia
  - Enucleation
- Toxoplasmosis (see *Neurological Disorders*).

Endocrine disorders

Neoplasia

- Adrenal neoplasia
- Adrenal hyperplasia
- Adrenal adenoma/carcinoma
- Pituitary gonadotroph adenomas
  (Schoemaker et al 2004)
- Insulinoma (see *Pancreatic Disorders*).

Other non-infectious problems

- Hyperoestrogenism (see *Reproductive Disorders*).

Findings on clinical examination

- Hyperadrenocortism
  - Symmetrical alopecia
  - Over 30% may be pruritic
  - Vulval swelling (also in spayed females)
  - Male behaviour in castrated males
  - Dysuria in males (urethral obstruction secondary to prostatic hyperplasia)
  - Splenomegaly
  - Enlarged adrenal glands may be palpable (not consistent).

Investigations

1. Radiography
2. Routine haematology and biochemistry
   a. Hyperadrenocortism
      i. Blood hormone levels (see Table 1.9) elevation varies between individuals; cortisol is the least likely to be raised and a diagnosis is more likely if androstenedione, oestradiol and hydroxyprogesterone are measured
      ii. Ideally blood samples for hyperadrenocortism should be taken under anaesthesia because manual restraint increases plasma cortisol and ACTH, but decreases alpha-melanocyte-stimulating hormone (α-MSH) production (Schoemaker et al 2003). However, it should be noted that isoflurane (but not medetomidine) anaesthesia increases the (α-MSH) from the pituitary gland which may subsequently affect the concentrations of adrenal hormones

Table 1.9   The ferret: Blood hormone levels

Parameter	Normal range	Hyperadrenocortism (mean values)
Androstenedione (nmol/L)	0–15	67
Dehydroepiandrosterone sulphate (µmol/L) (mean)	0.01	0.03
Oestradiol (pmol/L)	30–180	167
17-hydroxyprogesterone (nmol/L)	0–0.8	3.2
Cortisol (nmol/L)	0–140	
ACTH (ng/L)	13–98	
α-MSH (ng/L)	16–74	
Sodium (mmol/L)	137–162	
Potassium (mmol/L)	4.3–7.7	

Table 1.10 The ferret: Thyroid levels

	Male	Female
Thyroxine (T4) (nmol/L)	13.0–106.9	9.14–32.69
Tri-iodothyronine (T3) (nmol/L)	0.007–0.012	0.004–0.011

   iii. Pancytopaenia (severe cases)
   iv. Raised AST
   v. For suspect female ferrets, differentiate from ovarian remnant (or oestrus if entire) by giving 2 injections of 100 IU hCG 7 days apart. This should cause regression of vulval swelling unless the ferret has hyperadrenocortism
  b. Thyroid levels (Table 1.10)

Thyroid stimulation test (Keeble 2001)

1. TSH at 1.0 IU given i.v.
2. Blood for T4 taken at 120 min.

---

3. Culture and sensitivity
4. Endoscopy
5. Biopsy
6. Ultrasonography
  a. Enlarged adrenal gland
  b. Normal values left adrenal gland normally 6–8 mm length; right adrenal gland 8–11 mm length. Accessory nodules of adrenal tissue occur in some individuals.

Treatment/specific therapy

- Hyperadrenocortism
  - Surgical management (adrenalectomy)
  - Surgery is the treatment of choice, but in cases of bilateral adrenal disease then either completely remove one (the left is easiest) and perform a subtotal adrenalectomy on the other (right) one with subsequent medical management, or consider medical management only
  - If bilateral adrenalectomy, consider the use of supplementary glucocorticoids (prednisolone at 0.1 mg/kg p.o. s.i.d. (Martorell et al 2005) for several days post-surgery to prevent hypoadrenocortism. Monitor serum electrolyte ranges and titrate to effect; partial adrenalectomy or presence of accessory nodules may result in continued normal electrolyte levels without treatment
  - Temporary tube cystotomy may be beneficial in those cases with urinary obstruction from prostatic hyperplasia/prostatic cysts (Nolte et al 2002). Removal is after 5–10 days

- Medical management
  - Mitotane at 50 mg p.o. s.i.d. for 7 days, then a maintenance dose of 50 mg every 3rd day
  - Trilostane at 2 mg/kg s.i.d. p.o.
  - Leuprolide acetate at 100 µg/kg s.c. every 21–30 days
  - Ketoconazole ineffective at 15 mg/kg b.i.d. (cited in Keeble 2001)
  - Temporary cessation of clinical signs due to reduced hormone levels can be achieved with deslorelin, given as a single, slow-release 3 mg implant, with an average of 13.7 ± 3.5 months to recurrence of signs (Wagner et al 2005)
  - The disease is believed to be linked to luteinizing hormone (LH) effects on the sex steroid producing cells of the adrenal cortex (Schoemaker et al 2002), which in turn may explain the predisposing factor of early age of neutering
- Gonadotroph adenomas
  - Unknown significance.

Urinary disorders

Viral

- Aleutian disease (see *Systemic Disorders*).

Bacterial

- Cystitis.

Nutritional

- Urolithiasis (males>females) (see also *Reproductive System Disorders*).

Neoplasia

- Lymphoma (see *Systemic Disorders*)
- Transitional cell carcinoma
- Renal carcinoma.

Other non-infectious problems

- Chronic interstitial nephritis
- Hydronephrosis
- Renal cysts
- Prostatic hyperplasia (see 'Hyperadrenocortism', in *Endocrine Disorders*)
- Gentamicin toxicity.

Findings on clinical examination

- Depression
- Anorexia
- Weight loss
- Polydipsia/polyuria
- Oral ulceration
- Haematuria (urolithiasis, cystitis, neoplasia)
- Hind-leg weakness

- Melaena
- Dysuria/polyuria
- Urine dribbling, wet perineum, constant licking at genitalia (urolithiasis)
- Painful urination, stranguria (urolithiasis, cystitis)
- Death
- Palpable abnormalities
- Distended bladder (urethral obstruction)
- Cystic calculi/sand.

Investigations

1. Urinalysis (normal urine parameters, see Table 1.11)
   a. Magnesium ammonium phosphate (struvite) crystals (urolithiasis)
   b. Ketonuria (ketosis, see *Reproductive System Disorders*)
2. Radiography
   a. Useful to differentiate uncomplicated cystitis from urolithiasis
   b. Contrast studies (pyelography, double contrast bladder studies, pneumo-cystographies)
3. Routine haematology and biochemistry
   a. With renal disease, urea can be over 42.5 mmol/L in renal disease (normal 10–15 mmol/L) but creatinine rarely raised unless renal disease severe and long-standing
   b. Phosphorus often raised with renal disease
   c. Non-regenerative anaemia (advanced renal disease)
   d. GFR evaluation (from Hillyer 1997, see Table 1.12).

Table 1.11   The ferret: Normal urine parameters

Volume (mL/kg per h)	8–140
pH	6.0–7.5
Protein (mg/dL)	7–33
Ketones	Trace
Glucose	Negative
Crystals	Negative

Table 1.12   The ferret: GFR evaluation

Parameter	Normal (mean ± SD)
Exogenous creatinine clearance (mL/min per kg)	3.32 ± 2.16
Inulin clearance (mL/min per kg)	3.02 ± 1.78
Endogenous creatinine clearance (mL/min per kg)	2.5 ± 0.93

4. Cytology
   a. Renal casts, neoplastic cells
5. Culture and sensitivity
6. Endoscopy
7. Biopsy
8. Ultrasonography.

<h2>Management</h2>

1. Fluid therapy (see *Nursing Care*)
2. Appropriate antibiosis.

<h2>Treatment/specific therapy</h2>

- Renal cysts
  - No treatment
  - If large, painful and unilateral consider nephrectomy
- Hydronephrosis
  - Nephrectomy
  - Some cases may be linked to accidental ureteral occlusion during routine ovario-hysterectomy
- Urolithiasis
  - If urethral obstruction:
    - Attempt catheterization (can be difficult in males due to J-shaped os penis)
    - Cystocentesis
    - Surgical cystotomy
    - If unable to clear urethra, create a perineal urethrostomy
- Cystic calculi
  - Cystotomy
  - Submit any stones/sand for analysis
  - Antibiosis (usually has accompanying cystitis) and other supportive care
  - Note that diets high in plant protein (especially dog food or poor-quality cat food) may predispose ferrets to urinary calculi formation as well as urinary bacterial infections
  - Change diet to commercial ferret food or high-quality cat food
- Neoplasia
  - Transitional cell carcinoma of the bladder: surgery difficult because is often diffuse
  - Chemotherapy may prove useful
- Renal carcinoma
  - Nephrectomy.

<h2>Reproductive disorders</h2>

Ferrets are induced ovulators; ovulation occurs 30–40 h after copulation. Failure to mate can result in a prolonged oestrous (up to 6 months) and a resultant aplastic anaemia (see *Hyperoestrogenism* below). Oestrus is indicated by a pronounced swollen

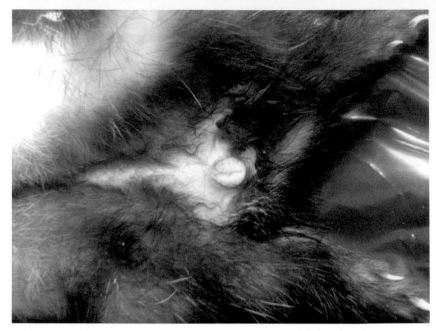

Fig. 1.2. Swollen vulval of a ferret in oestrus.

vulva (Fig. 1.2); any female in season for longer than 1 month is considered at risk of hyperoestrogenism
   Males have a J-shaped os penis.

Bacterial

- Prostatitis
- Metritis/pyometra
- Mastitis (*Staphylococcus spp*, coliforms)
- *Staphylococcus intermedius* (chronic mastitis).

Nutritional

- Ketosis/pregnancy toxaemia (in pregnant jills).

Neoplasia

- Hyperadrenocortism (see *Endocrine Disorders*)
- Prostatic hyperplasia and prostatic cysts
- Testicular neoplasia
- Sertoli cell tumours
- Interstitial cell tumours
- Prostatic carcinoma
- Ovarian stump neoplasia
- Undifferentiated carcinoma
- Leiomyoma

- Fibrosarcoma
- Ovarian teratoma
- Mammary cystic carcinoma
- Uterine adenoma.

Other non-infectious problems

- Hyperoestrogenism
- Failure to mate
- Adrenal neoplasia (see *Endocrine Disorders*)
- Ovarian remnant following ovario-hysterectomy
- Urolithiasis (in pregnant jills)
- Dystocia
  - Low litter size (unborn kits will die after 43 days' gestation)
  - Physical abnormalities
  - Large kits
  - Deformed/anasarca kits
  - Maternal pelvic abnormalities.

Findings on clinical examination

- Vulval hyperplasia (hyperoestrogenism, hyperadrenocortism, oestrus, ovarian remnant/neoplasia)
- Other signs of hyperoestrogenism include tachypnea, anaemia (pale mucous membranes), ecchymotic and petechial haemorrhages, melaena, weakness, hind limb paresis, secondary infections, alopecia at tail base
- Vaginal prolapse (may accompany rectal prolapse) (urolithiasis)
- Swollen uterus palpable; vaginal discharge may, but not always, be present (pyometra, metritis)
- Dysuria/stranguria (prostatic hyperplasia)
- Alopecia and pruritus in entire male ferret (Sertoli cell tumour)
- Swollen, painful, discoloured mammary glands (acute mastitis, neoplasia)
- Swollen but otherwise normal mammary glands (chronic mastitis)
- Lethargy dehydration in pregnant female (jill). Melaena may be present. Hair loss (pregnancy toxaemia).

Investigations

1. Radiography
   a. Prostatic hyperplasia (will also help differentiate from urolithiasis).
2. Routine haematology and biochemistry
   a. PCV (normal 46–61%). For hyperoestrogenism, PCV can be used as a prognostic indicator (from Keeble 2001, see Table 1.13)
   b. Other blood values consistent with hyperoestrogenism reflect a pancytopaenia and include a normocytic normochromic or macrocytic hypochromic anaemia plus a thrombocytopaenia, neutropaenia, eosinopaenia
   c. Pregnancy toxaemia/ketosis
   d. In addition to low blood glucose (< 2.8 mmol/L)and high blood urea, Batchelder et al (1999) report anaemia, hypoproteinaemia, hypocalcaemia, hyperbilirubinaemia and raised liver enzymes

Table 1.13 The ferret: PCV

PVC (%)	Prognosis	Treatment options
>25	Good	Ovario-hysterectomy
		HCG or GnRH injection
15–25	Guarded	HCG or GnRH injection
		Supportive care before surgery
<15	Poor	HCG or GnRH injection
		i.v. fluids
		Vitamin B
		Iron
		Prophylactic antibiotics
		Blood transfusion(s), then consider surgery

3. Urinalysis
   a. Ketonuria (ketosis)
4. Culture and sensitivity
5. Endoscopy
6. Biopsy
7. Ultrasonography
   a. Prostatic hyperplasia/cysts.

Management

1. Fluid therapy, including blood transfusions (see *Nursing Care*)
2. Vitamin B complex at 1–2 mg/kg thiamine content as needed, i.m.
3. Iron dextran at 10 mg/kg every 7 days
4. Prophylactic antibiotics.

Treatment/specific therapy

- Hyperoestrogenism
  - Ovario-hysterectomy
  - HCG at 100 IU/ferret. Repeat after 7 days if necessary
  - Gn-RH at 20 μg/ferret i.m./s.c. Repeat after 7–14 days if necessary
  - Prevention
    - Routine ovario-hysterectomy
    - Routine proligestone injections at 50 mg/kg i.m. once only before breeding season
    - Mate with vasectomized male
    - Altering and maintaining the photoperiod at 14 h light:10 h dark may prevent oestrus
- Prostatic hyperplasia
  - Often resolves following treatment of hyperadrenocortism

- Surgical debulking or marsupialization
- Appropriate antibiosis if prostatitis suspected
- Testicular neoplasia
  - Castration
- Metritis
  - Induce uterine contractions with 0.5 mg prostaglandin F_{2a}
  - Antibiosis
- Pyometra
  - Ovario-hysterectomy
  - Antibiosis
- Stump pyometra (following ovario-hysterectomy) may occur in some ferrets with hyperadrenocortism. These will require surgical removal of the stump as well treatment for adrenal disease
- Mastitis
  - Acute mastitis
    - Antibiosis and fluids
    - NSAIDs may have anti-endotoxin effects (see 'Analgesia', in *Nursing Care*)
    - Debride or surgically resect affected mammary tissue
    - Fostering kits may spread pathogens to other females
  - Chronic mastitis
    - Often non-responsive to therapy
  - Kits may need supplemental feeding (see *Neonatal Disorders*)
- Urolithiasis in pregnant jills
  - If possible undertake caesarean section with 24 h of parturition date
  - At same time perform cystotomy
  - For management of urolithiasis, see *Urinary Disorders*
- Ketosis
  - Usually linked to period of anorexia/starvation during pregnancy. This can be as little as 12–24 h
  - In some cases linked to large litters (15+)
  - Supportive treatment including fluids, warmth and i.v. glucose/force feeding (see *Nursing Care*)
  - Perform caesarean as soon as possible
  - Foster or euthanize young (<40 days) as ferret young hard to hand rear and recovering female unlikely to lactate
- Dystocia
  - Small litter size
  - Induce parturition at day 41 with 0.5 mg prostaglandin F_{2a}, followed by 0.2–3.0 units oxytocin 1–4 h later. Birth should be 2–12 h later. If not either repeat treatment or undertake caesarean
  - Large or deformed kits, pelvic abnormalities and other anomalies
  - Caesarean.

Neonatal disorders

Some normal parameters of Neonatal Kits (from Bell 1997, see Table 1.14)

Viral
- Rotavirus.

Table 1.14 The ferret: Neonatal kits normal parameters

Approximate weight at birth (g)	8–10
Approximate weight at 7 days (g)	30
Approximate weight at 14 days (g)	60–70
Approximate weight at 21 days (g)	100
Age of eyes opening (days)	30–35
Age of weaning (weeks)	6–8

Bacterial
- Eye infections prior to 35 days.

Other non-infectious problems
- Hypothermia (especially in first 2 weeks as kits unable to thermoregulate)
- Lack of maternal milk
- Mastitis (see *Reproductive System Disorders*)
- Maternal metritis (see *Reproductive System Disorders*)
- Maternal systemic illness
- Tangled umbilical cords.

Findings on clinical examination

- Lethargy
- Failure to feed
- History of lack of maternal care
- Failure to grow
- Diarrhoea (may not be apparent as female continually licks clean)
- Swelling of the unopened eyes in kits <3 weeks old.

Investigations

1. Weigh kits
2. Radiography
3. Routine haematology and biochemistry
4. Culture and sensitivity
5. Endoscopy
6. Biopsy
7. Ultrasonography.

Management

- Nursing care, especially provision of warmth and fluids is extremely important with neonates.

Treatment/specific therapy

- Rotavirus
  - Kits over 7 days old may not require treatment
  - Fluids as 0.5–1.0 mL saline s.c. repeated several times daily
  - Covering antibiosis
- Tangled umbilical cords
  - Gently disentangle from each other and associated nesting material, resecting umbilical cords where appropriate
- Lack of maternal milk production
  - Supplement with commercial puppy or kitten milk replacer enhanced with cream to give a fat content of around 20%, four times daily
  - Foster only if appropriate to do so (may transfer pathogens between females)
  - Investigate underlying problem in the dam
- Eye infections
  - Incise along the eyelid suture line
  - Flush out any debris or pus
  - Apply a topical ophthalmic antibiotic preparation b.i.d.

References

Batchelder M A, Bell J A, Erdman S E 1999 Pregnancy toxaemia. Lab Anim Sci 49(4): 372–379

Beck W 2007 Ectoparasites, endoparasites, and heartworm control in small animals. Comp Cont Edu Vet 29(5A):3–8

Bell J A 1997 Periparturient and neonatal diseases. In: Hillyer E V, Quesenberry K E (eds) Ferrets, rabbits, and rodents, 1st edn. Saunders, Philadelphia, p 60

Brown S A 1997 Neoplasia. In: Hillyer E V, Quesenberry K E (eds) Ferrets, rabbits, and rodents, 1st edn. Saunders, Philadelphia, p 108

Bublot I B, Randolph R W, Chalvet-Monfrey K et al 2006 The surface electrogram in domestic ferrets. J Vet Card 8:87–93

Erdman S E, Kanki P J, Moore F M et al 1996 Clusters of lymphoma in ferrets. Cancer Invest 14(3):225–230

Erdman S E, Reimann K A, Moore F M et al 1995 Transmission of a chronic lymphoproliferative syndrome in ferrets. Lab Invest 72(5):539–546

Govorkova E A, Rehg J E, Krauss S et al 2005. Lethality to ferrets of H5N1 influenza viruses isolated from humans and poultry in 2004. J Virol 79(4):2191–2198

Hanley C S, Wilson G H, Frank P et al 2004 T cell lymphoma in the lumbar spine of a domestic ferret (Mustela putorius furo). Vet Rec 155(11):329–332

Hillyer E V 1997 Urogenital diseases. In: Hillyer E V, Quesenberry K E (eds) Ferrets, rabbits, and rodents, 1st edn. Saunders, Philadelphia, p 47

Johnson-Delaney C A, Nelson W B 1992 A rapid procedure for filling fractured canine teeth of ferrets. J Small Exot Anim Med 1(3):100–102

Keeble E 2001 Endocrine diseases in small mammals. In Practice 23(10): 570–585

Larsen K S, Siggurdsson H, Mencke N 2005 Efficacy of imidacloprid, imidacloprid/permethrin and phoxim for flea control in the Mustelidae (ferrets, mink). Parasitol Res 97:S107–S112

Lu D, Lamb C R, Patterson-Kane J C et al 2004 Treatment of a prolapsed lumbar intervertebral disc in a ferret. J Small Anim Pract 45(10):501–503

Lunn J A, Martin P, Zaki S et al 2005. Pneumonia due to Mycobacterium abscessus in two domestic ferrets (Mustela putorius furo). Aust Vet J 83(9):542–546

Malik R, Alderton B, Finlaison D et al 2002 Cryptococcosis in ferrets: a diverse spectrum of clinical disease. Aust Vet J 80(12):749–755

Manning D D, Bell J A 1990 Lack of detectable blood groups in domestic ferrets: implications for transfusions. J Am Vet Med Assoc 197:84–86

Martorell J, Espada Y, Ramis A 2005 Bilateral adrenalectomy in a ferret (Mustela putorius furo) with hyperadrenocortism. Clin Vet Peq Anim 25(3):173–177

Miller D S, Eagle R P, Zabel S et al 2006 Efficacy and safety of selamectin in the treatment of Otodectes cynotis infestation in domestic ferrets. Vet Rec 159(22):748

Montiani-Ferreira F, Mattos B C, Russ H H 2006 Reference values for ophthalmic diagnostic tests in ferrets. Vet Ophthalmol 9(4):209–213

Moore G E, Glickman N W, Ward M P et al 2005. Incidence of and risk factors for adverse events associated with distemper and rabies vaccine administration in ferrets. J Am Vet Med Assoc 226(6):909–912

Mullen H 1997 Soft tissue surgery. In: Hillyer E V, Quesenberry K E (eds) Ferrets, rabbits, and rodents, 1st edn. Saunders, Philadelphia, p 143

Munday J S, Brown C A, Richey L J 2004 Suspected metastatic coccygeal chordoma in a ferret (Mustela putorius furo). J Vet Diagn Invest 16(5):454–458

Nolte D M, Carberry C A, Gannon K M et al 2002 Temporary tube cystotomy as a treatment for urinary obstruction secondary to adrenal disease in four ferrets. J Am Anim Hosp Assoc 38:527–532

Orcutt C J 1998 Emergency and critical care of ferrets. Vet Clin North Am Exot Anim Pract 1(1):99–126

Patterson M M, Rogers A B, Schrenzel M D et al 2003 Alopecia attributed to neoplastic ovarian tissue in two ferrets. Comp Med 53(2):213–217

Sasai H, Kato K, Sasaki T et al 2000 Echocardiographic diagnosis of dirofilariasis in a ferret. J Small Anim Pract 41, 172–174

Schoemaker N J, Mol J A, Lumeij J T et al 2003 Effects of anaesthesia and manual restraint on the plasma concentrations of pituitary and adrenocortical hormones in ferrets. Vet Rec 152:591–595

Schoemaker N J, van der Hage M H, Flik G et al 2004 Morphology of the pituitary gland in ferrets (Mustela putorius furo) with hyperadrenocortism. J Comp Path 130:255–265

Schoemaker N J, Teerds K J, Mol J A et al 2002 The role of luteinizing hormone in the pathogenesis of hyperadrenocortism in neutered ferrets. Mol Cell Endocrinol 197:117–125

Stamoulis M E, Miller M S, Hillyer E V 1997 Cardiovascular diseases. In: Hillyer E V, Quesenberry K E (eds) Ferrets, rabbits, and rodents, 1st edn. Saunders, Philadelphia, p 66

Une Y, Wakimoto Y, Nakano Y et al 2000 Spontaneous Aleutian disease in a ferret. J Vet Med Sci 62(5):553–555

Wagner R A, Piché CA, Jöchle W 2005 Clinical and endocrine responses to treatment with deslorelin acetate implants in ferrets with adrenocortical disease. Am J Vet Res 66(5):910–914

Rabbits

· ·

Table 2.1 The rabbit: Key facts

Average life span (years)	5–10
Weight (kg)	1.0 kg (Netherland dwarf) to 10 kg (giant breeds)
Body temperature (°C)	38–39.6
Respiratory rate (breaths/min)	30–60
Heart rate (beats/min)	120–325
Gestation (days)	28–35
Age at weaning (weeks)	4–6
Sexual maturity (months)	4.5–9

Consultation and handling

Rabbits are prey animals and, therefore, may exhibit extreme anti-predator behaviour, such as jumping from the examination table. During a clinical examination, movements should be moderated and deliberate with loud noises avoided as these may startle the rabbit. The scent of potential predators such as dogs, cats and ferrets may be stressful to some rabbits so these should be removed by cleaning your hands, examination table and equipment as best as possible prior to examination.

Always weigh the rabbit at every consultation; weight loss may be the first occult sign of chronic disease such as dental disease. Most rabbits can be examined on a table with minimal restraint. If lifted, then one hand is placed beneath the chest while the other supports the back-end and legs. Many rabbits can have their perineum and ventral surface examined by gently turning them upon their backs, such that the rabbit is held and supported upside-down between the examiner's chest and arm. The oral cavity can be examined with the use of an auroscope, although in the conscious rabbit this can never be regarded as a full oral examination.

Nursing care

Thermoregulation

This is one of the most crucial homeostatic mechanisms for rabbits (and other small mammals). They are susceptible to both hyperthermia and hypothermia (which acts as a general depressant and is also immunosuppressive). Body temperature is achieved and maintained at some cost to the rabbit, which must generate and maintain a high metabolic rate. However, their small size means that they have a large surface area compared with body mass with a consequent high potential for conductive, convective and radiative heat loss. In the conscious rabbit, heat loss is countered by a variety of mechanisms such as dense coats and subcutaneous fat (insulative layers) plus physiological methods – peripheral vasoconstriction/dilatation, piloerection and shivering. Behaviour also alters to either enhance or reduce heat loss. High respiratory rates secondary to stress can mean a significant evaporative heat loss.

Management of hyperthermia (see *Systemic Disorders*)

Management of hypothermia

1. Assess the rectal temperature of the rabbit. If in doubt, assume that the animal is hypothermic and that this should be corrected as soon as possible.
2. Applying insulation such as bubble wrap is often insufficient – collapsed or otherwise inactive rabbits are not generating heat and this may insulate it from a higher ambient temperature.
3. Place these animals on to a heat mat, on to which is placed an absorptive towel or other material to reduce the risk of localized burns.
4. Alternatives included heated operating tables, commercial warm air generators or incubators; 'hot-hands' (gloves filled with warm water) carry too high a risk of burns and cool too quickly.
5. Place insulative material over the animal and heat source.
6. Areas of the body where there is a high risk of radiative heat loss such as the pinnae or feet can be covered with aluminium foil to further conserve heat.
7. By either quickly raising the body temperature, or allowing the rabbit to maintain its core temperature with ease we remove the need for costly hyperthermic physiological processes, e.g. shivering.

Fluids

In small mammals the choice of fluid used is as indicated with other mammals. Venous access in the rabbit is via the cephalic, lateral saphenous and marginal ear vein (Fig. 2.1). Jugular cut down can be undertaken under general anaesthesia (GA), but may result in respiratory embarrassment. Fluids can be given i.v. either by bolus or by infusion.

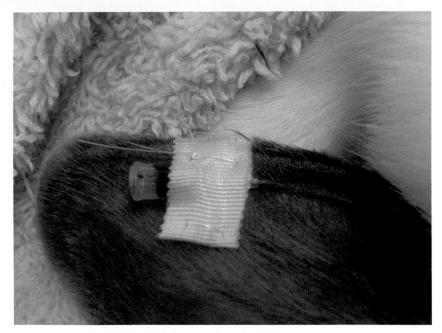

Fig. 2.1. Correct placement of a catheter into the marginal auricular vein.

In hypovolaemic patients vascular access may be impossible and it may be better to consider either i.p. or i.o. administration. For i.o. it is relatively simple under GA to insert either an intraosseous catheter or a hypodermic needle into the marrow of either the femur (via the greater trochanter) or tibia (through the tibial crest). Fluids, colloids and even blood can be i.o. if necessary.

Fluid administration

- All fluids should be warmed to 38°C.
- Daily fluid maintenance requirement for a rabbit is 100 mL/kg per day.
- Fluid replacement calculations are as for other species. Recommendations for rabbits are:
  - Crystalloids: For rabbits the maintenance fluid rate is 75–100 mL/kg per 24 h. Shock rate is up to 100 mL/kg over 1 h.
  - Colloids: A bolus of 10–15 mL/kg over 30 min can be given up to four times daily.
- Whole blood. Transfusions from other rabbits can be done, usually over a period of 20–30 mins. Transfusion reactions are rare but a major and minor cross-match are recommended.

Nutritional support

Many rabbits are presented as emergencies after a prolonged period of ill-health that will have affected their food intake, e.g. suffering from undiagnosed chronic dental disease. These animals are often hypoglycaemic, so testing beforehand (a commercial glucometer is suitable) is beneficial, followed by i.v. or i.p. glucose to those cases identified.

Longer-term support can be given by syringe feeding commercially available food supplements, e.g. Oxbow Critical Care and Supreme Recovery Diet. The following caveats apply:

- Use a relatively wide-bore syringe as blockage at the correct concentration is common. Feeding a dilute mixture may be counter productive.
- Naso-gastric tubes can be fitted but these are prone to block.
- If the rabbit is very debilitated then choking/failure to swallow may occur; in these cases concentrate on parenteral fluids, dextrose and B vitamin therapy.

Analgesia

Table 2.2 The rabbit: Analgesic doses

Analgesic	Dose
Buprenorphine	0.01–0.05 mg/kg s.c., i.m., i.v. every 6–12 h
Butorphanol	0.1–1.0 mg/kg s.c., i.m., i.v. every 2–4 h
Carprofen	1.0–2.0 mg/kg s.c. or p.o. b.i.d.
Ketoprofen	1.0 mg/kg i.m. b.i.d.
Meloxicam	0.1–0.3 mg/kg s.c. or p.o. s.i.d.
Morphine	2.0–5.0 mg/kg s.c. or i.m. every 4 h
Pethidine	5.0–10 mg/kg s.c. or i.m. every 2–4 h
Nalbuphine	1.0–2.0 mg/kg i.m., i.v. every 2–4 h

Anaesthesia

There are many safe anaesthetic techniques described for rabbits despite the fact that there is a persistent myth that rabbits do not survive anaesthesia. The author finds the following protocols of use:

Pre-anaesthetic protocol

1. Rabbits rarely vomit, so starving is not only unnecessary, but should be avoided due to their high metabolic rate.
2. Administering metoclopramide (0.5 mg/kg s.c. or p.o. q. 6–8 h) postoperatively will help to prevent a post-surgical ileus, especially following painful or abdominal surgery.
3. Monitor feeding and faecal output for 24 h following surgery.

Masking with volatile anaesthetics alone

The advantage of this technique is rapid recovery without the need to metabolize large amounts of drug, both of which can be important with rabbits that are catabolic, e.g. with chronic dental disease. Isoflurane appears to be less stressful for induction than halothane, based on lower corticosterone levels (González-Gil et al 2006).

Gaseous anaesthetic induction protocol

1. Preoxygenate rabbits before induction.
2. When masking down rabbits, breath holding is very common. This can lead to hypoxia, hypercapnia and bradycardia.
3. Monitor breathing closely and only increase anaesthetic concentration when seen breathing.
4. If rapidly increase the concentration, there is increased risk of inhalation of high concentrations of anaesthetic gas quickly, and increased risk of cardiovascular consequences once rabbit starts to breathe.
5. Once sufficiently anaesthetized, intubate – use an uncuffed endotracheal tube. Rabbits can exhibit laryngeal spasm so beware excessive trauma. Use local anaesthetic spray.

Blind intubation of rabbits

1. Spray glottis with local anaesthetic spray.
2. Place rabbit in sternal recumbency.
3. Run endotracheal (usually 2.0, 2.5 or 3.0 mm uncuffed) tube along midline of palate to back of pharynx.
4. Look for gagging reflex.
5. Listen for breaths.
6. Feel for exhalations.
7. Feel for sensation of tube passing over tracheal rings.
8. *Or* use laryngoscope with long blade.
9. Having an assistant hold the mouth open with pieces of bandage gauze behind the upper and lower incisors may be of some use.

Pre-medication protocol

1. Alternatively sedate with diazepam (0.2 mg/kg i.m. or i.v.) or midazolam (2.0 mg/kg i.m. or i.p.) or a combination of butorphanol (1.5 mg/kg) and medetomidine at 0.1 mg/kg. These may still not prevent breath holding.
2. Once sleepy, mask with isoflurane.
3. Spray glottis with local anaesthetic spray.
4. Intubate once able to and maintain with isoflurane.

• Oxygen can also be delivered via the nasal cavities – a small diameter catheter or tube is inserted into the ventral nasal meatus. Even moderate flow rates risk an explosive exit of such a tube! If necessary, a tracheotomy may need to be performed.

- Premedication with doxapram at 10 mg/kg i.p., i.v. or sublingually 5–10 min beforehand is occasionally recommended, but this will increase oxygen demand and the author finds it usually unnecessary.

Parenteral anaesthesia

- Ketamine/medetomidine/butorphanol given i.m. simultaneously:
  - Ketamine at 10 mg/kg
  - Medetomidine at 0.1 mg/kg
  - Butorphanol at 1.5 mg/kg.
- At end of procedure reverse medetomidine with atipamezole at 0.75 mg/kg.

Cardiopulmonary resuscitation

Respiratory arrest

1. Administer 100% oxygen.
2. Assist ventilation – compress thorax at around 60×/min.
3. Doxapram sublingual or at 10 mg/kg i.v. or i.p. *Note*: this will increase the animal's oxygen demand.
4. If appropriate, give atipamezole.

Cardiac arrest

As for respiratory arrest but also:
1. Compress thorax at around 90×/min.
2. If asystole – give adrenaline at 0.1 mg/kg of 1:10 000.
3. If ventricular fibrillation – lidocaine (lignocaine) at 1–2 mg/kg.

Skin disorders

Normally rabbits have a soft, short undercoat covered with larger guard hairs. Rex breeds have short guard hairs that do not exceed the undercoat while Angoran breeds have very long guard and undercoat hairs. Lionhead rabbits retain the long hair around the head, neck and rump area.

Satin breeds have altered hair fibre structure.

Findings on clinical examination

Signs of skin disease:
- Pruritus
  - Typically hairs will be damaged. There may be areas of reddened and inflamed skin

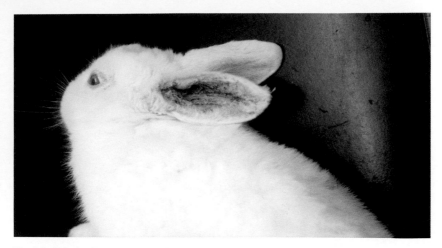

Fig. 2.2. Ear mite (*Psoroptes cuniculi*) infestation.

- Oedema may accompany a cellulitis
- Ectoparasites especially *Cheyletiella*, *Leporacarus* and *Psoroptes*. Occasionally fleas (rabbit flea *Spilopsyllus cuniculi* (Pinter 1999), cat and dog fleas *Ctenocephalides spp*), lice, sarcoptic and *Demodex* mites and blowfly maggots. *Cheyletiella* may act as a vector for myxomatosis
- Ear mites (*Psoroptes cuniculi*): inflammation and pruritus of the pinnae (Fig. 2.2). Can spread on to surrounding face and neck
- Bacterial disease, typically *Staphylococcus* and *Pasteurella* species (Fig. 2.3). *Pseudomonas* typically linked to moist dermatitis under chin (blue fur disease)
- Occasionally due to *Trichophyton*
- Alopecia
  - Self-mutilation secondary to pruritus
  - Sebaceous adenitis (Whitbread et al 2002)

Fig. 2.3. Severe bacterial dermatitis in a rabbit.

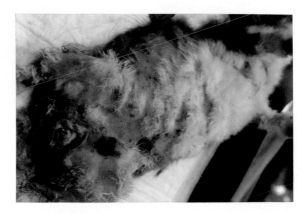

- Lack of dietary fibre can lead to 'barbering' if two or more rabbits present
    - Endocrinological
    - Cystic ovaries and other ovarian diseases
    - Suckling does will remove hair from around teats
    - Atypical myxomatosis
- Scaling and crusting
    - Ectoparasitic infestations especially *Cheyletiella*
    - Thickened crust-like material on pinnae and in ear canal strongly suggestive of *Psoroptes cuniculi*
    - Sebaceous adenitis
    - *Trichophyton mentagrophytes, Scopulariopsis brevicaulis* (Vangeel et al 2000) and rarely *Microsporum*
    - Myxomatosis lesions
    - Rabbit syphilis *Treponema cuniculi,* especially at mucocutaneous junctions. Vesicles may be present
    - Atypical myxomatosis
- Erosions and ulceration
    - Bacterial disease especially *Staphylococcus* and *Pseudomonas*
    - Myiasis
    - Cutaneous lymphosarcoma
    - Bites and lacerations (Fig. 2.4)
    - Pododermatitis
    - Atypical myxomatosis
    - Rabbit syphilis

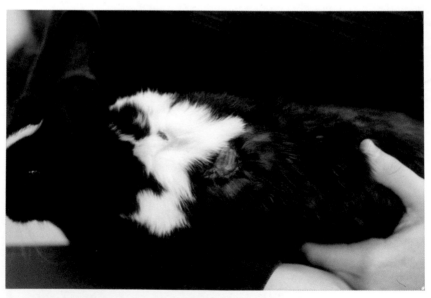

Fig. 2.4. Skin lacerations and subsequent dermal necrosis from fighting.

- Vaccine reactions. Can happen with oil adjuvanted vaccines, or if part of vaccine given intradermally (as manufacturer may recommend)
- Nodules, swellings and non-healing wounds
  - Abscess. If these are around the mouth strongly suspect underlying dental disease
  - Herpesvirus (circular, reddened skin lesions)
  - Poxvirus – initial nasal discharge and fever. Followed by generalized formation of papules and nodules. Oedema of the face and perineum
  - *Cuterebra* larvae
  - Mycobacteriosis
  - Myxomatosis (may see concurrent palpebral oedema, swollen pinnae, swelling of external genitalia and perineum)
  - Shope papilloma virus (papovavirus)
  - Shope fibroma virus (poxvirus)
  - Acrochordon
  - Lymphoma/lymphosarcoma
  - Other neoplastic diseases
    - Fibrosarcoma
    - Squamous cell carcinoma
    - Trichoepithelioma
    - Basal cell tumour
    - Lipoma
    - Apocrine adenocarcinoma (Miwa et al 2006)
- Excessively pronounced dewlap
  - Some breeds selected for this
  - More prominent in females
  - May be site of recurrent moist dermatitis, especially *Pseudomonas*, where the dewlap is consistently moist, e.g. from water bowls.

Investigations

1. Microscopy: examine fur pluck, acetate strips or skin scrapes to affected area and examine for ectoparasites
2. Examine material from ear canals for *Psoroptes cuniculi*
3. Examine teeth. Rabbits with dental disease may have difficulty grooming normally
4. Bacteriology and mycology: hair pluck or swab lesions for routine culture and sensitivity
5. Fine-needle aspirate followed by staining with rapid Romanowski stains
6. Biopsy obvious lesions
7. Ultraviolet (Wood's) lamp – positive for *Microsporium canis* only (not all strains fluoresce)
8. Routine haematology and biochemistry
9. Serology for *Treponema cuniculi* titre
10. Endocrine analysis (see *Endocrine Disorders*)
11. Normal plasma thyroid level: 22 nM/L (Hulbert 2000)
12. If barbering suspected, examine hair under microscope to see if chewed; separate from other rabbit; supply extra hay.

Management

1. Rabbits with dental disease, or those that have had incisor extractions are unable to groom and will require regular grooming by their owner.
2. Routine and regular examination of the perineum of pet rabbits is essential. The presence of caecotrophs adhered to the perineum will encourage myiasis (see *Failure to Caecotroph*).

Treatment/specific therapy

- Treat for any ectoparasites
  - Ivermectin at 200 µg/kg or as topical application (Xeno 450, Genitrix) works well for mites such as *Cheyletiella*, although treatment should be continued for greater than 6 weeks (life cycle = 5 weeks). Also for myiasis
  - Imidacloprid (Advantage, Bayer) applied as a 40 mg 'spot-on'. Can be applied weekly for lice and myiasis
  - Permethrin applied as either a dusting powder or shampoo
- Ear mites (*Psoroptes cuniculi*)
  - Ivermectin at 200 µg/kg or as topical application (Xeno 450, Genitrix)
  - Topical selamectin at 6–18 mg/kg (Hack et al 2002)
  - Topical 10% imidacloprid/1.0% moxidectin (Advocate, Bayer) at 10 mg/kg (imidacloprid) and 1 mg/kg (moxidectin) every 4 weeks for 3 treatments (Beck 2007)
  - Soften material in ear canal using either acaricidal ear drops or non-acaricidal products
  - After 5–7 days the crusty exudate should have softened sufficiently to allow atraumatic removal
- Myiasis
  - Initial treatment involves clipping of the fur and cleaning the affected area, with manual removal of maggots plus flushing with a dilute chlorhexidine or povidone-iodine cleanser. Supportive treatment should be aggressive with therapy for toxic shock plus ivermectin or imidacloprid to kill any maggots or emergent larvae that cannot be removed
  - The underlying cause of the caecotroph accumulation must be addressed (see *Failure to Caecotroph*) and regular perineal inspection and cleaning, plus protection from exposure to flies is crucial in preventing the condition
  - Topical cyromazine (Rearguard, Novartis) applied as a 6% solution topically every 6–10 weeks as a preventative for myiasis
  - *Cuterebra* larvae: either remove via the breathing hole, surgically or by using Ivermectin at 200 µg/kg or as topical application (Xeno 450, Genitrix)
- Pododermatitis
  - Commoner on large breeds
  - Typically on hocks
  - Can be linked to poor environment, e.g. moist flooring, slatted floors. Remove rabbit to solid flooring
  - May need repeated dressing (some rabbits may not tolerate such bandages)
  - IntraSite gel applied several times per day is beneficial
- Bacterial dermatitis and cellulitis
  - Topical and parenteral antibiotics
  - Cleaning with chlorhexidine solution may be beneficial

- Surgical removal of abscesses. Draining and flushing of rabbit abscesses rarely works
- Bites and lacerations
  - Clean and debride well. Prone to infection so may be better to surgically excise the lesion and heal by first intention
  - Covering broad-spectrum antibiosis
- Poxvirus, Shope fibroma virus
  - Supportive treatment only; usually spontaneously regress
- Shope papilloma virus
  - Can trigger warts especially on eyelids and ears
  - Consider surgical resection as may eventually become carcinomas
  - Spread by insect vector so anti-ectoparasiticidal treatment important adjunct
- Myxomatosis
  - Supportive therapy is required. Fluids, assisted feeding, covering antibiosis are essential if the rabbit is to stand any chance of survival
  - Spread by insect vectors so anti-ectoparasiticidal treatment important adjunct
  - Atypical myxomatosis. Three atypical forms have been described
    - Partially immune (vaccinated) rabbits may develop a papillomatous form that progresses to crusting lesions, especially on the eyelids and other muco-cutaneous junctions. These usually resolve with appropriate care
    - Papules and plaques appear in recently depilated areas. These progress to haemorrhagic and necrotic lesions. Recovery is spontaneous
    - Respiratory form
  - Vaccines are available
- Dermatophytosis
  - Griseofulvin at 25 mg/kg once daily for 4 weeks
  - Miconazole/chlorhexidine (Malaseb, Leo) shampoo – bath once daily
  - Itraconazole at 5.0 mg/kg s.i.d. for 30 days
- Treponema (Rabbit syphilis)
  - Responds well to penicillin at 50 000 IU given as once weekly for 3 weeks. In view of slight risk of inducing an enterotoxaemia, where possible always have serological test done first
  - Tetracyclines and chloramphenicol can also be effective
- Lymphoma/lymphosarcoma
  - See *Systemic Disorders*
- Neoplasia
  - Surgical debulking, resection or euthanasia
  - Accessible cutaneous tumours can be treated by injecting cisplatin directly into the tissue mass on a weekly basis as a debulking exercise
- Dewlap dermatitis
  - Clean with chlorhexidine solution
  - Antibiosis
  - Dewlap resection.

Respiratory tract disorders

Rabbits are obligate nasal breathers. The back of the pharynx is comparatively small and is occupied by the main body of the tongue, preventing easy visualization of the caudal pharynx.

Disorders of the upper respiratory tract

- Dental disease
- Pasteurellosis (includes atrophic rhinitis-like condition)
- Other bacterial infections
- Poxvirus
- *Treponema cuniculi*
- *Toxoplasmosis* (see *Neuromuscular Disorders*)
- Allergy.

Findings on clinical examination

- Nasal discharge
- Conjunctivitis (see *Ophthalmic Disorders*)
- Dacryocystitis (see *Ophthalmic Disorders*)
- Vesicles, erosions and crusty lesions (*Treponema cuniculi*)
- Fever (>40°C), oculo-nasal discharge, increased respiratory rate, CNS signs (toxoplasmosis).

Investigations and management

- See *Differential Diagnoses for Respiratory Disorders*

Treatment

- See also *Differential Diagnoses for Respiratory Disorders*
- Poxvirus – initial nasal discharge and fever. Followed by generalized formation of papules and nodules. Oedema of the face and perineum. Self-limiting.

Differential diagnoses for respiratory disorders

Viral

- Myxomatosis (see *Skin Disorders*)
- Viral haemorrhagic disease (VHD) (calicivirus)
- Herpesvirus
- Paramyxovirus (Sendai virus).

Bacterial

- Pasteurellosis (incl. *P. multocida*)
- *Bordetella bronchiseptica*
- *Staphylococcus aureus*
- *Streptococci spp*
- *Moraxella spp*
- *Pseudomonas aeruginosa*
- Mycobacteriosis
- Cilia-associated respiratory bacillus
- *Mycoplasma pulmonis*
- *Chlamydophila*

Protozoal
- Toxoplasmosis (see *Neuromuscular Disorders*).

Fungal

Neoplasia
- Lung metastases from uterine adenocarcinoma
- Thymomas.

Other non-infectious problems
- Allergic
- Congestive heart failure
- Traumatic tracheitis (secondary to endotracheal intubation)
- Heat stroke.

Findings on clinical examination

- Rhinitis
- Sinusitis
- Conjunctivitis
- Dacryocystitis (see *Ophthalmic Disorders*)
- Otitis
- Abscessation (can involve skin and variety of organs or joints due to bacteraemic spread)
- Increased respiratory noise
- Dyspnoea/tachypnoea
- Fever
- Bilateral exophthalmia (thymomas)
- Anorexia and weight loss
- Loss of exercise tolerance
- Associated cardiovascular disease, e.g. pericarditis with *Pasteurella* bacteraemia (see *Cardiovascular Disorders*).

Investigations

1. Auscultation
   a. Rales and rattles. Differentiate between upper respiratory tract disease and lower respiratory tract (pneumonia)
   b. Areas of consolidation may be silent
2. Radiography
   a. Skull (dental disease, bulla abscessation, turbinate atrophy)
   b. Contrast studies on nasolacrimal ducts
   c. Spine (disco-spondylitis)
   d. Thorax (lung metastases, cardiac disease, consolidated lung tissue, effusion lines)
3. Routine haematology and biochemistry
   a. Look for alterations in heterophil/lymphocyte ratios
4. Serology for *Pasteurella*, *Mycoplasma pulmonis*, *Chlamydophila*, myxomatosis.
5. Culture and sensitivity (including from tracheal wash)
   a. Always have anaerobic culture performed as well as aerobic

6. *Chlamydophila* PCR
7. Cytology from tracheal wash
8. Pleural tap and cytology
9. Endoscopy
10. Ultrasonography
    a. Thymoma
11. Biopsy.

Management

1. Give supportive treatment, e.g. covering antibiosis
2. Reduce stress levels. Hospitalize away from dogs and noisy cats; keep in darkened position
3. Supply oxygen, preferably via an 'oxygen-tent'
4. Mucolytics may be useful, e.g. bromhexine, N-acetyl-cysteine.

Treatment/specific therapy

- Viral haemorrhagic disease (VHD)
  - No treatment; supportive treatment only
- Pasteurellosis and other bacterial infections – broad-spectrum antibiotics plus anaerobic cover, e.g. metronidazole at 20 mg/kg b.i.d. p.o.
- Surgical removal or debridement of abscesses often necessary
- If surgery is not practical, then some abscesses may be allowed to heal by second intention. Daily topical applications of IntraSite Gel (Smith and Nephew Health) are helpful. Topical Manuka honey is also said to be useful
- Heat stroke – see *Systemic Diseases*
- Thymoma
  - Radiation therapy; 24 Gy given in 3 fractions of 8 Gy on days 0, 7 and 21 (Sanchez-Migallon et al 2006).

Dental disorders

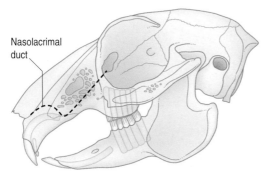

Nasolacrimal
duct

Fig. 2.5. A diagram of a rabbit skull showing position of teeth and track of nasolacrimal duct.

- The permanent dental formula of the rabbit (Fig. 2.5) is:

> **Permanent dental formula of the rabbit**
>
> $$I : \frac{2}{1}, C : \frac{0}{0}, PM : \frac{3}{2}, M : \frac{3}{3}$$

Protozoal

- *E. cuniculi* (meningitis may produce abnormal chewing muscle movements; partial paralysis of tongue secondary to hypoglossal nerve damage).

Nutritional

- Lack of long fibre, e.g. hay, in diet
- Inappropriate nutrition.

Neoplasia

- Osteosarcoma of the mandible.

Other non-infectious problems

- Congenital incisor malocclusion (esp. brachycephalic breeds such as Netherland dwarf, lionhead and mini-lops).

Findings on clinical examination

- Incisor malocclusion (Fig. 2.6)
- Mandibular swelling (unilateral or bilateral) due to bone remodelling to accommodate tooth root overgrowth
- Gross swelling, typically in the mandibular area (Fig. 2.7) but can be at maxilla, secondary to tooth root abscess
- Excessive salivation/moist fur on chin and ventral neck
- Weight loss
- Anorexia (may be intermittent)

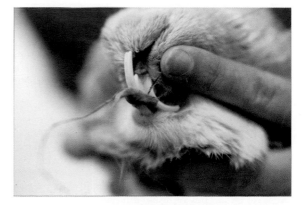

Fig. 2.6. Overgrown maxillary and mandibular incisors, with hair matted around the lower teeth.

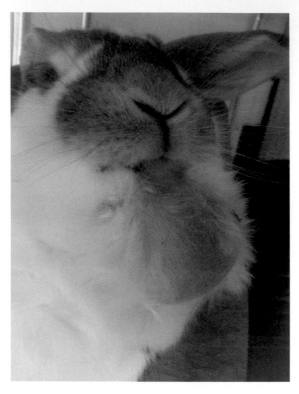

Fig. 2.7. Mandibular tooth root abscess.

- Perineal accumulations of caecotrophs
- Ectoparasitic disease
- Dacryocystitis
- Conjunctivitis
- Exophthalmus (secondary to retrobulbar abscess) (see *Ophthalmic Disorders*).

Investigations

1. Otoscopic examination
   a. Spurs on cheek teeth (tend to be lingual on the mandibular cheek teeth and buccal on the maxillary)
   b. Lingual tilting of mandibular cheek teeth and buccal tilting of maxillary cheek teeth (Fig. 2.8)
   c. Ulceration of tongue and cheeks
   d. Purulent material in mouth
   e. Otoscopic examination does not constitute a complete examination of the oral cavity as structures at the back of the pharynx can be difficult to see due to its depth and the large size of the tongue
2. Radiography
   a. Lateral, DV views of skull. *Note* skulls often appear osteoporotic. Probably due to an atrophy of disuse but has been linked to hypocalcaemia

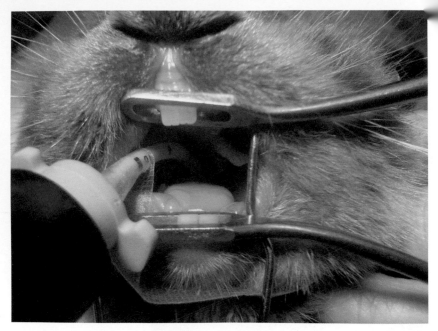

Fig. 2.8. Buccal tilting and overgrowth of the upper first premolar.

    b. Left and right lateral oblique views of skull to allow assessment of individual tooth roots. Any divergence of maxillary or mandibular tooth roots away from each other suggests abnormal root elongation (Figs 2.9, 2.10)

    c. Contrast study on nasolacrimal ducts

3. Check patency of nasolacrimal ducts (Fig. 2.11)
4. Routine haematology and biochemistry

Fig. 2.9. Right lateral oblique skull showing osteolysis around the root of the left first mandibular premolar associated with a tooth root abscess; there is also overgrowth of the second premolar, first molar and incisor roots.

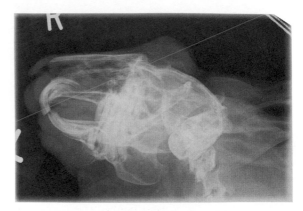

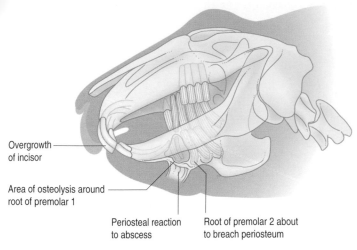

Overgrowth of incisor

Area of osteolysis around root of premolar 1

Periosteal reaction to abscess

Root of premolar 2 about to breach periosteum

Fig. 2.10. Explanatory diagram of Figure 2.9.

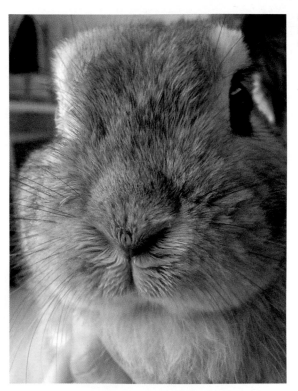

Fig. 2.11. Fluorescein can be used to check nasolacrimal duct patency.

a. Concerns that rabbits with dental disease are hypocalcaemic are ill-founded. Calcium levels are readily responsive to dietary levels and calcium status is monitored with ionized calcium (total calcium 3.0–4.0 mmol/L; ionized 1.57–1.83 mmol/L)
5. Culture and sensitivity
   a. Aerobic and anaerobic culture of abscesses
6. Endoscopy
7. Examination of oral cavity under GA
8. Biopsy (osteosarcoma).

Management

1. Chronic cases often cachexic – may need parenteral fluid support. Check blood glucose levels (normal range 6.0–8.9 mmol/L)
2. Syringe feeding with commercial feed suspensions, e.g. Critical Care (Oxbow) or Recovery diet (Supreme Petfoods). May require nasogastric tube
3. Flushing of nasolacrimal ducts and antibiosis.

Treatment/specific therapy

- Regular coronal reduction
  - Always burr overgrown incisors in preference to clipping due to risk of fracture, pulpal haemorrhage and infection
  - For cheek teeth, this will likely necessitate heavy sedation or a GA. 'Concious' dental work on the cheek teeth is stressful to the rabbit and risks serious traumatic back injuries, including fracture of lumbar vertebrae (see *Neuromuscular Disorders*)
  - Often coronal reduction alone is insufficient; often by the time of presentation, dental disease has progressed to a quite advanced stage
  - Use of a dental drill or equivalent is essential; dental spurs can be clipped but the teeth must be burred down but clipping is likely to fracture the tooth
- Incisor extraction
- Cheek teeth extraction
- Surgical debridement of tooth root abscesses including removal of infected bone and affected tooth roots, followed by:
  - Packing with antibiotic-impregnated methyl-methacrylate (bone cement or similar) *and/or*
  - Marsupialization leaving ostium for recurrent povidone-iodine/antibiotic application during second intention healing
  - Antibiosis
    - Usually a broad-spectrum such as enrofloxacin at 5 mg/kg s.i.d. p.o. or co-trimoxazole at 30 mg/kg b.i.d. p.o. *plus*
    - anaerobic antibiosis, e.g. metronidazole at 10–20 mg/kg p.o. s.i.d. or procaine G benzylpenicillin at 20 000–60 000 IU/kg s.i.d. i.m., s.c.
- Drilling out of tooth root apices to initiate tooth root death where extraction is not viable
- Analgesia, e.g. meloxicam at 0.3 mg/kg p.o. s.i.d. – can be given for many weeks
- Where possible, wean rabbit on to a diet high in long fibre, i.e. grass and hay, as this encourages normal chewing and dental wear on the back teeth
- Osteosarcoma. Treatment is difficult even with surgical debridement and chemotherapy – consider euthanasia.

Gastrointestinal tract disorders

Viral

- Rotavirus
- Papillomatosis
- Viral haemorrhagic disease (VHD).

Bacterial

- The normal gut flora of the rabbit is predominantly G +ve. Typical inhabitants include *Bacteroides spp., Propionibacterium spp., Butyrivibrio spp.* plus G −ve oval and fusiform rods. Also present are large ciliated protozoa (*Isotricha*) and yeasts (*Cyniclomyces guttulatus*). Coliforms are not present in healthy animals
- *E. coli*
- *Staphylococcus* (enteritis in newborn/suckling rabbits)
- *Clostridium spiroforme*
- *Clostridium piliforme* (Tyzzer's disease)
- *Salmonellosis*
- *Klebsiella pneumoniae* (Coletti et al 2001)
- *Pseudomonas*
- *Mycobacterium avium paratuberculosis* (Greig et al 1997).

Fungal

Protozoal

- Intestinal coccidiosis (especially *Eimeria perforans, E. magna, E. media* and *E. irresidua*)
- Hepatic coccidiosis *Eimeria stiedae*
- *Cryptosporidium* (young rabbits)
- *Giardia duodenalis* (non-pathogenic)
- *Monocercomonas cuniculi* (non-pathogenic)
- *Retortamonas cuniculi* (non-pathogenic)
- *Entamoeba cuniculi* (non-pathogenic)
- The commensal yeast (*Cyniclomyces guttulatus*) should not be mistaken for *Eimeria* oocysts.

Parasitic

- Nematodes
  - Pinworms (*Passalurus ambiguus*)
  - Trichostrongyle *Obeliscoides cuniculi*
- Cestodes
  - *Cittotaenia variablis*
  - *Mosgovoyia pectinata americana, M. perplexa*
  - *Monoecocestus americana*
  - *Ctenotaenia ctenoids*
- Trematodes
  - *Hasstilesia tricolor*
  - *Fasciola hepatica*
  - Cystercercosis (see *Liver Disease*).

Nutritional

- Insufficient fibre in diet, especially long fibre (grass and hay)
- Excessive carbohydrate intake (predisposes to *Clostridial* overgrowth)
- Selective feeding out of mixed pellet and grain diets is an unsubstantiated but possible problem.

Neoplasia

- Adenocarcinomas
- Leiomyomas
- Leiomyosarcoma
- Metastases from uterine adenocarcinoma
- Rectal papillomas
- Inflammatory fibroid polyps.

Other non-infectious problems

- Gastric trichobezoars (usually secondary to gut motility problems, lack of dietary fibre or dehydration)
- Caecoliths
- Mucoid enteropathy
- Dysautonomia
- Dental disease (see *Dental Disease*)
- Iatrogenic enterotoxaemia secondary to antibiotic use. Problem antibiotics include clindamycin, erythromycin, lincomycin, ampicillin and amoxicillin. Less likely, but capable of causing problems is the cephalosporin family of antibiotics. Antibiotics that rarely if ever cause problems include the fluoroquinolones such as enrofloxacin and marbofloxacin, the potentiated sulfonamide drugs and the aminoglycosides
- Failure to caecotroph
- Gastric stasis and bloat
- Foreign body
- Ingestion of toxin
- Intussusception (can be secondary to severe coccidiosis, caecal polyp).

Findings on clinical examination

- Diarrhoea (may be haemorrhagic (coccidiosis, *Klebsiella*), green (rotavirus))
- Abnormal faeces (jelly-like mucus with mucoid enteropathy, dysautonomia)
- Lack of faeces (gut stasis, occasionally mucoid enteropathy, dysautonomia)
- Depression
- Dehydration
- Perineal accumulations of caecotrophs (see *Failure to Caecotroph*)
- Anorexia, weight loss
- Abdominal distension (gastric bloat, ileus, gut stasis)
- Collapse, hypothermia
- Hepatomegaly, ascites, jaundice (*E. stiedae*, liver neoplasia, cystercercosis)
- Fever, diarrhoea abortions, sudden death (salmonellosis)
- Small white growths on ventral tongue (papillomatosis).

Investigations

1. Radiography
   a. Lateral and DV. Normal rabbit abdomen very variable in appearance
   b. Contrast studies. Can be complicated by re-ingestion of caecotrophs
2. Microscopy
3. Parasitology
4. Gram stain
5. Staining/cytology
6. Routine haematology and biochemistry
   a. Slightly raised liver enzymes (cystercercosis)
7. Serological test for rotavirus, VHD, *Clostridium piliforme*
8. Culture and sensitivity
9. Endoscopy
   a. Gastroscopy
10. Laparoscopy
11. Ultrasonography
12. Exploratory laparotomy and biopsy
13. Postmortem.

Management

1. Fluid therapy (see *Nursing Care*)
2. High-fibre diet
3. May need to syringe feed
4. Probiotics
   a. May be of benefit – the natural low pH of the rabbit stomach may reduce the amount of probiotics gaining access to the large intestine/caecum
   b. Transfaunation, using caecotrophs from a healthy rabbit may help natural gut flora to re-establish
5. Only use antibiotics if indicated. Many cases do not require their use, which can be counterproductive
6. Gut motility modifiers
   a. Metoclopramide at 0.5 mg/kg s.c. or p.o. q. 6–8 h.
   b. Cisapride 0.5 mg/kg s.i.d. or b.i.d.
7. Analgesics can be necessary but avoid those likely to exacerbate GIT ulceration, e.g. flunixin.

Treatment/specific therapy

1. Rotavirus
   a. Usually just in young rabbits
   b. Supportive treatment
2. Papillomatosis
   a. Covering antibiotics and analgesia if required. Usually self-limiting (<145 days)
3. Viral haemorrhagic disease
   a. Supportive treatment only (see *Systemic Disorders*)

4. Bacterial enteritis
   a. Appropriate antibiosis based upon culture and sensitivity
   b. Cholestyramine at 2 g/20 mL water orally s.i.d. for 14 days for *Cl. spiroforme* infections
5. Coccidiosis
   a. Usually seen in young rabbits below 12–14 weeks of age
   b. Cotrimoxazole at 30 mg/kg b.i.d.
   c. Sulphadimidine in drinking water 0.2% 100–233 mg/L over 3 days
   d. Improve hygiene to prevent ingestion of contaminated faeces
6. *Cryptosporidium*
   a. Potentiated sulphonamides at 30 mg/kg p.o. b.i.d., may be of use
   b. Nitazoxanide may prove useful
7. Pinworms and *Obelisciodes*
   a. Ivermectin at 200 µg/kg or as topical (450 µg/tube) spot on (Xeno450, Genitrix)
   b. Fenbendazole at 10–20 mg/kg; repeat after 2 weeks
8. Cestodes, including cystercercosis
   a. Praziquantel at 5–10 mg/kg as a single dose
9. Trematodes
   a. *Hasstilesia tricolor*. Usually non-pathogenic. Intermediate host is snails
   b. *Fasciola hepatica*. Intermediate host is aquatic snails; infected from foods collected from wet meadows and stream-sides
   c. Praziquantel at 5–10 mg/kg as a single dose
10. Trichobezoars – usually symptomatic of gut motility problem or dehydration
    a. Aggressive fluid therapy
    b. Analgesia
    c. Gut motility modifiers, e.g. metoclopramide at 0.2–1.0 mg/kg and cisapride at 0.5–1.0 mg/kg
    d. The use of enzyme papain, bromelin or pineapple juice (10 mL p.o. t.i.d.) to break down hair accretions often unsuccessful
    e. Avoid surgery unless absolutely necessary
11. Mucoid enteropathy and dysautonomia
    a. Usually seen in young rabbits 4–14 weeks old
    b. Fluid therapy, high-fibre diet, gut motility modifiers and analgesics
12. Intussusception
    a. Surgical correction
    b. May be due secondary to caecal fibroid polyp (Pizzi et al 2007)
13. Gastric stasis and bloat
    a. Decompress by passing stomach tube (insert and maintain in diastema as may bite through tube with incisors)
    b. Cimetidine at 5–10 mg/kg b.i.d. – t.i.d. p.o., s.c., i.v., i.m.
    c. Nursing care as under *General Management* above
    d. Investigate underlying aetiology, e.g. foreign body.

Failure to caecotroph

Nutritional
- High plane of nutrition
- Obesity

- Excess caecotroph production (low-fibre, high-protein and high-carbohydrate diet)
- Unpalatable caecotrophs (diet high in protein and carbohydrate) (Richardson 2001).

Neoplasia

Other non-infectious problems
- Dental disease
- Incisor extraction
- Spondylosis
- Spondylitis
- Other illness.

Findings on clinical examination

- Faecal accumulation or impaction around the perineum, especially in the skin folds either side of the genitalia
- Underlying skin is sore – liable to tear under mild traction to remove overlying faeces
- Maggots (see *myiasis* in *Skin Disorders*)
- Overt dental disease, e.g. incisor malocclusion, bilateral mandibular swelling (see *Dental Disease*)
- The rabbit may appear overtly overweight.

Investigations

1. Radiography
   a. Include full spinal radiography lateral and DV
   b. Skull radiography for dental disease
2. Routine haematology and biochemistry
3. Culture and sensitivity
4. Cytology
5. Endoscopy
6. Ultrasonography
7. Exploratory laparotomy
8. Biopsy.

Management

1. Gentle removal of impacted faecal material. May require anaesthetic as skin very friable around perineum
2. Cleaning of underlying skin with dilute chlorhexidine or povidone-iodine solution. Topical antibiotics may be used if there is an underlying dermatitis
3. Re-evaluation of diet – consider switching to a lower energy diet with high-fibre intake to encourage normal caecotrophy.

Treatment/specific therapy

- Spondylosis/spondylitis. NSAIDs, e.g. meloxicam at 0.3 mg/kg p.o. s.i.d. plus appropriate antibiosis if necessary. Spondylitis may be present as part of a bacteraemic spread
- Weight reduction (see *Re-evaluation of diet*)
- Dental disease (see *Dental Disease*).

Nutritional disorders

- Hypovitaminosis A
  - Reproductive disorders including infertility, fetal resorptions and abortion
  - High neonatal mortality and morbidity
  - Central nervous abnormalities including hydrocephalus
  - Supplement with commercial vitamin A preparations
- Hypovitaminosis E
  - Reproductive disorders including infertility, fetal resorptions and abortion
  - High neonatal mortality and morbidity
  - Muscular dystrophies
  - Supplement with commercial vitamin E preparations
- Hepatic lipidosis
  - Linked to obesity
  - Can predispose to diabetes mellitus and ketosis
  - Ketones in blood and urine (ketonuria)
  - Treatment – see *Systemic Disorders*
- Lack of dietary fibre
  - Increased risk of gastrointestinal disease secondary to altered gut motility and gut environment/commensal flora
  - Barbering of conspecifics
  - Supplement with long fibre (grass and hay)
- Copper deficiency
  - Anaemia in weanlings, decreased growth, hairloss, dry scaly skin and greying of black hairs
  - Recommended daily intake is 2.7 mg, and foods should have an absolute minimum of around 8 mg copper/kg
- Excess calcium intake
  - Calcium levels are readily responsive to dietary levels and there is a theoretical risk of hypercalcaemia. This has been linked to urolithiasis and arteriosclerosis
  - Total calcium 3.0–4.0 mmol/L; ionized 1.57–1.83 mmol/L.

Hepatic disorders

Viral
- Viral haemorrhagic disease (calicivirus) (see *Systemic Disorders*).

Bacterial
- Bacterial hepatitis.

Fungal

Protozoal

- *Eimeria stiedae.*

Parasitic

- Cystercercosis.

Nutritional

- Hepatic lipidosis
- Aflatoxicosis.

Neoplasia

- Bile duct adenoma
- Bile duct adenocarcinoma
- Metastatic spread of uterine adenocarcinoma.

Other non-infectious problems

- Heart disease (see *Cardiovascular Disorders*).

Findings on clinical examination

- Reduced or loss of appetite
- Vague signs of ill-health
- Abnormal faeces
- Hepatomegaly
- Jaundice
- Ascites.

Investigations

1. Radiography
   a. Hepatomegaly
   b. Ascitic fluid
2. Routine haematology and biochemistry
   a. Raised liver enzymes
3. Culture and sensitivity
4. Cytology
5. Peritoneal tap
6. Endoscopy
7. Laparoscopy
8. Ultrasonography
9. Biopsy
10. Postmortem
    a. Demonstration of *E. stiedae* oocysts from characteristic yellow coloured liver lesions or distended bile ducts
11. Feed analysis. Food concentrations of aflatoxin B1>100 ppm are toxic.

Management

1. Fluid therapy (see *Nursing Care*)
2. Lactulose at 0.5 mL/kg p.o. b.i.d.
3. Milk thistle (*Silybum marianum*) is a hepatoprotectant. Dose at 4–15 mg/kg b.i.d. or t.i.d.

Treatment/specific therapy

- Bacterial hepatitis
  - Appropriate antibiosis
- *E. stiedae*
  - Usually seen in young rabbits below 12–14 weeks of age
  - Toltrazuril at 7.0 mg/kg daily for 2 days. Repeat after 12 days
  - Cotrimoxazole at 30 mg/kg b.i.d.
  - Often have concurrent gastric bloat and gut stasis so treat as for *Management of Gastrointestinal Tract Disorders*
  - Improve hygiene to prevent ingestion of contaminated faeces
- Cystercercosis
  - Praziquantel at 5 mg/kg s.c. or p.o.
  - Regular worming of in-contact dogs and cats
- Neoplasia
  - No treatment.

Pancreatic disorders

Non-infectious problems

- Diabetes mellitus (see *Endocrine Disorders*).

Cardiovascular disorders

Viral

- Coronavirus (pleural effusion/dilated cardiomyopathy, DCM).

Bacterial

- Pericarditis and endocarditis (esp. *Pasteurella*, *Staphylococcus* species, *Salmonella* species, *Streptococcus viridans*).

Protozoal

- *Encephalitozoon cuniculi* (myocarditis)
- *Trypanosoma cruzi* (ventricular hypertrophy and dilatation).

Nutritional

- Hypovitaminosis E (myocardial muscular dystrophy).

Neoplasia

- Thymomas (exophthalmos).

Other non-infectious problems

- Congenital
  - Ventricular septal defects
  - Atrial septal defects
  - Valvular cysts
- Hypertrophic cardiomyopathy (HCM)
- Dilated cardiomyopathy (DCM)
- Bicuspid valve insufficiency
- Mitral valve insufficiency
- Coronary atherosclerosis
- Doxorubicin administration (DCM)
- Alpha agonist drugs (myocardial fibrosis)
- Catecholamines (coronary vasoconstriction with resultant myocardial fibrosis)
- Arteriosclerosis (possibly linked to hypercalcaemia)
- Atherosclerosis (possibly linked to hyperlipidaemia).

Findings on clinical examination

- Cyanosis or pallor of the mucous membranes
- Slow capillary refill time
- Exophthalmos (venous congestion of retrobulbar venous plexus)
- Dyspnoea (normal respiratory rate = 30–60/min)
- Precordial thrill
- Dysrhythmia (normal rate = 180–250 b.p.m.; excited healthy rabbits increase to 330 b.p.m.)
- Lack of thoracic percussion with auscultation
- Abnormal lung sounds
- Abnormal heart sounds
- Exercise intolerance
- Ascites
- Weight loss.

Investigations

1. Routine haematology and biochemistry
   a. Renal and hepatic parameters may be raised due to congestion and/or poor perfusion
   b. Raised cholesterol (0.1–2.0 mmol/L) and triglycerides (2.67–4.29 mmol/L)
2. *E. cuniculi* serology
3. Blood plasma K-tocopherol (vitamin E). Should be >0.5 µg/mL
4. Blood calcium (total calcium 3.0–4.0 mmol/L; ionized 1.57–1.83 mmol/L)
5. Serology for coronavirus
6. Pleural tap
   a. Cytology of effusions
7. ECG
   a. P waves are positive in standard limb leads
   b. Normal ECG values (from Reusch & Boswood 2003, see Table 2.3)

Table 2.3 The rabbit: Normal lead II ECGs

ECG Parameter (lead II)	Value
Heart rate (bpm)	198–330
P-wave duration (s)	0.01–0.05
P-wave amplitude (mV)	0.04–0.12
P–R interval (s)	0.04–0.08
QRS duration (s)	0.02–0.06
R-wave amplitude (mV)	0.03–0.39
Q–T interval (s)	0.08–0.16
T-wave amplitude (mV)	0.05–0.17
Mean electrical axis (°)	−43–+80

8. Radiography
   a. Lateral and DV views
   b. Note thymus persistent into adulthood
   c. Lateral view: normal heart around two rib spaces; 2.5–3 rib spaces suggests cardiomegaly (Fig. 2.12)
9. Echocardiography
   a. Normal values for echocardiographic parameters in rabbits (from Marini et al 1999, see Table 2.4)
10. Table 2.5 (Fontes-Sousa et al 2006) give these values for two-dimensional, M-mode, and Doppler echocardiographic variables in male New Zealand white rabbits anaesthetized with a combination of ketamine and medetomidine
11. Blood pressure (cited in Reusch 2005, Table 2.6).

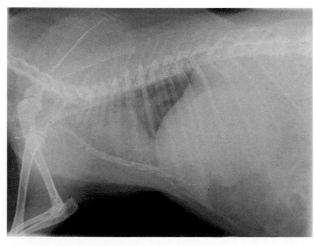

Fig. 2.12. Cardiomegaly.

Table 2.4 The rabbit: Normal echocardiographic values

Measurement	Cardiac timing	Mean ± SD
Left ventricular internal diameter (cm)	Diastole	1.17 ± 0.19
	Systole	0.70 ± 0.09
Left ventricular free wall (cm)	Diastole	0.31 ± 0.08
Interventricular septum (cm)	Diastole	0.25 ± 0.05
Fractional shortening (%)		39.5 ± 5.39
E-point septal separation (cm)	Diastole	0.05 ± 0.05
Aorta (cm)	Diastole	0.67 ± 0.10
Left atrial dimension (cm)	Systole	0.17 ± 0.41
Right ventricular outflow tract velocity (m/s)		0.83 ± 0.10
Left ventricular outflow tract velocity (m/s)		0.65 ± 0.14
Body weight (kg)		2.32 ± 0.36

Table 2.5 Echocardiographic variables in male New Zealand white rabbits anaesthetized with a combination of ketamine and medetomidine

Variable	Mean ± SD	Range
Body weight (kg)	2.59 ± 0.25	2.2–3.2
Thickness of the IVS in diastole (mm)	2.03 ± 0.37	1.43–3.10
Thickness of the IVS in systole (mm)	3.05 ± 0.45	2.17–4.03
LVID in diastole (mm)	14.37 ± 1.49	11.87–19.06
LVID in systole (mm)	10.05 ± 1.22	7.83–13.53
Thickness of the LVFW in diastole (mm)	2.16 ± 0.25	1.60–2.80
Thickness of the LVFW in systole (mm)	3.48 ± 0.55	2.43–4.55
Fractional shortening (%)	30.13 ± 2.98	22.60–36.83
Ejection fraction (%)	61.29 ± 4.66	49.07–70.0
Ao = Aortic diameter (mm)	8.26 ± 0.76	6.73–9.80
Left atrial appendage diameter (mm)	9.66 ± 1.14	7.53–12.0
Left atrium: Aortic diameter	1.17 ± 0.14	0.94–1.54
Mitral valve E-point–septal separation interval (mm)	1.71 ± 0.29	1.20–2.33
Doppler heart rate (beats/min)	155 ± 29	115–234
Maximal aortic outflow velocity (m/s)	0.85 ± 0.11	0.56–1.06
Maximal pulmonary artery outflow velocity (m/s)	0.59 ± 0.10	0.34–0.84
Maximal mitral E-wave velocity (m/s)	0.59 ± 0.10	0.41–0.83
Maximal mitral A-wave velocity (m/s)	0.28 ± 0.07	0.19–0.44
Mitral E:A	2.19 ± 0.46	1.34–3.55

Table 2.6 The rabbit: Blood pressure

	Normal range (mmHg)
Mean arterial pressure	80–91
Systolic pressure	92.7–135
Diastolic pressure	64–75

Management

1. Reduce stress, e.g. keep in a cool, shaded or darkened area away from dogs, cats, ferrets and other 'predators'.
2. Monitor closely – diuretics can produce a dehydration, which in rabbits can present as a gastric or caecal impaction.
3. Supply oxygen.

Treatment/specific therapy

- Cardiomyopathy
  - Taurine at 100 mg/kg s.i.d. for 8 weeks
- Arrhythmias
  - Digoxin at 0.003–0.03 mg/kg p.o. every 12–48 h
  - Lidocaine 1–2 mg/kg i.v. or 2–4 mg/kg i.t.
- Congestive heart failure
  - Furosemide 0.3–4 mg/kg p.o., s.c., i.m., i.v. s.i.d., b.i.d.
  - Enalapril 0.1–0.5 mg/kg p.o. every 24–48 h. Beware hypotensive side-effects
  - Glyceryl trinitrate ointment (2%) at 3 mm applied topically to the inner pinna every 6–12 h
- Other medications
  - Atenolol 0.5–2 mg/kg p.o. s.i.d.
  - Verapamil 0.2 mg/kg p.o., s.c., i.v. t.i.d.
  - Diltiazem 0.5–1 mg/kg p.o. b.i.d., s.i.d.
  - Atropine 0.05–0.5 mg/kg s.c., i.m. Note that rabbits have high tissue and serum atropinase levels
  - Glycopyrronium (glycopyrrolate) 0.01–0.1 mg/kg s.c., i.m., i.v.
  - Pimobendan at 0.2 mg/kg s.i.d.
  - Benazepril at <0.1 mg/kg p.o. s.i.d. Note rabbits appear very susceptible to the hypotensive side-effects of benazepril.

Systemic disorders

Viral
- Viral haemorrhagic disease (VHD). Calicivirus.

Bacterial
- Salmonellosis.

Fungal

Protozoal

Parasitic

Nutritional

Neoplasia

* Lymphosarcoma/lymphoma (Gómez et al 2002).

Other non-infectious problems

* Hypoglycaemia (especially with chronic dental disease)
* Heat stroke
* Pregnancy toxaemia/ketosis
* Severe cardiovascular disease.

Findings on clinical examination

* Anorexia. A recent history of anorexia, e.g. with dental disease or other ill-health suggests hypoglycaemia or ketosis
* Weight loss/poor physical condition
* Marked dental disease
* Lethargy
* Ataxia, convulsions (ketosis)
* Collapse
* Pale mucous membranes (lymphosarcoma)
* Hyperthermia (>40.5°C) (heat stroke)
* Lymphadenopathy (lymphosarcoma)
* Tachypnea/dyspnea (heat stroke, lymphosarcoma)
* Obesity (ketosis)
* Late pregnancy (pregnancy toxaemia)
* Acute onset epistaxis and/or respiratory signs and/or diarrhoea (VHD)
* High mortalities (VHD)
* Fever, diarrhoea, abortion, sudden death (salmonellosis, VHD)
* Dyspnoea.

Investigations

1. Radiography
2. Routine haematology and biochemistry
   a. White cell count and differentiation
   b. Blood glucose levels (normal glucose 5.0–9.0 mmol/L)
   c. Ketosis
3. Serology for VHD
4. Urinalysis
   a. Ketonuria (ketosis/pregnancy toxaemia)
   b. Aciduria pH 5–6 (ketosis)
5. Culture and sensitivity

6. Cytology
7. Bone marrow aspirate/biopsy
8. Laparoscopic endoscopy
9. Ultrasonography
10. Biopsy
    a. Multi-organ biopsies for lymphosarcoma
11. Necropsy
    a. Hepatic necrosis, haemorrhagic viscera (VHD)
    b. Hepatomegaly, splenomegaly, mesenteric lymphadenopathy (lymphosarcoma).

Management

1. Supportive therapy – parenteral fluids, assisted feeding
2. May require additional heat if recumbent.

Treatment/specific therapy

- Lymphosarcoma
  - The author has found that a chemotherapy regime, modified from that used for ferrets (Brown 1997), can be beneficial (Table 2.7)
- Hypoglycaemia
  - i.v. glucose by bolus and infusion
  - Assisted feeding
- Hepatic lipidosis/ketosis/pregnancy toxaemia
  - Aggressive fluid therapy
  - Parenteral nutrition with glucose and vitamins
  - Assisted feeding either by syringe or nasogastric tube. Calcium gluconate p.o. or propylene glycol p.o. may be of use
  - Dexamethasone at 0.2 mg/kg i.v., s.c. or p.o.
- Heat stroke
  - Monitor core body temperature

Table 2.7 The rabbit: Chemotherapy protocol

Week	Day	Drug	Dose
1	1	Vincristine	0.1 mg/kg i.v.
		Prednisolone	1 mg/kg p.o. b.i.d. throughout therapy
1	3	Cyclophosphamide	10 mg/kg p.o.
2	8	Vincristine	0.1 mg/kg i.v.
3	15	Vincristine	0.1 mg/kg i.v.
4	22	Vincristine	0.1 mg/kg i.v.
4	24	Cyclophosphamide	10 mg/kg p.o.
7	46	Cyclophosphamide	10 mg/kg p.o.
9		Prednisolone	Begin to wean off prednisolone over the next 4 weeks

- Cool (not cold) body, e.g. damp towels, water bath
- Dexamethasone at 2–4 mg/kg given i.v. once only
- Supportive treatment such as cool intravenous fluids; heat stroke may have unforeseen sequelae, e.g. gut stasis
- Viral haemorrhagic disease. Supportive treatment only
  - 0.5% sodium hypochlorite will inactivate virus
  - Virus can survive for some time in environment and can be carried on fomites
  - Vaccine available; recommended annual vaccination. Vaccinated rabbits can develop a subclinical infection.

Neuromuscular disorders

Viral

- Herpes simplex
- Rabies.

Bacterial

- Pasteurellosis (otitis media/interna, encephalitis)
- Other bacteria frequently isolated from otitis media are *Staphylococcus aureus* and *Bordetella bronchiseptica*
- Disco-spondylitis
- Osteomyelitis
- *Listeria monocytogenes.*

Fungal

Protozoal

- *E. cuniculi*
- *Toxoplasma gondii*
- *Sarcocystis* (myositis).

Parasitic

- *Baylisascaris procyonis*
- Other aberrant migrant parasites, e.g. *Ascaris spp*
- *Psoroptes cuniculi* (predisposes to otitis media).

Nutritional

- Hypovitaminosis A (hydrocephalus and other CNS defects)
- Hypovitaminosis E (muscular dystrophy).

Neoplasia

- Osteosarcomas
- Osteochondromas
- CNS metastases.

Other non-infectious problems

- Trauma
  - Vertebral fracture – typically L6 or L7
  - Other fractures

- Electrocution (lumbar or pelvic fractures following spasm of lumbar musculature)
  - Intervertebral disc disease
  - Metastatic calcification of cerebral vasculature/arteriosclerosis
- Atherosclerosis
- Splay leg – autosomal recessive defect (unable to adduct one or more limbs, accompanies distortion of joints and long bones)
- Idiopathic epilepsy
- Intoxication
  - Heavy metals
  - Fertilizers, herbicides, insecticides
  - Fipronil application.

Findings on clinical examination

- Otitis media/externa (see also 'Ear mites' in *Skin Disorders*)
- Mild head tilt or torticollis
- Nystagmus (only in acute disease)
- Extreme twisting of the body along the longitudinal axis.
- Hind limb paresis or paralysis
- Paresis or paralysis of one or more legs
- Seizures
- Anorexia
- Fever (>40°C), oculo-nasal discharge, increased respiratory rate (toxoplasmosis)
- Ophthalmic disease (see *Ophthalmic Disorders*).

Investigations

1. Neurological examination
2. Radiography
   a. Skull – check tympanic bullae
   b. Lateral and DV spinal radiographs
   c. Myelography
   d. Ingested metal in gut
3. Routine haematology and biochemistry
   a. Triglycerides and cholesterol for atherosclerosis
   b. Blood lead levels; basophilic stippling of RBCs
4. Serology for *E. cuniculi, Toxoplasma gondii, Pasteurella, Sarcocystis, Rabies*
5. Culture and sensitivity
   a. Swab if perform bulla osteotomy
6. Cytology from CSF tap (Table 2.8)

Collection of CSF

- Collect as from the cat.
- Undertake ventral flexion of neck.
- Collect from the atlanto-occipital joint, using a 22 gauge needle, and direct towards nose.

NORTHEAST COMMUNITY COLLEGE LIBRARY

Table 2.8 The rabbit: CSF parameters (adapted from Weisbroth et al)

Parameter	Value	*E. cuniculi* infected
WBC (per μL)	0–4	5–78
Glucose (mmol/L)	4.2	
Urea nitrogen (mmol/L)	10.8	
Creatinine (mmol/L)	1.5	
Cholesterol (mmol/L)	0.858	
Total protein (g/L)	0.13–0.31	0.31–1.54
ALP (U/L)	50.0	
CO_2 (mL%)	41.2–48.5	
Na (mmol/L)	149	
K (mmol/L)	3.0	
Cl (mmol/L)	127	
Ca (mmol/L)	1.35	
Mg (mmol/L)	1.1	
PO_4 (mmol/L)	0.74	
Lactic acid (mmol/L)	0.16–0.44	
Non-protein nitrogen (mmol/L)	4.0–12	

7. Toxicology
8. Endoscopy of ear canal
9. Ultrasonography
10. Exploratory laparotomy
11. Biopsy.

Management

1. May require food and fluid support if unable to feed. Consider fluid therapy, syringe feeding or nasogastric tube
2. Supportive harnesses may be useful where there is hind limb paresis/paralysis
3. Nursing care to prevent pressure sores, urine scalding and perineal caecotroph accumulation.

Treatment/specific therapy

- Otitis media. Treat with appropriate antibiotics both topical and systemic. Ensure eardrum is intact before treatment
- Otitis interna
  - Covering antibiotics
  - May require bulla osteotomy. Swab for culture and sensitivity if do so
- *E. cuniculi*
  - Co-trimoxazole at 30 mg/kg b.i.d. p.o. for at least 3 weeks

- Albendazole at 10 mg/kg p.o. for 6 weeks
- Fenbendazole at 10–20 mg/kg p.o. for 1 month
- Also treatment protocol for *Toxoplasma* effective (see *Toxoplasma gondii*)
- *Toxoplasma gondii*
  - Combination therapy consisting of:
    - Co-trimoxazole at 30 mg/kg b.i.d. p.o.
    - Pyrimethamine at 0.5 mg/kg b.i.d. p.o.
    - Folic acid at 3.0–5.0 s.i.d.
  - Rabbits with acute toxoplasmosis have congested tissues and marked splenomegaly
  - Avoid access to soil/food contaminated with Toxoplasma oocysts
- Sarcocystis
  - Treat with trimethoprim sulphamethoxazole and pyrimethamine at Toxoplasma dose rates
  - The Virginia opossum is the primary host; cockroaches can act as paratenic hosts
- *Baylisascaris procyonis*
  - Adults found in raccoon (*Procyon lotor*)
  - Attempt treatment with Fenbendazole at 20 mg/kg p.o. daily for 5 days, plus supportive therapy. Consider euthanasia
- Vertebral fracture – usually requires euthanasia
- Other fractures especially long-bone fractures usually respond well to orthopaedic procedures. Because they are relatively light, external fixation techniques are especially useful providing chewing can be avoided
- Intervertebral disc disease
  - Spondylitis – antibiotics and NSAIDs, e.g. meloxicam at 0.3 mg/kg p.o. s.i.d.
  - Intervertebral disc prolapse – may require surgery, e.g. disc fenestration. Guarded prognosis
- Metastatic calcification of cerebral vasculature/arteriosclerosis
  - Guarded prognosis. Consider cerebral vasodilators such as nicergoline and propentofylline
- Atherosclerosis
  - Switch to a lower fat/carbohydrate diet
- Toxin ingestion
  - Supportive therapy. Antidote if applicable, e.g. Ca EDTA for lead poisoning at 27.5 mg/kg q.i.d. for 5 days; repeat after week if required
- Fipronil application
  - Supportive therapy only
- Rabies: euthanasia
- Idiopathic epilepsy/control of seizures
  - Phenobarbitone at 1–4 mg/kg p.o.

Ophthalmic disorders

The rabbit eye differs from that of carnivores in several respects. A tapetum is absent and there is a merangiotic retina with a horizontal band of myelinated nerve fibres and blood vessels. These provide a horizontal, photoreceptor rich, macula-like region. It may be that, combined with lateral positioning of eyes, a band of high-resolution vision across the whole horizon is produced. There is a large ventral retrobulbar venous sinus which can cause serious intraoperative complications during enucleation.

Differential diagnoses of ocular disorders

Viral

- Myxomatosis.

Bacterial

- Retrobulbar abscess (often secondary to dental disease)
- *Staphylococcus spp, Pasteurella, Haemophilus*
- *Treponema cuniculi.*

Fungal

Protozoal

- *E. cuniculi* (uveitis).

Neoplasia

- Thymoma.

Other non-infectious problems

- Glaucoma in New Zealand white rabbits (autosomal recessive disorder)
- Corneal occlusion syndrome – aberrant covering of cornea by conjunctiva
- Entropion
- Foreign bodies
- Diabetes mellitus (cataracts).

Findings on clinical examination

- Ulceration
- Severe blepharitis and whitish ocular discharge (myxomatosis). Look for other signs of myxomatosis (see *Skin Disorders*)
- Conjunctivitis (distinguish from dacryocystitis)
- Dacryocystitis is common in rabbits (often secondary to dental disease as the nasolacrimal duct runs close to roots of incisor teeth and premolars)
- Microabscesses in eyelid margins – often a sequel to severe or chronic periocular infection
- Nasal discharge
- Uveitis
- Corneal oedema, hypopyon, and synechiae. May see large iridial abscesses. Occasionally secondary cataracts
- Exophthalmus
- Third eyelid may be prolapsed and swollen
- Megaglobus/glaucoma
- Cataracts.

Investigations

1. Ophthalmic examination
   a. Conjunctivitis is common in rabbits, often associated with dacryocystitis. Differentiate from dacryocystitis by cannulation of nasolacrimal duct (single ventral nasolacrimal punctum at medial canthus) (Fig. 2.13)
   b. Topical fluorescein to assess extent of ulceration (Fig. 2.14)

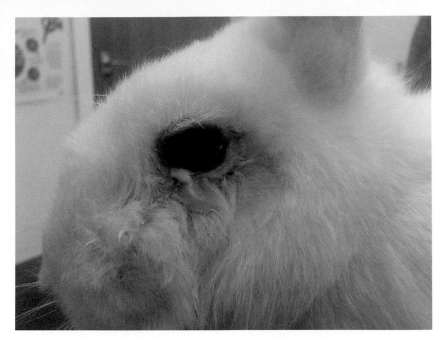

Fig. 2.13. Proliferative lymphatic tissue response of the conjunctiva in a chronic dacryocystitis.

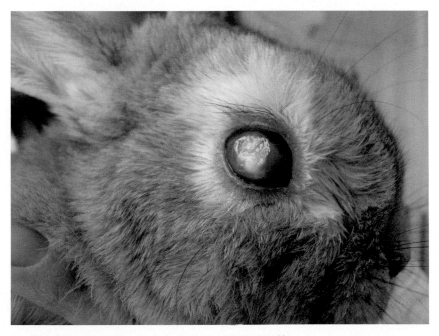

Fig. 2.14. Fluorescein positive corneal ulcer in a rabbit with keratitis.

2. Schirmer tear test 2.0–11.0 mm/min (Biricik et al 2005)
3. Phenol red thread test 15–27 mm/15 s
4. Tonometry
   a. Normal intraocular pressure is 15–23 mmHg. With hereditary glaucoma in New Zealand white rabbits = 26–48 mmHg
5. Radiography
   a. Assess tooth roots for underlying dental disease
   b. Contrast studies of nasolacrimal duct to determine if occluded
6. Cannulate and flush the nasolacrimal duct to collect sterile samples for culture, sensitivity and cytology if appropriate
7. Ultrasonography.

Treatment/specific therapy

- Corneal ulceration
  - Topical and systemic antibiosis
  - Once infection cleared, treat as for other small animals, e.g. scarification to encourage healing, conjunctival grafts, etc. Note third eyelid may not cover whole cornea if attempt a third eyelid flap
- Dacryocystitis
  - Topical ophthalmic antibiotic preparations. Conjunctival bacterial flora can be both G +ve and G −ve so select antibiotic according to sensitivity results
  - Regularly cannulate and flush the nasolacrimal ducts
  - Incisor or premolar extraction if linked to nasolacrimal disease
- *Encephalitozoon cuniculi*
  - Can cause cataracts or even lens capsule rupture, producing a phacoclastic uveitis.
  - Co-trimoxazole at 30 mg/kg b.i.d. p.o. for at least 3 weeks
  - Albendazole at 10 mg/kg p.o. for 6 weeks
  - Fenbendazole 10–20 mg/kg p.o. for 1 month
  - Combination therapy consisting of:
    - Co-trimoxazole at 30 mg/kg b.i.d. p.o.
    - Pyrimethamine at 0.5 mg/kg b.i.d. p.o.
    - Folic acid at 3.0–5.0 s.i.d.
  - Consider lens removal, preferably by phacoemulsification
- Retrobulbar abscess
  - Start on antibiotics – treat for anaerobic as well as aerobic; see under 'Treatment' in *Dental Disorders*
  - Remove affected teeth
  - May require enucleation. Haemorrhage is likely to be a significant complication due to the large retrobulbar abscess
  - Dental disease. Treat as under *Dental Disorders*
- Corneal occlusion syndrome. Surgery and topical cyclosporin
- Diabetes mellitus (see *Endocrine Disorders*).

Endocrine disorders

- Diabetes mellitus
- Adrenal disease
- Hypertestosteronism in castrated males secondary to adrenal hyperplasia/neoplasia.

Findings on clinical examination

- Sudden-onset cataracts
- Polydipsia
- Polyuria
- Weight loss despite good appetite
- Increased aggression and sexual behaviour in castrated male rabbits (hypertestosteronism).

Investigations

1. Radiography
2. Routine haematology and biochemistry
   a. High blood glucose usually associated with stress; for diabetes mellitus correlate with glycosuria, polydipsia and polyuria. Normal glucose is 5.0–9.0 mmol/L
   b. Normal rabbit fructosamine is 289–399 µmol/L

ACTH stimulation test

- Cortisol (resting) 1.0–2.04 µg/dL.
- ACTH at 6.0 µg/dL i.m.
- Resample after 30 min: cortisol 12.0–27.8.
- Note that corticosterone is the principle adrenocortical hormone in rabbits, with an approximate ratio of 20:1 corticosterone:cortisol.

3. Blood testosterone levels
   a. Normal intact New Zealand white rabbits (reported in Lennox & Chitty 2006) = 0.51–9.16 ng/mL. Castrated males have significantly lower testosterone levels >0.1 ng/mL
4. Urinalysis – should be glucose negative, but can also occur after periods of stress and certain diseases, e.g. ketosis
5. Cytology
6. Endoscopy
7. Ultrasonography
8. Biopsy.

Treatment/specific therapy

- Diabetes mellitus
  - Insulin usually not required
  - Maintain on a high-fibre, low-carbohydrate diet
- Hypertestosteronism secondary to adrenal hyperplasia/neoplasia
  - Adrenalectomy
  - Trilostane
  - The poor result of trial treatment with leuprolide acetate described in Lennox & Chitty (2006) suggests that hormonal antagonism as a treatment is likely to be of limited value.

Urinary disorders

Bacterial

- Pyelonephritis (*Staphylococcus aureus, Pasteurella multocida*)
- Cystitis (*Staphylococcus aureus, Pasteurella multocida*).

Protozoal

- *E. cuniculi.*

Nutritional

- Urolithiasis (usually combined with a cystitis)
- Renal calcinosis (hypercalcaemia, hypervitaminosis D)
- Fatty degeneration.

Neoplasia

- Embryonal nephroma
- Renal carcinoma
- Renal leiomyoma.

Other non-infectious problems

- Congenital abnormalities
- Renal
- Inguinal hernias
- Poor mobility, e.g. discospondylitis contributes to calciuria/urolithiasis.
- Haemolytic anaemias
- Nephrotoxic drugs (gentamicin, zolazepam).

Findings on clinical examination

- Polydipsia, polyuria
- Urinary tenesmus
- Apparent haematuria (uterine adenocarcinoma, endometrial venous aneurysms, porphyrinuria). Differentiate from porphyrinuria by either urinalysis dipstick test or expose to ultra-violet light: porphyrins fluoresce a purple-like colour
- Anorexia
- Depression
- Urolithiasis
- 'Sand'-like material in the urine
- Small stones present in the urine or lodged in the penis.

Investigations

1. Urinalysis (Table 2.9)
   a. Culture and sensitivity
   b. Sediment examination/cytology
2. Urolith analysis
3. Radiography
   a. Uroliths or calciuria in the renal pelvices, ureters, bladder or urethra

Table 2.9 The rabbit: Typical urinalysis values

Volume	20–350 mL/kg per 24 h
s.g.	1.003–1.036, but can be difficult to measure due to crystals
pH	≈8.2. Can fall to 6.0 in anorectic or fasted animals
Colour	Cloudy, pale to dark yellow BUT may be pink/rust/red due to porphyrins (see *Findings*)
Protein	Negative to trace
Casts	None
Crystals	Triple phosphate, $CaCO_3$
Epithelial cells	None or rare
Bacteria	None or rare
Glucose	Negative
Ketones	Negative
WBC	Rare
RBC	Rare

   b. Radio-dense lesions in the kidney (*E. cuniculi*)
   c. Intravenous urograms
4. Routine haematology and biochemistry
   a. Renal parameters may be raised, i.e. raised urea, creatinine, calcium, phosphate and potassium
5. Serology for *E. cuniculi*, *Pasteurella*
6. Endoscopic laparotomy
7. Ultrasonography
8. Exploratory laparotomy
9. Biopsy.

Management

1. Fluid therapy if appropriate
2. Consider if diet too high in calcium; dietary modification alone unlikely to resolve or prevent recurrence of excess sand/urolithiasis.

Treatment/specific therapy

- Acute and chronic renal failure
  - Fluid therapy
  - Daily fluid maintenance requirement for a rabbit is 100 mL/kg per day
  - Recommended approximate volumes for fluid replacement therapy (mL) are 10–15 mL/kg s.c. in divided sites or 15 mL/kg i.p. Fluids can also be given i.v. either by bolus or by infusion
- Pyelonephritis
  - Appropriate antibiosis (avoid aminoglycosides and other known nephrotoxic drugs)
  - Fluid therapy

- Calciuria
  - Catheterization and flushing of the bladder under anaesthetic may work
  - Cystotomy, removal of sand and flush
- Urolithiasis
  - Surgery to remove stones (White 2001)
  - Antibiosis as often accompanied by cystitis
- *E. cuniculi*
  - Co-trimoxazole at 30 mg/kg b.i.d. p.o. for at least 3 weeks
  - Albendazole at 10 mg/kg p.o. for 6 weeks
  - Fenbendazole at 10–20 mg/kg p.o. for 1 month.

Reproductive disorders

Viral

- Myxomatosis (see *Skin Disorders*)

Bacterial

- *Pasteurella*
- *Staphylococcus*
- *Streptococcus*
- Mycoplasmosis (esp. *Mycoplasma pulmonis*)
- Enteric bacteria
- *Leptospira interrogans* (Boucher et al 2001)
- Rabbit syphilis, *Treponema cuniculi*.

Nutritional

- Hypovitaminosis A (see *Nutritional Disorders*)
- Hypovitaminosis E (see *Nutritional Disorders*).

Neoplasia

- Uterine adenocarcinoma. (common in entire does over age of 3–4 years old) (Fig. 2.15)
- Testicular neoplasia (5-year plus bucks)
- Ovarian tumours
- Mammary adenocarcinomas
- Hypertestosteronism (see 'Adrenal hyperplasia/neoplasia', in *Endocrine Disorders*).

Other non-infectious problems

- Ovarian cysts
- Endometrial hyperplasia
- Uterine polyps
- Vaginal prolapse
- Uterine torsion
- Hydrometra
- Pseudopregnancy
- Dystocia
- Cystic mastitis (may progress to mammary adenocarcinomas).

Fig. 2.15. Uterine adenocarcinoma.

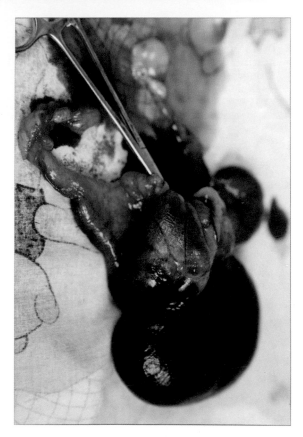

Findings on clinical examination

- Septic mastitis: swollen, painful mammary glands. Abnormal milk
- Cystic mastitis: glands swollen, firm, not painful. May have a clear or serosanguineous discharge
- High temperature
- Anorexia
- Vaginal discharge
- Apparent haematuria (uterine adenocarcinoma, endometrial venous aneurysms, porphyrinuria)
- Pyometra
- Enlarged palpable viscus (pyometra, uterine adenocarcinoma)
- Epididymitis
- Orchitis

- Vesicles, ulcers and crusty lesions on the external genitalia; may also be present at the mouth and nares (*T. cuniculi*)
- Poor reproductive performance
- Increased aggression and sexual behaviour in castrated male rabbits (hypertestosteronism).

Investigations

1. Radiography
   a. Include thoracic radiographs for metastases from uterine or mammary adenocarcinomas
2. Routine haematology and biochemistry
3. Serology for *T. cuniculi, Mycoplasma pulmonis*
4. Culture and sensitivity
5. Cytology
6. Endoscopy
7. Laparoscopy
8. Ultrasonography
9. Exploratory laparotomy
10. Biopsy.

Treatment/specific therapy

- Rabbit syphilis – see *Skin Disorders*
- Mastitis
  - Septic mastitis (typically *Staphylococcus, Pasteurella* and *Streptococcus spp*)
    - Appropriate antibiosis
    - Supportive care including parenteral fluids, analgesia, fostering or hand rearing of young
    - Surgical mastectomy
  - Cystic mastitis
    - Ovariohysterectomy
    - Surgical mastectomy as may progress to adenocarcinomas)
    - Can be associated with uterine hyperplasia and adenocarcinoma
- Metritis and pyometra (typically *Pasteurella,* mycoplasmosis; occ. *T. cuniculi* and enteric bacteria)
  - Appropriate antibiosis
  - Supportive care
  - Ovario-hysterectomy
- Endometrial venous aneurysms
  - Ovario-hysterectomy
- Orchitis, epididymitis
  - Appropriate antibiosis
  - Castration
- Uterine adenocarcinoma
  - Ovario-hysterectomy
  - V poor prognosis if metastatic spread
  - Can be seen in neutered females if significant uterine stump remains
  - Recommend routine ovario-hysterectomy at 4 months of age

- Ovarian tumours or cysts
  - Ovario-hysterectomy
- Testicular neoplasia
  - Castration
- Vaginal prolapse
  - Fluid therapy
  - Surgical replacement or resection of prolapse
  - Consider ovario-hysterectomy
- Pseudopregnancy
  - Will usually resolve spontaneously within 2–3 weeks
  - Hormonal treatment, e.g. proligestone at 10 to 30 mg/kg once only
  - Cabergoline at 5 µg/kg s.i.d. for 4–6 days
- Dystocia
  - If no obvious obstruction, oxytocin at 1–2 IU i.m., s.c.
  - Uterine inertia, 5–10 mL calcium gluconate p.o. 30 min prior to oxytocin
  - Caesarean section.

References

Beck W 2007 Ectoparasites, endoparasites, and heartworm control in small mammals. Comp Cont Edu Vet 29(5A):3–8

Boucher S, Gracia E, Villa A et al 2001 Pathogens in the reproductive tract of farm rabbits. Vet Rec 149:677–678

Biricik H S, Oguz H, Sindak N et al 2005 Evaluation of the Schirmer and phenol red thread tests for measuring tear secretion in rabbits. Vet Rec 156:485–487

Brown S A 1997 Neoplasia. In: Hillyer E V, Quesenberry K E (eds) Ferrets, rabbits, and rodents, 1st edn. Saunders, Philadelphia, p 108

Coletti M, Passamonti F, Del Rossi E 2001 Klebsiella pneumoniae infection in Italian rabbits. Vet Rec 149:626–627

Fontes-Sousa A P N, Brás-Silva C, Moura C et al 2006 M-mode and Doppler echocardiographic reference values for male New Zealand white rabbits. Am J Vet Res 67(10): 1725–1729

Gómez L, Gázquez A, Roncero V et al 2002 Lymphoma in a rabbit: histopathological and immunohistochemical findings. J Small Anim Pract 43:224–226

González-Gil A, Silván G, García-Partida P et al 2006 Serum glucocorticoid concentrations after halothane and isoflurane anaesthesia in New Zealand white rabbits. Vet Rec 159:51–52

Greig A, Stevenson K, Perez V et al 1997 Paratuberculosis in wild rabbits (Oryctolagus cuniculus). Vet Rec 140:141–143

Hack R J, Walstrom D J, Hair J A 2002 Efficacy and safety of two different dose rates of selamectin against natural infestations of Psoroptes cuniculi in rabbits. Clinical Research Abstracts presented at BSAVA Congress 2001. J Small Anim Pract 43:ix

Hulbert A J 2000 Thyroid hormones and their effects: a new perspective. Biol Rev 75:519–631

Lennox A M, Chitty J 2006 Adrenal neoplasia and hyperplasia as a cause of hypertestosteronism in two rabbits. J Exot Pet Med 15(1):56–58

Marini R P, Li X, Harpster N K et al 1999 Cardiovascular pathology possibly associated with ketamine/xylazine anaesthesia in Dutch belted rabbits. Lab Anim Sci 49:153–160

Miwa Y, Mochiduki M, Nakayama H et al 2006 Apocrine adenocarcinoma of possible sweat gland origin in a male rabbit. J Small Anim Pract 47:541–544

Pinter L 1999 Leporacarus gibbus and Spilopsyllus cuniculi infestation in a pet rabbit. J Small Anim Pract 40:220–221

Pizzi R, Hagan R U, Meredith A L 2007 Intermittent colic and intussusception due to a caecal polyp in a rabbit. J Exot Pet Med 16(2):113–117

Reusch B 2005 Investigation and management of cardiovascular disease in rabbits. In Practice 27:418–435

Reusch B, Boswood A 2003 Electrocardiography of the normal domestic pet rabbit (Abstract). J Small Anim Pract 44:514

Richardson V 2001 Rabbits. The digestive system. UK Vet 6(4):72–76

Sanchez-Migallon D G, Mayer J, Gould J et al 2006 Radiation therapy for the treatment of thymoma in rabbits (Oryctolagus cuniculus). J Exot Pet Med 15(2):138–144

Vangeel I, Pasmans F, Vanrobaeys M et al 2000 Prevalence of dermatophytes in asymptomatic guinea pigs and rabbits. Vet Rec 146:440–441

Whitbread T J, Genovese L, Hargreaves J et al 2002 Sebaceous adenitis in the rabbit, a presentation of three cases and comparison with sebaceous adenitis in the dog and the cat. Clinical Research Abstracts presented at BSAVA Congress 2001. J Small Anim Pract 43:ix

White R N 2001 Management of calcium ureterolithiasis in a French Lop rabbit. J Small Anim Pract 42:595–598

Guinea pigs, chinchillas and degus

3

Many of the pet rodents presented to the veterinarian belong to the group known as hystricomorphs. The following species are the commonest as household pets:

* Guinea pig (*Cavia porcellus*)
* Chinchilla (*Chinchilla laniger*) – the commonest species kept as pets
* Short-tailed chinchilla (*C. brevicaudata*)
* Degu (*Octodon degus*).

Table 3.1 Guinea pigs, chinchillas and degus: Key facts

		Guinea pig	Chinchilla	Degu
Average life span (years)		3–8	8–20	5–9
Weight (g)	Female	600–900	400–600	250
	Male	700–1200	400–500	
Body temperature (°C)		37.2–39.5	35.4–38	38
Respiratory rate (per min)		42–150	45–65	75
Heart rate (beats/min)		230–380	100	100–150
Gestation (days)		59–72	111 (*C. laniger*)	90–93
			124–128 (*C. brevicaudata*)	
Age at weaning		14–21 days	6–8 weeks	4–6 weeks
Sexual maturity		2–3 months (female)	4–12 months	6 months
		3–4 months (male)		

Consultation and handling

Hystricomorph rodents are prey animals so some may respond poorly to handling. All of these rodents are likely to struggle vigorously and care should be taken to gently restrain them. Always weigh the rodent at every consultation. The earliest sign of dental disease may be weight loss. Guinea pigs and chinchillas rarely bite, although there are always individual exceptions to this; degus are inclined to bite. 'Fur slip' in chinchillas is an anti-predator response whereby stressed individuals will shed clumps of hair while being handled.

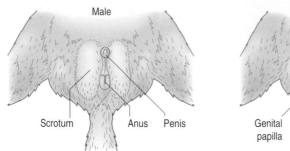
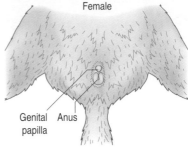

Fig. 3.1. Sexing of chinchillas.

Although both rabbits and guinea pigs are social animals, generally the keeping of guinea pigs with rabbits is not recommended because:

1. Rabbits are often aggressive to guinea pigs and may bite and harass them. Much of this activity occurs at night and may not be noticed by the owner.
2. Guinea pigs require dietary vitamin C (see *Nutritional Disorders*) and may suffer hypovitaminosis if fed on commercial rabbit food only.
3. Rabbits harbour *Bordetella* in their respiratory tract which can be a significant respiratory pathogen in guinea pigs.

Sexing of chinchillas can be problematic as the female has a pronounced genital papilla that can be easily mistaken as a penis. The vulva lies immediately caudal to this papilla (Fig. 3.1).

Nursing care

For general concepts, see *Nursing Care* in *Rabbits*.

Fluid therapy

Small rodents by virtue of their size and the high risk of predation are forced to obtain most of their water from preformed (food) and metabolic sources. Dehydration can be critical for hystricomorphs rodents, especially at higher environmental temperatures. For an adult chinchilla, 55.5% of its daily water loss is as urine; 16.7% evaporates form its skin; 22.2% evaporates from its lungs and 5.6% is lost in the faeces. Therefore, 38.9% of its water loss is insensible.

Table 3.2 Guinea pigs, chinchillas and degus: Fluid therapy

	Guinea pig	Chinchilla	Degu
Daily fluid maintenance requirements mL/kg per day	80–100	36	
Subcutaneous (mL/kg) (in divided sites)	10–20	20	10
Intraperitoneal (mL/kg)	20	20	10–15
Shock (mL/kg)	70	70	

Table 3.3 Guinea pigs, chinchillas and degus: Sites for fluid administration

Intravenous (guinea pig)	Lateral or medial saphenous and cephalic vein.
Intravenous (chinchilla)	Femoral, lateral saphenous and cephalic vein. Ear veins can be used for i.v. in some cases, and the use of EMLA cream greatly aids this, but is inappropriate if the chinchilla is considered hypothermic.
Intra-peritoneal (all three species)	Hold the patient vertically downward and inject into the lower left quadrant.
Intra-osseous (all three species)	Under GA to insert either an intraosseous catheter or a hypodermic needle into the marrow of either the femur (via the greater trochanter) or tibia (through the tibial crest). Fluids, colloids and even blood can be i.o. if necessary.

Fluids can be given s.c., i.p. or i.o. – indeed if there is marked dehydration, then i.p. or i.o. is preferable to s.c. Fluids can be given i.v. either by bolus or by infusion and all fluids should be warmed to 38°C. For sites for fluid administration see Table 3.

Jugular catheterization can be attempted in all species, but it is difficult and may result in respiratory embarrassment. Many of these sites may also require anaesthesia and surgical cut down. In hypovolaemic patients, vascular access may be impossible. It is better to consider either i.p. or i.o. administration.

Thermoregulation and hypothermia

Use a heat source, e.g. electric heat mat plus insulation such as silver foil (reduces heat lost by conduction) and bubble wrap (reduces heat lost by convection). Pay particular attention to the pinnae of chinchillas as these are significant organs of heat loss. Alternatively, maintain in warm air, e.g. incubator, or use commercial medical warm air generator. If body temperature falls too low, consider the risk of enterotoxaemia following massive gut bacterial die-off.

Nutritional status

Many small mammals are presented as emergencies after a prolonged period of ill-health that will have affected their food intake, e.g. chinchillas and guinea pigs suffering from undiagnosed chronic dental disease. These rodents are often hypoglycaemic – testing with a commercial glucometer on a small sample of blood – and i.v. or i.p. glucose can be given to these cases once identified.

Analgesia

Table 3.4 Guinea pigs, chinchillas and degus: Analgesic doses

Analgesic	Dose		
	Guinea pig	Chinchilla	Degu
Buprenorphine	0.01–0.05 mg/kg s.c. every 6–12 h	0.01–0.05 mg/kg s.c. every 6–12 h	0.05 mg/kg s. c. every 8–12 h
Butorphanol	0.2–2.0 mg/kg s.c. every 4 h	0.2–2.0 mg/kg s.c. every 4 h	
Carprofen	1.0–4.0 mg/kg s.c., p.o every 12–24 h	1.0–2.0 mg/kg s.c., p.o every 12–24 h	4.0 mg/kg s.c, p.o. s.i.d.
Ketoprofen	1.0 mg/kg s.c., i.m. every 12–24 h	1.0 mg/kg s.c., i.m. every 12–24 h	
Meloxicam	0.1–0.3 mg/kg s.c., p.o. s.i.d.	0.1–0.3 mg/kg s.c., p.o. s.i.d. Chinchillas particularly like meloxicam oral suspension.	
Morphine	2.0–10.0 mg/kg s.c., i.m. every 4 h		
Pethidine	10–20 mg/kg s.c, i.m. every 2–3 h		
Nalbuphine	1.0–2.0 mg/kg i.m. every 2–4 h		

Anaesthesia

Beware of subclinical respiratory infections. There is no need to starve; prolonged fasting can lead to hypoglycaemia.

Keep the animal warm; as they have a large surface area compared with volume this results in significant heat loss during surgery and hypothermia acts as a general depressant and is also immunosuppressive. Merely applying insulation such as bubble wrap is often insufficient – inactive, anaesthetized rodents are not generating heat and you may be insulating it from a higher ambient temperature. Place these animals onto a heat mat, onto which is placed an absorptive towel or other material to both protect the mat from becoming wet, and reduce the slight risk of localized burns.

Gaseous anaesthesia

1. Masking down or placing in an induction chamber is often the safest way to induce anesthesia in hystricomorph rodent.
2. Guinea pigs will often hypersalivate in response to isoflurane; atropine at 0.1–0.2 mg/kg s.c. may reduce this.
3. Intubation is extremely difficult due to the narrow caudal pharynx, large tongue and small glottis. Makeshift endotracheal tubes using intravenous catheters readily block with respiratory secretions. It is often more expedient to maintain on a mask, or intubate by a tracheotomy if thought necessary.

Parenteral anaesthesia

1. Ketamine/medetomidine/butorphanol given i.m. simultaneously:
   a. Ketamine at 10 mg/kg
   b. Medetomidine at 0.1 mg/kg
   c. Butorphanol at 1.5 mg/kg.
2. At end of procedure, reverse medetomidine with atipamezole at 0.75 mg/kg.
3. Administering metoclopramide (0.5 mg/kg s.c. or p.o. q. 6–8 h) postoperatively will help to prevent a post-surgical ileus, especially following painful or abdominal surgery.
4. Monitor feeding and faecal output for 24 h following surgery.

Cardiopulmonary resuscitation

Respiratory arrest

1. Administer 100% oxygen.
2. Assist ventilation – compress thorax at around 60×/min.
3. Doxapram sublingual or at 10 mg/kg i.v. or i.p. – *Note*: this will increase the animal's oxygen demand.
4. If appropriate, give atipamezole.

Cardiac arrest

1. As for respiratory arrest.
But also:
2. Compress thorax at around 90×/min.
3. If asystole – give adrenaline at 0.1 mg/kg of 1:10 000.
4. If ventricular fibrillation – lidocaine (lignocaine) at 1–2 mg/kg.

Skin disorders

Chinchillas have extremely dense fur, an attribute that has probably been enhanced by artificial selection. This may be why external parasites are uncommon in the chinchilla.

Pruritus

* Guinea pig
  * *Trixacaris caviae* (sarcoptid mite) (Fig. 3.2). Commonly associated with immunosuppression associated with pregnancy/parturition
  * Other sarcoptids *Sarcoptes muris*, *Notoedres muris*
  * *Chirodiscoides caviae* and *Myocoptes musculinus* (fur mites).

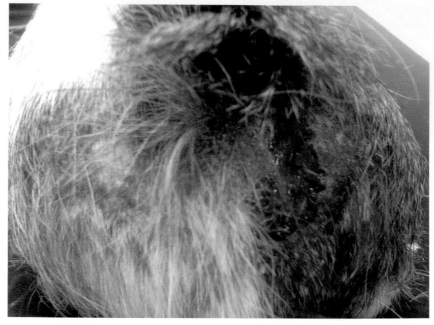

Fig. 3.2. Severe self-inflicted trauma; pruritus secondary to *Trixacarus*.

Alopecia

- Parasitic
  - Mites:
    - *Trixacara caviae* (sarcoptid mite) (guinea pigs). Commonly associated with immunosuppression associated with pregnancy/parturition
    - Other sarcoptids *Sarcoptes muris, Notoedres muris*
    - *Cheyletiella parasitivorax*
    - *Chirodiscoides caviae* and *Myocoptes musculinus* (fur mites)
    - *Demodex caviae* (significance uncertain)
    - Storage mites *Acarus farris* (Linek & Bourdeau 2005)
  - Lice:
    - *Gyropus ovalis, Gliricola porcelli* (chewing lice) and *Trimenopon hispidum* (sucking louse). Usually asymptomatic; if heavy infestation, may cause alopecia and a rough coat
- Bacterial
  - Pyoderma (often secondary infection from scratching)
  - Salmonellosis (Singh et al 2005)
- Fungal
  - Dermatophytosis (*Trichophyton mentagrophytes, Microsporum spp*). Can be asymptomatic
  - *Scopulariopsis brevicaulis* – usually asymptomatic
- Nutritional
  - Hypovitaminosis C (rough hair coat/hair loss in guinea pigs)

- Fatty acid deficiency (chinchillas) (see *Nutritional Disorders*)
- Pantothenic acid deficiency (chinchillas). May be complicated by zinc deficiency (see *Nutritional Disorders*).

Other

- Fur slip – improper handling/anti-predator response seen in chinchillas)
- Cystic ovarian disease (guinea pigs – see *Reproductive Tract Disorders*)
- Hyperadrenocortism (Cushing's disease) – see *Endocrine Disorders*
- Barbering/fur chewing (for chinchillas – see also *Endocrine Disorders*). May be linked to lack of dietary fibre
- Very low environmental humidity, e.g. central heating.(chinchillas)
- Linked to intensive breeding of female guinea pigs.

Scaling and crusting

- Dermatophytosis (*Trichophyton mentagrophytes, Microsporum spp*)
- *Scopulariopsis brevicaulis.*

Seborrhea

- Dermatophytosis (*Trichophyton mentagrophytes, Microsporum spp*).

Sebaceous secretions

- Excessive accumulation around the perineal and perianal region in older guinea pig boars.

Erosions and ulceration

- Pododermatitis (*Staphylococcus aureus* and *S. epidermidis*)
- *Cryptococcus neoformans*
- Frost bite (chinchillas).

Swellings, nodules and non-healing wounds

- Abscess
- Mycobacteriosis
- Aural haematoma (chinchillas)
- Hypovitaminosis E (chinchillas; distinct swellings on abdomen – see *Nutritional Disorders*)
- Cutaneous cysts.

Changes in pigmentation

- Yellow ears (chinchillas) (see *Nutritional Disorders*).

Neoplasia

- Trichofolliculoma
- Fibrosarcoma
- Sebaceous adenoma
- Lipoma
- Mammary fibroadenoma
- Mammary fibrocarcinoma
- Mammary adenocarcinoma
- Cutaneous papilloma of the foot pad
- Cutaneous haemangioma (Hammer et al 2005).

Other abnormalities

- Bites to pinnae (chinchillas, guinea pigs kept with rabbits)
- Cotton fur syndrome (chinchillas) (see *Nutritional Disorders*)
- Degloving of tail in chinchillas and degus (improper handling).

Findings on clinical examination

- Areas of alopecia – may be bilateral (hormonal) or patchy (fatty acid deficiency, pantothenic acid deficiency in chinchillas)
- Swellings, often firm consistency even if abscess. Displacement of normal outline of coat may indicate swelling
- Texture of hair coat may alter, becoming rougher
- Cuts and abrasions: these may be self-inflicted in cases of severe pruritus. In guinea pigs such lesions tend to be over the shoulders and back of the neck where the guinea pig scratches with its hind claws
- Extreme pruritus
- Seizures may follow episodes of extreme pruritus (guinea pigs with ectoparasites)
- Pododermatitis
    - Ulcerations, erythema, callouses, nail distortions and abnormalities. Related lymph nodes may be enlarged (especially guinea pigs).
- Systemic signs
    - Linked to amyloidosis in liver, kidneys, pancreas, spleen, adrenal glands.
- Overgrown claws.
- Degloved tip of tail (chinchillas and degus).

Investigations

1. Radiography
    a. Pododermatitis – often underlying osteoarthritis
2. Routine haematology and biochemistry
    a. Eosinophilia (ectoparasitism)
3. Bacteriology and mycology: hair pluck or swab lesions for routine culture and sensitivity
4. Faecal swab for salmonellosis
5. Cytology
    a. Fine-needle aspirate followed by staining with rapid Romanowsky stains
    b. Gram stain
6. Microscopy: examine fur pluck, acetate strips or skin scrapes to affected area and examine for ectoparasites
7. Examine teeth. Rodents with dental disease may have difficulty grooming normally
8. Biopsy obvious lesions
9. Ultraviolet (Wood's) lamp – positive for *Microsporium canis* only (not all strains fluoresce)
10. Endocrine analysis: thyroxine, oestradiol (see *Endocrine Disorders*)
11. If barbering suspected, examine hair under microscope to see if chewed; separate from other animals; supply extra hay.

Treatment/specific therapy

- Treat for any ectoparasites
  - Ivermectin at 200 µg/kg or as topical application (Xeno 450, Genitrix); 3 treatments given 2 weeks apart
  - Imidacloprid (Advantage, Bayer) applied as a 40 mg 'spot-on'
  - 40 mg imidacloprid/4.0 mg moxidectin (Advocate, Bayer) at 0.1 mL per guinea pig (Beck 2007)
  - Permethrin applied as either a dusting powder or shampoo
- *Chirodiscoides caviae*
  - Ivermectin at 0.4–0.5 mg/kg
  - Selamectin at 12 mg/kg, 2 treatments, 2 weeks apart
- *Demodex*
  - Ivermectin at 0.4–0.5 mg/kg s.c. or topically every 7 days
  - Amitraz washes at 250 mg/L every 7 days
  - If very pruritic, consider use of NSAIDs
- Pododermatitis
  - Chronic infections lead to persistent swelling of the feet and gross abnormalities of the feet
  - *Note*: may also induce amyloidosis in internal organs (see *Hepatic Disorders, Pancreatic Disorders, Endocrine Disorders*)
  - Amelioration of underlying factors, e.g. removal from mesh floorings
  - Topical and systemic antibiosis
  - Analgesia, such as meloxicam at 0.3 mg/kg p.o. s.i.d.
  - Amputation of chronic, resistant infections to prevent risk of amyloidosis
- Abscessation
  - Surgical removal (with swab for culture and sensitivity) plus appropriate antibiosis
  - Lancing, debriding and cleaning of abscesses gives poor results compared to surgical resection
- Salmonellosis
  - Vitamin supplementation (1 g/kg feed) or 50–100 mg/kg p.o.
  - Appropriate antibiosis
- Cysts – surgical resection; may respond to local draining
- Dermatophytosis, *Scopulariopsis* and *Cryptococcus*
  - Griseofulvin at 15–25 mg/kg once daily for 4 weeks. Toxic to immature and fetal guinea pigs so use on adult, non-pregnant guinea pigs only
  - Miconazole/chlorhexidine (Malaseb, Leo) shampoo – bath once daily
  - Itraconazole at 15 mg/kg given daily to effect (Van Gestel & Engelen 2004)
  - Lufenuron was found to be ineffective (Van Gestel & Engelen 2004)
  - Often found in young guinea pigs (< 6 months old)
- Seborrhoea
  - Miconazole/chlorhexidine (Malaseb, Leo) shampoo – bath once daily
- Excessive perianal sebaceous secretion accumulation in older boars
  - Remove manually. Clean regularly with chlorhexidine scrub
- Neoplasia
  - Surgical resection where possible
- Lacerations/bites to the pinnae
  - If fresh attend to haemostasis

- Debride, clean up and apply topical amorphous hydrogel dressings to encourage secondary healing, e.g. IntraSite Gel (Smith and Nephew Healthcare Ltd.)
  - If cartilage is torn then suturing is unlikely to work
- Frostbite: debride, clean, dry thoroughly and apply antibiotic ointment
- Haematomas
  - Drain the haematoma
  - If necessary apply sutures to hold the stretched skin against the pinnal cartilage
  - Do not use steroids
- Fur chewing
  - Can be related to poor environmental conditions, e.g. high temperatures, high humidity. In rabbits it is often related to lack of provision of long fibre such as hay
  - Fur chewing chinchillas often have hyperthyroidism and hyperactive adrenal glands (see *Endocrine Disorders*)
  - If behavioural, consider fluoxetine at 5–10 mg/kg s.i.d.
  - Treatment involves elimination of other possible aetiologies correction of environmental conditions
  - Shaving of the remaining dark-coloured short undercoat often encourages regrowth
- Degloving of tail
  - Apply topical antibacterial preparation if infected. Otherwise encourage granulation using IntraSite Gel or Dermisol cream (Pfizer)
  - Extensive lesions may require amputation.

Respiratory tract disorders

See also *Cardiovascular and Haematological Disorders.*

Viral

- Adenovirus (guinea pigs)
- Paramyxoviruses including Sendai virus
- Simian virus 5 (SV5)
- Pneumonia virus of mice (PVM).

Bacterial

- *Bordetella bronchiseptica*
- *Chlamydophila psittaci* (see also *Ophthalmic Disorders*)
- *Mycoplasma caviae* (usually asymptomatic)
- *Mycoplasma pulmonis*
- *Pasteurella*
- *Pneumocystis carnii* (usually asymptomatic except with severe immunosuppression)
- *Pseudomonas*
- *Streptobacillus moniliformis*
- *Streptococcus equi zooepidemicus* (pleuritis, hydrothorax, pericarditis)
- *Streptococcus pneumoniae*
- *Streptococcus pyogenes.*

Fungal

- *Histoplasma capsulatum* (see *Systemic Disorders*).

Protozoal

● *Toxoplasma gondii* (see *Neurological Disorders*).

Nutritional

● Hypovitaminosis C (see *Nutritional Disorders*).

Neoplasia

● Bronchogenic and alveologenic papillary adenomas (may be secondary to foreign body inhalation).

Other non-infectious problems

● Trauma (improper handling)
● Pneumothorax
● Diaphragmatic hernia
● Gastric tympany/torsion (see *Gastrointestinal Tract Disorders*)
● Heat stress (see *Systemic Disorders*)
● Dental disease (may resemble upper respiratory tract disease in chinchillas; see *Dental Disorders*)
● Choke (especially chinchillas)
● Cardiovascular disease (see *Cardiovascular and Haematological Disorders*)
● Inappropriate bedding – wood shavings and sawdust can be a source of irritant essential oils.

Findings on clinical examination

● Dyspnoea/tachypnoea
● Open-mouth breathing
● Cyanosis.
● High temperature
● Increased respiratory sounds
● Anorexia
● Weight loss
● Severe distress (choke)
● Conjunctivitis
  ● Chlamydophila rarely causes respiratory disease other than conjunctivitis, however can occur alongside bacterial pneumonia
● Nasal discharge
● Vaginal discharge from metritis (guinea pigs with bordetellosis). Pregnant sows may abort
● Swollen submandibular lymph nodes (*Streptobacillus moniliformis*).

Investigations

1. Radiography
   a. Lateral and DV radiographs
2. Routine haematology and biochemistry
   a. Serology for *Chlamydophila, Bordetella, Adenovirus,* Sendai virus, Simian Virus 5, Pneumonia virus of mice, *Mycoplasma pulmonis*
3. PCR for *Chlamydophila*

4. Culture and sensitivity
5. Cytology
   a. Transtracheal wash
   b. Gram-stain
6. Pleural tap and cytology
7. Endoscopy
8. Ultrasonography
9. Biopsy
   a. Intranuclear inclusions (adenovirus)
10. Necropsy.

Management

1. Supplement with vitamin C (guinea pigs, degus)
2. Parenteral fluids
3. Gentle soaking and removal of encrusted oculo-nasal discharges
4. Provide oxygen via mask or chamber
5. Covering or specific antibiosis. Consider nebulization
6. Syringe feeding (beware aspiration pneumonia)
7. NSAIDs, e.g. meloxicam 0.3 mg/kg p.o. s.i.d. may reduce lung damage
8. Mucolytics such as bromhexine and N-acetyl-cysteine may be useful
9. Change bedding to paper-based zsubstrate.

Treatment/specific therapy

- Bordetellosis
  - Appropriate antibiosis
  - *Note* that it is found asymptomatically in the upper respiratory tract of rabbits, which may, therefore, act as a reservoir of infection for guinea pigs when kept with rabbits
  - Vaccination with canine Bordetella vaccine at 0.2 mL per individual either s.c. or p.o.; repeat after 2–3 weeks then given annual or 6-monthly booster according to risk (Huerkamp et al 1996)
- Streptococci
  - Appropriate antibiosis
- *S. pyogenes* may be spread by biting insects
  - *S. pneumoniae* is spread by aerosol transmission
- Sendai virus, Simian virus 5 and pneumonia virus of mice are usually asymptomatic
- Adenovirus. Treat symptomatically
- Mycoplasmosis
  - Appropriate antibiosis
- Choke
  - Often die before treatment initiated
  - Remove or dislodge foreign body (often food item) wedged over glottis.

Dental disorders

> ### Permanent dental formula of the guinea pig and chinchilla
>
> $$I : \frac{1}{1}, C : \frac{0}{0}, PM : \frac{1}{1}, M : \frac{3}{3}$$

Nutritional
- Lack of long fibre, e.g. hay, in diet
- Hypovitaminosis C (guinea pigs, possibly degus – see *Nutritional Disorders*)
- Inappropriate nutrition.

Neoplasia
- Oral neoplasia causing differential wear.

Other non-infectious problems
- Fractured incisors (trauma)
- Congenital malocclusion
- Genetic predisposition.

Findings on clinical examination

- Chinchilla and degu incisor teeth are naturally highly coloured orange or yellow; this often fades with dental disease. Such fading may indicate a hypovitaminosis A (see *Nutritional Disorders*)
- Incisor malocclusion
  - Chewing in rodents involves a significant rostrocaudal movement of the mandibles, therefore, the lower incisors in particular are naturally quite long; this should not be mistaken for an abnormality. Compare where possible with another individual
- Mandibular swellings (unilateral or bilateral) due to bone remodelling to accommodate tooth root overgrowth
- Maxillary swellings rostral to eye; painful on palpation – maxillary root overgrowth (especially chinchillas)
- One or more incisors shortened fractured
- Excessive salivation/moist fur on chin and ventral neck (slobbers)
- Weight loss
- Anorexia
- Ectoparasitic disease
- Dacryocystitis/conjunctivitis
- Seizures (due to hypoglycaemia).

Investigations

1. Otoscopic examination of oral cavity
   a. Normal guinea pig or chinchilla always has a significant amount of food/cae-cotrophic material in its mouth obscuring the dental arcades; if this is not the case then it is likely to be eating very poorly
   b. Lingual tilting of mandibular cheek teeth and buccal tilting of maxillary cheek teeth (Fig. 3.3)
   c. The mandibular premolars may form a partial or complete arch over the tongue (guinea pig)
   d. Otoscopic examination does not constitute a complete examination of the oral cavity as structures at the back of the pharynx can be difficult to see due to its depth and the large size of the tongue
   e. Spurs on cheek teeth. Often rostral facing on first lower premolars (chinchil-las, degus)
   f. Ulceration of tongue
   g. Purulent material in mouth
2. Radiography
   a. Lateral and DV views of skull. *Note* skulls often appear osteoporotic (Figs 3.4, 3.5)
   b. Left and right lateral oblique views of skull to allow assessment of individual tooth roots. Any divergence of maxillary or mandibular tooth roots away from each other suggests abnormal root elongation
   c. Contrast study on nasolacrimal ducts. Difficult in small hystricomorphs

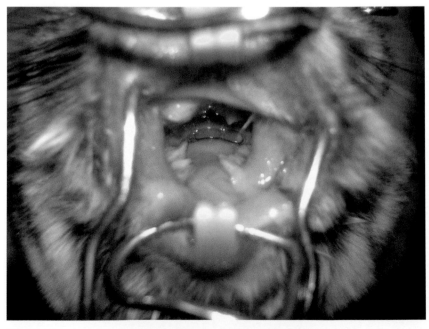

Fig. 3.3. Lingual spurs on the lower premolars and molars of a chinchilla.

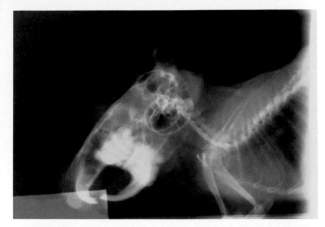

Fig. 3.4. Lateral radiograph of a chinchilla with dental disease. *Note* the divergence of the maxillary tooth roots and the (palpable) bony remodelling of the mandibles associated with cheek tooth root overgrowth.

3. Routine haematology and biochemistry
4. Culture and sensitivity
    a. Aerobic and anaerobic culture of abscesses
5. Examination of oral cavity under GA
6. Endoscopy.

Management

1. Chronic cases often cachexic – may need parenteral fluid support
2. Check blood glucose levels: (guinea pig 3.36–7.8 mmol/L) (chinchilla 3.36–6.72 mmol/L)

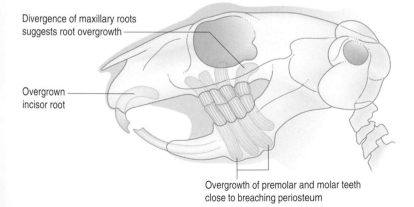

Divergence of maxillary roots suggests root overgrowth

Overgrown incisor root

Overgrowth of premolar and molar teeth close to breaching periosteum

Fig. 3.5. Explanatory diagram of skull shown in Figure 2.14.

3. Syringe feeding with commercial feed suspensions, e.g. Critical Care (Oxbow) or Recovery diet (Supreme Petfoods). May require nasogastric tube or tube feeding
4. Flushing of nasolacrimal ducts where possible
5. Only use antibiotics if indicated. Many cases do not require their use, which can be counterproductive
6. Gut motility modifiers
7. Metoclopramide at 0.5 mg/kg s.c. or p.o. q. 6–8 h
8. Cisapride 0.5 mg/kg s.i.d. or b.i.d.

Treatment/specific therapy

- Regular coronal reduction
  - Always burr overgrown incisors in preference to clipping due to risk of fracture, pulpal haemorrhage and infection
  - For cheek teeth, this will likely necessitate heavy sedation or a GA. 'Concious' dental work on the cheek teeth is stressful to the rodent and risks serious traumatic to the oral cavity and spine
  - Often coronal reduction alone is insufficient; often by the time of presentation, dental disease has progressed to a quite advanced stage
  - Use of a dental drill or equivalent is essential; dental spurs can be clipped but the teeth must be burred down; clipping is likely to fracture the tooth
- Incisor extraction
- Cheek teeth extraction
- Surgical debridement of tooth root abscesses including removal of infected bone and affected tooth roots, followed by:
  - Packing with antibiotic-impregnated methyl-methacrylate (bone cement or similar) *and/or* marsupialization leaving ostium for recurrent povidone-iodine/antibiotic application during second intention healing
  - Antibiosis
    - Usually a broad-spectrum such as enrofloxacin at 5 mg/kg s.i.d. p.o. or co-trimoxazole at 30 mg/kg b.i.d. p.o. *plus*
    - Anaerobic antibiosis, e.g. metronidazole at 20 mg/kg p.o. s.i.d.
  - Drilling out of tooth root apices to initiate tooth root death where extraction is not viable. *Note* that aggressive dental work in guinea pigs can trigger neuronal degeneration of afferent nerves in the periodontal ligament with subsequent degeneration of the mesencephalic trigeminal nucleus resulting in dysphagia, postural abnormalities and death (Azuma et al 1999, Kimoto 1993) See *Neurological Disorders* and *Cardiovascular and Haematological Disorders*
  - Analgesia, e.g. meloxicam at 0.3 mg/kg p.o. s.i.d. – can be given for many weeks
- Where possible, wean the animal on to a diet high in long fibre, i.e. grass and hay, as this encourages normal chewing and dental wear on the back teeth. Provision of a pumice stone may encourage gnawing behaviour
  - *Note* that many chinchillas with dental disease have adrenal hyperplasia (Crossley 2001) (see *Endocrine Disorders*)
- Fractured incisors
  - Burr and file back to both the affected tooth and the contralateral to allow normal even wear to occur.

Gastrointestinal tract disorders

It is normal for guinea pigs, chinchillas and degus to coprophage, especially at night (Kenagy et al 1999).

Disorders of the oral cavity

- Dental disease (see *Dental Disorders*)
- Foreign bodies especially cheek impactions or under tongue
- Choke (see *Respiratory Disorders*)
- Parotid salivary gland abscessation
- Investigation requires sedation or anaesthesia for thorough examination of the oral cavity
- Foreign bodies and choke requires removal of the problem material
- Parotid salivary gland abscessation requires surgical resection of the abscess; consider bacteriological culture and sensitivity from the abscess
- Crusty lesions at corner of mouth (guinea pigs)
  - Hypovitaminosis C (see *Nutritional Disorders*)
  - Secondary bacterial/fungal infection
  - Chewing on sharp foods or cage mesh.

Differential diagnoses for gastrointestinal disorders

Viral

- Coronavirus (guinea pigs).

Bacterial

- *Clostridium difficile*
- *Clostridium perfringens* Type E (guinea pigs)
- *Clostridium perfringens* Type D (occasionally Type A) (chinchillas)
- *Clostridium piliforme* (Tyzzer's disease)
- *E. coli*
- *Listeria monocytogenes* (can be asymptomatic in chinchillas, but also has visceral and neurological presentations – see *Neurological Disorders*)
- *Campylobacter spp* (asymptomatic)
- *Citrobacter freundii*
- *Yersinia pseudotuberculosis*
- *Salmonella spp*
- *Corynebacterium spp.*

Fungal

- *Torulopsis pintolopesii.*

Protozoal

- Guinea pig
  - *Eimeria caviae*
  - *Eimeria spp* (cross infection with rabbit *Coccidia*)
  - *Cryptosporidium muris* and *C. wrairi*
  - *Entamoeba caviae*

- *Tritrichomonas caviae*
- *Giardia caviae*
- *Balantidium caviae*
- Chinchilla
  - *Giardia*
  - *Trichomonas* (haemorrhagic typhilitis)
  - *Balantidium* (haemorrhagic colitis)
  - *Cryptosporidium*
  - *Eimeria chinchillae.*

Parasitic

- Guinea pig
  - *Paraspidodera uncinata* (heterakid nematode)
  - Cestodes (from wild rodents)
    - *Fasciola hepatica*
    - Fasciola giganticus
- Chinchilla
  - Physaloptera
  - *Hymenolepis spp*
  - *Haemonchus contortus.*

Nutritional

- Sudden influx of greens or fruit in diet, probably a carbohydrate overload and fermentation producing gastric dilatation, dysbiosis
- Hypovitaminosis C in guinea pigs (malabsorption, pyogranulomatous enteritis) (see *Nutritional Disorders*)
- Constipation (degus and chinchillas on poor diet, possibly too low in short length fibre).

Neoplasia

Other non-infectious problems

- Iatrogenic dysbiosis (e.g. from antibiotics, especially penicillin, procaine, erythromycin, lincomycin, clindamycin, streptomycin, erythromycin, aureomycin, bacitracin and spiramycin). Such dysbiosis can result in clostridial overgrowth
- Intestinal obstruction
  - Neoplasia, foreign body, abscess, impaction
- Colorectal impaction (guinea pigs)
- Caecal impaction
- Caecal dilatation/tympany
- Rectal prolapse
- Gastric ulceration (chinchillas)
- Gastric torsion
- Gastric dilatation
- Aerophagy during anaesthetic induction and recovery
- Pregnant, unfasted females especially at risk of dilation/torsion
- Sudden influx of greens in diet (probably carbohydrate overload and fermentation).

Findings on clinical examination

- History of poor diet, e.g. excessive fruit or greens (diarrhoea, dysbiosis); course or mouldy feeds (gastric ulceration)
- Diarrhoea
  - Watery diarrhoea (*Cl. Piliforme*, hypovitaminosis C)
- Decreased faecal output
  - Constipation
  - Gut stasis
  - Colorectal impaction
  - Obstruction
  - Foreign body
  - Caecal impaction
- Frank blood in faeces (severe enteritis)
- Occult blood in faeces (hypovitaminosis C)
- Depression
- Hypothermia
- Gut stasis; gastric bloat
- Weight loss
- Impacted rectum; may find inspissated faeces, wood shavings, trichobezoars (guinea pigs)
- Flaccid hind limb paralysis
- Subcutaneous inguinal oedema (*Cl. piliforme* in guinea pigs)
- Dyspnoea (compression of thoracic cavity with gastric dilatation, gastric torsion, caecal dilatation)
- Death.

Investigations

1. Radiography
   a. Trichobezoars and caecal impactions likely linked to either foreign bodies or poor gut motility
   b. Assess lumbar spine for lesions in cases of colorectal impaction
2. Routine haematology and biochemistry
3. Serology for *Cl. piliforme*, coronavirus
4. Culture and sensitivity
5. Faecal examination
   a. Light microscopy (parasites)
   b. Gram stain
   c. Normal gastrointestinal flora is G +ve, i.e. *Bifidobacterium spp, Bacteroides spp, Eubacterium spp* and *Lactobacillus spp*
   d. Giemsa or acid-fast staining (*Cryptosporidium*)
6. Cytology
7. Electron microscopy
8. Endoscopy
   a. Gastroscopy, colonoscopy
   b. Endoscopic laparoscopy
9. Ultrasonography
10. Biopsy.

Management

1. Fluid therapy (see *Nursing Care*)
2. High-fibre diet
3. May need to syringe feed
4. Probiotics. These may be of benefit, but often species specific. One study found no benefit in administering oral *Lactobacillus spp* as an aid to antibiotic-induced enteritis in guinea pigs (Wasson et al 2000)
5. Transfaunation, using caecotrophs from a healthy rodent may help natural gut flora to re-establish
6. Only use antibiotics if indicated. Many cases do not require their use, which can be counterproductive
7. Analgesics can be necessary, but avoid those likely to exacerbate GIT ulceration, e.g. flunixin.

Treatment/specific therapy

- Clostridial overgrowth and Tyzzer's disease.
  - Covering antibiotics especially cephalosporins, metronidazole (20 mg/kg p.o. s.i.d.) vancomycin (20 mg/kg s.i.d. p.o.)

plus:

  - Cholestyramine at 100 mg/mL in drinking water
  - Vaccination with clostridial toxoids reduces mortalities (chinchillas)
- Corona virus – supportive care only
- *Torulopsis pintolopesii*
  - Nystatin at 100 000 units/kg b.i.d. p.o.
- *Eimeria spp*
  - Sulphonamides, e.g. cotrimoxazole at 30 mg/kg b.i.d.
- *Giardia*
  - Metronidazole 20 mg/kg p.o. s.i.d.
- *Cryptosporidium*
  - Potentiated sulfonamides may be of use
  - Nitazoxanide (Alinia) may prove useful
- Nematodes
  - *Paraspidodera uncinata*. Fenbendazole 20 mg/kg s.i.d. p.o. for 5 days
- Cestodes and trematodes
  - Praziquantel 5–10 mg/kg p.o., s.c., i.m. Repeat after 10 days
- Simple constipation
  - Liquid paraffin or syrup-of-figs
  - Increase fibre in diet
  - Consider other aetiologies
- Trichobezoars and caecal impactions
  - *Note:* can be symptomatic of foreign body, gut motility problem or dehydration
  - Aggressive fluid therapy
  - Analgesia
  - Gut motility modifiers, e.g. metoclopramide at 0.2–1.0 mg/kg and cisapride at 0.5–1.0 mg/kg
  - Avoid surgery unless absolutely necessary

- Colorectal impactions
  - Frequent removal of impacted faeces
  - Supplement with B vitamins and vitamin K as caecotrophy will be compromised
- Rectal prolapse
  - Give fluids and covering antibiosis
  - Moisten, lubricate and replace
  - Keep in place with purse-string suture
  - May require resection of devitalized area and anastomosis of cut ends
  - Withhold high-fibre foods for a few days
- Gastric dilatation
  - Tympany: consider gut motility enhancers such as metoclopramide at 0.5 mg/kg s.c. or p.o. q. 6–8 h, offering or syringe feeding a high-fibre diet, e.g. Supreme Recovery or Oxbow Critical Care. Decompress by stomach tube or by paracentesis if severe
  - Torsion: immediate decompression by stomach tube or paracentesis but trans-abdominal decompression highly likely to initiate a peritonitis. May require surgical correction
  - Fluid therapy
  - Feed high-fibre, low-carbohydrate foods
  - Cimetidine at 5–10 mg/kg q. 6–12 h p.o., s.c. i.m.
  - Probiotics (see *Management*)
  - Gut stasis, gastric dilation accompanied by hind-limb paralysis in lactating chinchillas often the result of hypocalcaemia; usually seen in lactating chinchillas at 2–3 weeks postpartum. Calcium gluconate i.v. or i.p. at 94–140 mg/kg (see *Systemic Disorders*)
- Gastric ulceration
  - Cimetidine at 5–10 mg/kg q. 6–12 h p.o., s.c. i.m.
- Intestinal obstruction
  - Fluid therapy
  - Covering antibiosis
  - Enemas using warm soapy water
  - Surgical correction/removal of foreign body.

Nutritional disorders

- Hypovitaminosis A (chinchillas) (see *Ophthalmic Disorders*)
- Hypovitaminosis C (scurvy) (guinea pigs, not proven but often suggested for degus)
- Hypervitaminosis C (may cause heterotrophic bony metaplasia and calcification (metastatic calcification) (guinea pigs)
- Hypovitaminosis E (nutritional muscular dystrophy – see *Musculoskeletal Disorders*)
- Hypovitaminosis E or choline or methionine deficiency linked with yellow discolouration of pinna, and raised, pigmented lesions in the perineal area and ventral abdomen in chinchillas
- Thiamine deficiency (chinchillas)
- Fatty acid deficiency (chinchillas)
- Pantothenic acid deficiency
- 'Cotton fur' (chinchillas)
- Nutritional metabolic bone disease (chinchillas)
- Hepatic lipidosis (see *Hepatic Disorders*).

Findings on clinical examination

- Vague ill-health including weight loss and dehydration
- Dental disease (hypovitaminosis C in guinea pigs)
- Motor abnormalities including trembling, paralysis and convulsions
- Pain
- Spontaneous fractures (hypovitaminosis C in guinea pigs)
- Ocular and nasal discharges
- Abortions and still-births
- Soft stools/diarrhoea (hypovitaminosis C in guinea pigs)
- Spontaneous haemorrhage (hypovitaminosis C in guinea pigs)
- History of guinea pig fed on rabbit food (hypovitaminosis C in guinea pigs)
- Coat abnormalities (cotton-like appearance of fur (cotton fur) and hypovitaminosis A in chinchillas)
- Alopecia (chinchillas) (fatty acid deficiency, pantothenic acid deficiency)
- Polydipsia (hepatic lipidosis)
- Oedema (hypovitaminosis C, hepatopathy, cardiovascular disease).

Investigations

1. Radiography
   a. Enlarged joints and costochondral junctions, epiphyseal and long bone malformations, pathological fractures (hypovitaminosis C)
   b. Dental abnormalities (hypovitaminosis C) (see also *Dental Disorders*)
2. Routine haematology and biochemistry
   a. Anaemia
   b. Clotting disorders
3. Culture and sensitivity
4. Cytology
5. Endoscopy
6. Ultrasonography
7. Biopsy.

Treatment/specific therapy

- Hypovitaminosis C
  - Supplement with vitamin C (ascorbic acid) at 50–100 mg/kg daily
  - Feed with food commercial guinea pig food supplemented with vitamin C. Maintenance requirements are 10 mg/kg for adults, 30 mg/kg during pregnancy (Huerkamp et al 1996)
  - Rabbit food fed to rabbit/guinea pig combinations is likely to induce hypovitaminosis in the guinea pig
  - Guinea pig food that is out of date or has been poorly stored is likely to contain insufficient levels of vitamin C
  - Degus should be fed either a dedicated degu diet or a vitamin C-supplemented guinea pig food
- Cotton fur. Excessive protein intake. Alter rations to lower protein (15%) diet
- Fatty acid deficiency

- Supplement with unsaturated fatty acids, especially linoleic and arachidonic acid
- Recommend feeding 5–10 mg/kg evening primrose oil (Richardson 2003)
- Monitor food storage facilities to prevent rancidity
- Pantothenic acid deficiency (may be complicated by zinc deficiency)
  - Supplement with dietary pantothenic acid and zinc
- Nutritional metabolic bone disease
  - Calcium gluconate i.m. at 94–140 mg/kg i.v. or i.p.
  - Investigate and correct calcium/phosphorus imbalance in diet.

Hepatic disorders

Bacterial

- Hepatitis
- Yersiniosis (see *Systemic Disorders*).

Fungal

- Ingestion of aflatoxins and mycotoxins in food
- Histoplasmosis (see *Systemic Disorders*).

Protozoal

- *Cryptosporidium* (chinchillas) (see *Gastrointestinal Disorders*).

Parasitic

Nutritional

- Hepatic lipidosis (especially degus).

Neoplasia

- Lymphosarcoma
- Other hepatic and biliary tumours.

Other non-infectious problems

- Amyloidosis (secondary to chronic infection especially pododermatitis (guinea pigs).

Findings on clinical examination

- Diarrhoea
- Weight loss
- Jaundice
- Polydipsia/polyuria
- Poor blood clotting (hepatic lipidosis)
- Hepatomegaly.

Investigations

1. Radiography
   a. Routine haematology and biochemistry
   b. Liver parameters raised
   c. Hyperlipidaemia (hepatic lipidosis)

    d. Anaemia
    e. Ketones in blood
2. Urinalysis
    a. Ketonuria (hepatic lipidosis)
3. Culture and sensitivity
4. Cytology
5. Endoscopy
6. Ultrasonography
    a. Hepatomegaly (hepatic lipidosis)
7. Biopsy.

Management

1. Fluid therapy
2. Milk thistle (*Silybum marianum*) is hepatoprotectant; dose at 4–15 mg/kg b.i.d. or t.i.d.
3. Lactulose at 0.5 mL/kg b.i.d. p.o.

Treatment/specific therapy

- Hepatic lipidosis
  - Aggressive fluid therapy
  - Parenteral nutrition with glucose and vitamins
  - Assisted feeding by syringe. Calcium gluconate p.o. or propylene glycol p.o. may be of use
  - Dexamethasone at 0.1–0.6 mg/kg i.m.
- Mycotoxicosis
  - General management of liver disease
  - Prevent exposure to sources of contamination, usually old foods with fungal contamination
- Neoplasia
  - Lymphosarcoma (see *Cardiovascular and Haematological Disorders*)
  - Hepatic neoplasia
  - Poor prognosis. In some cases surgery may be possible but euthanasia more practicable.

Pancreatic disorders

Nutritional
- Congenital manganese deficiency (diabetes mellitus).

Neoplasia
- Islet tumours (benign).

Other non-infectious problems
- Amyloidosis (secondary to chronic infection especially pododermatitis (guinea pigs)
- Diabetes mellitus (esp. degus).

Findings on clinical examination

- Weight loss
- Polydipsia/polyuria
- Bilateral cataracts
- Infertility and other reproductive abnormalities
- Cystitis.

Investigations

1. Radiography
2. Routine haematology and biochemistry
   a. Hyperlipidaemia
   b. Hyperglycaemia (Table 3.5)
3. Glucose tolerance test.

Glucose tolerance test for guinea pigs

1. 18 h fast.
2. Take baseline blood glucose sample.
3. Give oral glucose 1.75 g/kg.
4. Repeat blood glucose after 4 h.
5. Normal blood glucose <1.5 baseline glucose; diabetic = 2× baseline glucose.

4. Urinalysis (see *Urinary Disorders*)
   a. Note that ascorbic acid can interfere with urinary glucose testing
   b. Glycosuria, ketoacidosis (rare)
5. Cytology
6. Endoscopy
7. Ultrasonography
8. Biopsy.

Treatment/specific therapy

- Diabetes mellitus
  - Place on a high-fibre (e.g. hay), low-carbohydrate diet
  - Insulin usually not required in guinea pigs

Table 3.5 Guinea pigs, chinchillas and degus: Hyperglycaemia

Species	Normal range for blood glucose (mmol/L)	Diabetic blood glucose (mmol/L)
Guinea pig	3.36–7.8	>20
Chinchilla	3.36–6.72	22
Degu	4.44–5.55	–

- Spontaneous remissions are common in guinea pigs
- *Note* that an undiagnosed infectious agent has been linked to induction of diabetes mellitus in Abyssinian guinea pigs (cited in Huerkamp et al 1996)
- For chinchillas, if unable to stabilize by dietary management alone, insulin initiated at 1 IU/kg b.i.d. and adjusted at 0.1 IU/kg as required, dependant upon twice daily urine analysis (Keeble 2001)
- For degus, place on a low-sugar (carbohydrate) diet and substitute vegetables for fruit. Avoid obesity; recommended to keep breeding female degus at around 250 g body weight (Najecki & Tate 1999).

Cardiovascular and haematological disorders

See also *Respiratory Disorders*.

Viral

- Type C retrovirus.

Bacterial

- Endocarditis
- *Streptococcus equi zooepidemicus* (pleuritis, hydrothorax, pericarditis)
- *Streptococcus pneumoniae* (haemopericardium, pericarditis, pleuritis)
- *Streptococcus pyogenes* (haemopericardium, pericarditis, pleuritis)
- *Haemobartonella caviae* (Rickettsial).

Nutritional

- Hypovitaminosis C (see *Nutritional Disorders*)
- Copper deficiency
- Heterotrophic bony metaplasia and calcification (see *Systemic Disorders*).

Neoplasia

- Lymphosarcoma/leukaemia (usually B cell)
- Mesenchymomas of right atrium
- Cardiac fibrosarcomas
- Splenic haematoma
- Splenic haemangioma.

Other non-infectious problems

- Cardiomyopathies (esp. chinchillas)
- Poor blood clotting (hepatic lipidosis, see *Hepatic Disorders*)
- 90% of guinea pigs with postural abnormalities following extreme dental extractions showed T-wave inversion on ECG (Azuma et al 1999).

Findings on clinical examination

- Dyspnoea
- Abnormal respiratory sounds
- Weight loss
- Dysphagia. Cardiomegaly can produce a difficulty swallowing

- Cardiac arrhythmias
- Tachycardia or bradycardia
- Abnormal heart sounds (not always present)
- Spontaneous haemorrhage; bleeding disorders (hypovitaminosis C, copper deficiency, hypokalaemia)
- Central nervous signs (leukaemia).

Investigations

1. Radiography
2. Routine haematology and biochemistry
   a. Intraerythrocytic inclusions, anaemia, hypoproteinaemia, reticulocytosis, increased clotting time (*Haemobartonella caviae*)
   b. Marked lymphocytosis ($\geq 25 \times 10^9$/L) (leukaemia/lymphosarcoma)
3. Culture and sensitivity, including blood culture
4. Cytology
   a. Intraerythrocytic inclusions (*Haemobartonella caviae*)
   b. Bone marrow aspirate
5. Endoscopy
6. ECG
7. Ultrasonography
   a. Measure cardiac parameters
   b. Echocardiographic measurements from healthy chinchillas (Linde et al 2004, see Table 3.6)
   c. Hepatosplenomegaly (lymphosarcoma).
8. Biopsy
   a. Liver/lymph node (lymphosarcoma)
   b. Bone marrow biopsy.

Treatment/specific therapy

- Bacterial diseases
  - Appropriate antibiosis. For *S. pneumoniae* and *S. pyogenes* consider chloramphenicol at 30–50 mg/kg b.i.d.
- Lymphosarcoma
  - Females>males; usually 2+ years old
  - Cyclophosphamide as described in *Rabbits* may induce remission
  - Vincristine, methotrexate and prednisolone reported as ineffective
- Cardiomyopathies and other heart abnormalities
  - Manage as for other species
  - Examples of suitable medications include taurine at 100 mg/kg s.i.d. for 8 weeks
- Arrhythmias
  - Digoxin at 0.003–0.03 mg/kg p.o. every 12–48 h
  - Lidocaine 1–2 mg/kg i.v. or 2–4 mg/kg i.t.
- Congestive heart failure
  - Furosemide 0.3–4 mg/kg p.o., s.c., i.m., i.v. s.i.d., b.i.d.
  - Enalapril 0.1–0.5 mg/kg p.o. every 24–48 h
  - Glyceryl trinitrate ointment (2%) at 3 mm applied topically to the inner pinna every 6–12 h

Table 3.6 Echocardiographic measurements from healthy chinchillas

Variable	Anaesthetized		Awake	
	Range	Mean ± SD	Range	Mean ± SD
Interventricular septum in diastole (cm)	0.15–0.25	0.18 ± 0.03	0.16–0.25	0.20 ± 0.03
Left ventricular free wall in diastole (cm)	0.23–0.32	0.26 ± 0.03	0.18–0.31	0.24 ± 0.04
Left ventricular diastolic dimension (cm)	0.47–0.69	0.64 ± 0.05	0.43–0.75	0.59 ± 0.08
Left ventricular systolic dimension (cm)	0.23–0.45	0.38 ± 0.05	0.18–0.40	0.29 ± 0.06
Fractional shortening (%)	32–51	40 ± 5	35–64	50 ± 8
E-point septal separation (cm)	0.00–0.06	0.03 ± 0.02	0.00–0.09	0.04 ± 0.03
Left atrial diameter (cm)	0.37–0.60	0.49 ± 0.06	0.45–0.67	0.53 ± 0.06
Aortic diameter (cm)	0.27–0.48	0.36 ± 0.05	0.36–0.49	0.41 ± 0.04
Left atrium diameter: Aortic diameter ratio	1.03–1.66	1.38 ± 0.20	1.02–1.52	1.28 ± 0.13
Heart rate (beats/min)	130–220	170 ± 22	130–235	169 ± 32
Aorta peak flow velocity (m/s)	0.33–0.75	0.46 ± 0.10	0.40–1.33	0.81 ± 0.26
Aorta ejection time (ms)	150–225	175 ± 20	110–160	131 ± 13
Pulmonary artery peak flow velocity (m/s)	0.37–1.00	0.61 ± 0.16	0.53–1.47	0.97 ± 0.32
Pulmonary artery ejection time (ms)	125–225	192 ± 34	105–150	129 ± 12
Mitral valve inflow summated (m/s)	–	–	0.50–0.90	0.74 ± 0.10
Mitral valve, E-wave peak flow velocity (m/s)	0.35–0.60	0.48 ± 0.08	–	–
Mitral valve, A-wave peak flow velocity (m/s)	0.17–0.40	0.29 ± 0.07	–	–

- Other medications
  - Atenolol 0.5–2 mg/kg p.o. s.i.d.
  - Verapamil 0.2 mg/kg p.o., s.c., i.v. t.i.d.
  - Diltiazem 0.5–1 mg/kg p.o. b.i.d., s.i.d.
  - Atropine 0.05–0.5 mg/kg s.c., i.m.
  - Glycopyrronium (glycopyrrolate) 0.01–0.1 mg/kg s.c., i.m., i.v.
  - Pimobendan at 0.2 mg/kg b.i.d.
  - Benazepril at <0.1 mg/kg p.o. s.i.d.

Systemic disorders

Viral

- Lymphocytic choriomeningitis (LCM).

Bacterial

- *Pseudomonas aeruginosa*
- *Corynebacterium kutscheri*
- *Corynebacterium pyogenes*
- *Listeria monocytogenes* (chinchilla; see *Neurological Disorders*)
- Salmonella
- *Streptobacillus moniliformis*
- *Streptococcus equi zooepidemicus*
- *Streptococcus equi equisimilis*
- *Yersinia pseudotuberculosis.*

Fungal

- *Histoplasma capsulatum.*

Protozoal

- *Toxoplasma gondii* (chinchillas; see also *Neurological Disorders*).

Nutritional

- Hypovitaminosis C (see *Nutritional Disorders*)
- Heterotrophic bony metaplasia and calcification (metastatic calcification) (guinea pigs). Often secondary to high phosphorus, low magnesium and potassium diets (may be linked to hypervitaminosis C in guinea pigs)
- Hypervitaminosis C. Possible cause of heterotrophic bony metaplasia and calcification (see *Nutritional Disorders*)
- Hypocalcaemia (lactating chinchillas) (see also *Gastrointestinal Tract Disorders, Neurological Disorders* and *Reproductive Tract Disorders*).

Neoplasia

- Lymphoma/leukaemia (see *Cardiovascular and Haematological Disorders*).

Other non-infectious problems

- Hypoglycaemia (especially following chronic dental disease)
- Aggressive treatment of dental disease (see *Dental Disorders*)
- Ketosis
- Heat stress (temperatures >27°C).

Findings on clinical examination

- Anorexia/poor physical condition/weight loss
- Fever
- Lethargy
- Conjunctivitis (Salmonella, histoplasmosis – see *Ophthalmic Disorders*)
- Marked dental disease/recent history of dental work (guinea pigs)

- Ataxia/weakness
- Central nervous signs (toxoplasmosis, listeriosis)
- Diarrhoea (occasionally with salmonellosis)
- Tachypnea, hypersalivation (heat stress, ketosis)
- Hyperthermia (rectal temperature above 41°C)
- Hepatosplenomegaly and enlarged mesenteric lymph nodes palpable (salmonellosis, streptococci, yersiniosis)
- Swollen submandibular lymph nodes (*Streptobacillus moniliformis*, streptococci, *Yersinia*)
- Sudden death (septicaemia, ketosis, heterotrophic bony metaplasia and calcification)
- Multiple signs including respiratory, mastitis, metritis CNS signs, ocular disease (*Streptococci*)
- Haemorrhagic discharge from nares, mouth and vagina (*Streptococcus equi equisimilis*)
- Disseminated granulomatous disease on postmortem *(Yersinia, Histoplasma)*
- Periparturient female guinea pig (ketosis)
- Prolonged anorexia, especially in obese guinea pigs (ketosis)
- Seizures
- Abortion
- Organ-specific diseases (heterotrophic bony metaplasia and calcification, metastatic calcification).

Investigations

1. Radiography
   a. Signs of heterotrophic bony metaplasia and calcification may be visible
2. Routine haematology and biochemistry
   a. Hypoglycemia (guinea pig normal range 3.36–7.8 mmol/L) (chinchilla 3.36–6.72 mmol/L)
   b. Hyperkalaemia (guinea pig normal range 4.0–5.0 mmol/L) (chinchilla 5–6.5 mmol/L)
   c. Hyponatraemia (guinea pig normal range 120–152 mmol/L) (chinchilla 130–155 mmol/L)
   d. Hypochloraemia (guinea pig normal range 90–115 mmol/L) (chinchilla 105–115 mmol/L)
   e. Hyperlipidaemia
   f. Hypokalaemia (guinea pigs; linked with heterotrophic bony metaplasia and calcification)
   g. Hypocalcaemia (guinea pig 2.0–3.0 mmol/L) (chinchilla 2.5–3.75 mmol/L) (lactating chinchillas).
   h. Lymphocytosis ($\geq 25 \times 10^9$/L) (leukaemia/lymphosarcoma).
3. Serology for LCM, toxoplasmosis
4. Culture and sensitivity
   a. May need repeated or bulk faecal samples to isolate intermittent Salmonella excreters
5. Cytology
   a. Gram stain smears from swollen submandibular glands (*Streptococci*: G +ve; *Yersinia*: G −ve)

6. Endoscopy
   a. Gastric ulceration (ketosis)
7. Ultrasonography
8. Biopsy.

Management

- Supportive treatment, including fluid therapy.

Treatment/specific therapy

- Bacterial disease
  - Appropriate antibiosis
  - Carrier animals may exist with Salmonellosis
  - Swollen submandibular lymph nodes may require surgical intervention
  - Yersiniosis – transmitted from faecal contamination from wild birds and rodents
  - Pseudomoniasis. Reduce water contamination by acidifying water to pH 2.5–2.8 or chlorination at 12 mg/L (cited in Strake et al 1996)
- Histoplasmosis
  - May be linked to soil contaminated with bird droppings
  - Amphotericin B at 0.1–1.0 mg/kg i.v. by infusion s.i.d. 5 days per week for 3 weeks
  - Ketoconazole at 10.0 mg/kg e.o.d. <1 year
- Hypoglycaemia
  - i.v. glucose by bolus and infusion
  - Assisted feeding
  - Investigate underlying causes, e.g. dental disease
- Ketosis
  - Fluid therapy
  - Calcium gluconate, i.v. or i.p. at 94–140 mg/kg
  - Dexamethasone at 0.1–0.6 mg/kg i.m.
  - Pregnant female guinea pig – consider caesarian/ovario-hysterectomy
  - Gradual weight reduction using low-calorie, high-fibre diet, e.g. hay
- Heat stress
  - Monitor core body temperature: guinea pig 37.2–39.5°C, 99–103.1°F; chinchilla 37–38°C, 98.6–100.4°F; degu 38°C, 100°F
  - Cool (not cold) body, e.g. damp towels, water bath. The pinnae in chinchillas are designed for radiative heat loss so these can be targeted especially
  - Dexamethasone at 0.1–0.6 mg/kg given i.v. once only
  - Supportive treatment such as cool intravenous fluids; heat stroke may have unforeseen sequelae, e.g. gut stasis
- Heterotrophic bony metaplasia and calcification
  - No treatment
  - Prevention is by providing an appropriate diet. Dietary recommendations (Huerkamp et al 1996) are:
    - 0.9–1.1% calcium; 0.6–0.7% phosphorus; Ca:P: 1.5:1.0
    - 0.3–0.4% magnesium, 0.4–1.4% potassium

- Associated hypokalaemia: daily supplement with 0.5–1.0 mg/kg potassium p.o.
- Heterotrophic bony metaplasia and calcification may be linked to a hypervitaminosis C
- Hypocalcaemia
  - Usually seen in lactating chinchillas at 2–3 weeks postpartum. May be accompanied by gut stasis
  - Calcium gluconate i.v. or i.p. at 94–140 mg/kg
- Lymphocytic choriomeningitis
  - Potential zoonosis. No treatment. Consider euthanasia.

Musculoskeletal disorders

Bacterial

- Septic arthritis (streptococci, mycoplasmosis).

Fungal

- *Histoplasma capsulatum* (see *Systemic Disorders*).

Nutritional

- Hypovitaminosis C (see *Nutritional Disorders*)
- Hypovitaminosis E (nutritional muscular dystrophy)
- Nutritional metabolic bone disease (see *Nutritional Disorders*).

Neoplasia

- Osteosarcoma.

Other non-infectious problems

- Osteoarthritis
- Fractures.

Findings on clinical examination

- Pain (osteosarcoma, hypovitaminosis C)
- Swellings associated with limbs and joints
- Abnormal gait
- Lameness
- Infertility problems (hypovitaminosis E)
- Severe muscle spasms of the hind limbs, fore limbs and face (nutritional metabolic bone disease).

Investigations

1. Radiography
   a. Fractures (trauma, hypovitaminosis C, osteosarcoma)
   b. Long bone and epiphyseal abnormalities (hypovitaminosis C)
   c. Lytic lesions in bone (osteosarcoma)

2. Routine haematology and biochemistry
   a. High CK levels (hypovitaminosis E)
3. Serology for mycoplasmosis
4. Culture and sensitivity
5. Cytology
6. Endoscopy
7. Ultrasonography
8. Biopsy
   a. Muscle biopsy and liver biopsy and vitamin E analysis (hypovitaminosis E).

Treatment/specific therapy

- Septic arthritis
  - Appropriate antibiosis
  - Joint lavage may be appropriate
- Hypovitaminosis E
  - Supplement with vitamin E at 5–10 mg/kg
  - Normal dietary levels should be 50 mg/kg
- Osteoarthritis; meloxicam 0.3 mg/kg s.i.d. p.o.
- Nutritional metabolic bone disease (see *Nutritional Disorders*)
- Fractures
  - Traumatic fractures can be managed:
    - Conservatively by strict rest in confinement, possibly with supportive dressings – although these rodents will tend to gnaw through dressings
    - Surgical repair.

Neurological disorders

Viral

- Lymphocytic choriomeningitis (LCM) (arenavirus).

Bacterial

- Otitis media/interna (*Streptococcus equi, Streptococcus pneumoniae, Bordetella bronchiseptica*, Klebsiella, Pseudomonas, other coliforms). *Pasteurella/Actinobacillus spp* may be encountered
- *Listeria monocytogenes.*

Fungal

- Ingestion of aflatoxins and mycotoxins (liver damage).

Protozoal

- *Encephalitozoon cuniculi*
- *Toxoplasma gondii* (see *Neurological Disorders*)
- *Frenkelia spp* (Meingassner & Burtscher 1977).

Parasitic

- *Trixacaris caviae*: intense pruritus may trigger seizure-like spasms) (guinea pigs)
- *Baylisascaris procyonis* (cerebral nematodiasis).

Nutritional

- Eclampsia in periparturient guinea pigs (see *Reproductive Tract Disorders*)
- Thiamine deficiency (chinchillas) (see *Nutritional Disorders*).

Neoplasia

Other non-infectious problems

- Heavy metal poisoning
- Neuronal degeneration in the mesencephalic trigeminal nerve nucleus following dental work (guinea pigs) (Kimoto 1993)
- Lymphosarcoma (meningeal infiltration – see *Cardiovascular and Haematological Disorders*)
- Renal disease
- Hypocalcaemia in lactating chinchillas (see *Systemic Disorders* and *Gastrointestinal Disorders*)
- Epilepsy-like conditions.

Findings on clinical examination

- Central nervous signs
- Progressive flaccid paralysis
- Closure of the ear canal with debris and inflammatory tissue (otitis media)
- Otitis interna evidenced by torticollis, rolling and nystagmus
- Drooping ears (chinchillas)
- Seizures
- Pneumonia
- Progressive deterioration following dental work, accompanied by ataxia, postural abnormalities, dysphagia/inability to chew (guinea pigs) (trigeminal motor neuron degeneration) (Azuma 1999)
- Self-inflicted lesions especially over the shoulders (*Trixacaris caviae*).

Investigations

1. Otoscopic examination of the ear canals
2. Radiography
   a. Skull radiography to assess tympanic bullae for otitis interna
3. Routine haematology and biochemistry
   a. Blood levels for heavy metals, e.g. zinc and lead
4. Serology for LCM, *E. cuniculi*, *Toxoplasma*
5. Culture and sensitivity
6. Cytology
7. Endoscopy
   a. Examination of the ear canal
8. Ultrasonography
9. Biopsy
   a. Heavy metal levels in liver tissue
10. Postmortem.

Management

- Supportive treatment including fluid therapy, assisted feeding and covering antibiosis.

Treatment/specific therapy

- Otitis media/interna
  - Very guarded prognosis – treatment often unsuccessful
  - Appropriate antibiosis
  - Bulla osteotomy
- *Listeria* monocytogenes
  - Usually poor response to therapy
  - Prophylactic treatment of in-contact chinchillas with autogenous vaccine or antibiotics
  - Trigeminal mesencephalic neuron degeneration following dental work in guinea pigs
  - Supportive treatment only. Usually require euthanasia
- *E. cuniculi*
  - Co-trimoxazole at 30 mg/kg b.i.d. p.o. for at least 3 weeks
  - Albendazole at 10 mg/kg p.o. for 6 weeks
  - Fenbendazole at 10 mg/kg p.o. for 1 month
- Toxoplasma and *Frenkelia spp*
  - Co-trimoxazole at 30 mg/kg b.i.d. p.o. for at least 3 weeks
- *Trixacaris caviae* (see *Skin Disorders*)
- *Baylisascaris procyonis* (cerebral nematodiasis)
  - Treatment difficult – consider ivermectin as anthelminthic plus NSAID, e.g. meloxicam at 0.1 mg/kg s.i.d.
  - Adult roundworms found in raccoon
- Hypocalcaemia
  - Gut stasis and gastric dilation and hind-limb paralysis in lactating chinchillas often the result of hypocalcaemia; usually seen in lactating chinchillas at 2–3 weeks postpartum. Calcium gluconate i.v. or i.p. at 94–140 mg/kg (see *Systemic Disorders*)
- Lymphocytic choriomeningitis
  - No treatment. Consider euthanasia
- Thiamine deficiency
  - Supplement with thiamine at 1 mg/kg food
- Heavy metal poisoning
  - Calcium disodium edetate at 30 mg/kg b.i.d. for 5 days (Richardson 2003)
- Epilepsy-like conditions
  - Epilepsy is a diagnosis of exclusion. Attempt to control with paediatric phenobarbitone preparations at 1–3 mg/kg b.i.d. (Richardson 2003).

Ophthalmic disorders

Bacterial

- *Chlamydophila psittaci*
- *Streptococcus equi zooepidemicus*
- Salmonella.

Fungal

- Histoplasma capsulatum (see *Systemic Disorders*).

Protozoal

- *Encephalitozoon cuniculi* (uveitis).

Nutritional

- Protein deficiency (cataracts) (guinea pigs)
- Fed on cow's milk (cataracts) (guinea pigs)
- Hypovitaminosis A (chinchillas)
- Hypervitaminosis C (heterotrophic bony metaplasia and calcification).

Neoplasia

Other non-infectious problems

- Diabetes mellitus (cataracts) (see *Pancreatic Disorders*)
- Ageing changes (cataracts and asteroid hyalosis in chinchillas).

Findings on clinical examination

- Conjunctivitis (*Chlamydophila*, Salmonella, hypovitaminosis A in chinchillas)
- Panophthalmitis/uveitis
- Exophthalmos (retrobulbar abscess/retro-orbital lymphadenopathy (*S. e. zooepidemicus*))
- Cataracts (chinchillas: hypovitaminosis A)
- Systemic signs (Salmonellosis, hypovitaminosis A in chinchillas)
- Bony spicules surrounded by fibrous tissue present in the ciliary body (hypervitaminosis C).

Investigations

1. Full ophthalmic examination
2. Radiography
3. Routine haematology and biochemistry
4. Serology for *E. cuniculi*
5. PCR for *Chlamydophila*
6. Culture and sensitivity
7. Cytology
   a. Gram stain
8. Endoscopy
9. Ultrasonography
10. Biopsy.

Treatment/specific therapy

- Chlamydophila
  - Enrofloxacin at 5 mg/kg s.i.d.
  - Ofloxacin ophthalmic drops topically

- Chlortetracycline ointment topically
- Other bacterial causes
  - Appropriate topical and systemic antibiosis
- *E. cuniculi*
  - Co-trimoxazole at 30 mg/kg b.i.d. p.o. for at least 3 weeks
  - Albendazole at 10 mg/kg p.o. for 6 weeks
  - Fenbendazole at 10 mg/kg p.o. for 1 month
- Hypovitaminosis A
  - Supplement with vitamin A at 2000 IU/chinchilla/day for 7 days, then every 7–14 days
- Heterotrophic bony metaplasia and calcification of the ciliary body. No treatment. Assess vitamin C status
- Other nutritional causes – identify and correct.

Endocrine disorders

- Amyloidosis of the adrenal glands and pancreatic islets (secondary to chronic infection especially pododermatitis (guinea pigs)
- Diabetes mellitus (see *Pancreatic Disorders*)
- Cystic ovarian disease (see *Reproductive Tract Disorders*)
- Hyperadrenocortism (see also *Skin Disorders*)
- Adrenal hyperplasia often accompanies dental disease and fur chewing in chinchillas (Crossley 2001)
- Thyroid hyperplasia can be associated with fur chewing in chinchillas.

Findings on clinical examination

- Alopecia (see *Skin Disorders*)
- Bilateral symmetrical often non-pruritic (guinea pigs) (cystic ovarian disease, hyperadrenocortism)
- Fur chewing (chinchillas) (possibly associated with thyroid hyperplasia or adrenal hyperplasia).

Investigations

1. Blood cortisol levels (guinea pig)
   a. These are biphasic in guinea pigs. Peaks at 1600 and 0400 hours; low points at 0800 and 2400 hours (Fujieda et al 1982)
   b. Normal free plasma cortisol = 0.6–5.8 μg/dL. This represents 6.1–14.5% of total cortisol levels (Fujieda et al 1982)
   c. Mean salivary cortisol = 6.6 ± 3.4 ng/mL. After ACTH stimulation 157 ± 53 ng/mL (Zeugswetter et al 2007).

ACTH response test in guinea pigs

1. Collect blood or saliva for basal cortisol.
2. Inject 20 IU ACTH i.m.
3. Repeat blood or saliva collection at 4 h post-ACTH.

2. Thyroid hormone levels (guinea pig)
   a. Total serum T4 = 2.5 ± 0.3–3.2 ± 0.8 µg/dL (Castro et al 1986)
   b. Free T4 = 1.26–2.03 ng/dL (%free T4 = 0.046–0.068%)
   c. Total T3 = 39–44 ng/dL
   d. Free T3 = 0.221–0.260 ng/dL (%free T3 = 0.521–0.638%)
3. Radiography
4. Routine haematology and biochemistry
   a. Low potassium levels (guinea pig normal levels 4.5–8.8 mmol/L)
5. Culture and sensitivity
6. Endoscopy
7. Biopsy
8. Ultrasonography
   a. Guinea pig: normal size adrenal glands around 14 × 4 mm (left); 13 × 6 mm (right) (Zeugswetter et al 2007). Enlarged adrenal glands were 15 × 7 mm (left) and 16 × 9 mm (right).

Treatment/specific therapy

- Hyperadrenocortism
  - Trilostane at 2–4 mg/kg p.o. s.i.d.
  - Attempt management and treatment as in other species.

Urinary disorders

Bacterial

- Cystitis
- *Streptococcus pyogenes*, staphylococci, faecal coliforms
- Pyelonephritis may follow metritis or abortion.

Protozoal

- *Klossiella cobayae* (*caviae*).

Neoplasia

Other non-infectious problems

- Amyloidosis (often linked to chronic inflammatory conditions, e.g. pododermatitis)
- Urethral obstruction with coagulated seminal vesicle secretions or other proteinaceous concretions in males (guinea pigs)
- Urinary calculi (triple phosphate, $CaCO_3$, $CaPO_4$, Ca oxalate) (guinea pigs)
- Hydronephrosis
- Idiopathic glomerulonephropathy
- Hypertensive nephrosclerosis (linked to Ca:P imbalance – see text on *heterotrophic bony metaplasia and calcification* above)
- Chronic renal failure
- Balanoposthitis (see *Reproductive Tract Disorders*)
- Diabetes mellitus (see *Pancreatic Disorders*).

Findings on clinical examination

- Polydipsia/polyuria
- Perineal dermatitis (urine scalding)
- Urinary tenesmus
- Obvious pain and discomfort; vocalization (guinea pigs)
- Haematuria
- Glycosuria, ketonuria (diabetes mellitus)
- Haemorrhagic discharge from vagina
- Anorexia, listlessness
- Weight loss
- Gross swelling of the abdomen (urinary retention/obstruction)
- Cystitis may be asymptomatic.

Investigations

1. Urinalysis (Table 3.7)
2. Culture and sensitivity
3. Sediment examination/cytology
4. Radiography
   a. Lateral and VD views
   b. Contrast studies
   c. IPV
5. Routine haematology and biochemistry
   a. Raised renal parameters
6. Endoscopy
7. Laparoscopic endoscopy
8. Ultrasonography
9. Biopsy
   a. Renal biopsy.

Table 3.7 Normal urine parameters for guinea pigs and chinchillas

Value	Guinea pig	Chinchilla
Volume (mL/adult per day)	20–25	
pH (average)	9.0	8.5
Urine gravity	>1.045	
Protein	Negligible	
Crystals	Triple phosphate, CaCO3	
Glucose	Negative (mild glycosuria may be masked by ascorbic acid excretion)	
Ketones	Negative	
Other	The cysts of Klossiella cobayae may occasionally be observed	

Management

- Fluid therapy
- Covering broad-spectrum antibiosis if appropriate, e.g. enrofloxacin at 5 mg/kg s.i.d. p.o., s.c.

Treatment/specific therapy

- Urinary calculi
- Surgical removal via cystotomy
- Predisposed by reduced fluid intake, nutritional imbalance, bacterial cystitis and anatomical abnormalities
- Ureteral calculi advanced gently into bladder for removal via cystotomy
- Triple phosphate calculi may be prevented by high supplementation with ascorbic acid to acidify the urine
- Oxalates: avoid high oxalate foods, e.g. rhubarb
- Select a lower calcium diet. Calcium requirement = 4 mg/kg per day
- Supplement with magnesium hydroxide at 4 mg/kg may protect against calcium uroliths (cited in Huerkamp et al 1996)
- Cystitis
  - Appropriate antibiosis
  - Supplement with vitamin C
  - Exacerbated by diabetes mellitus.

Reproductive tract disorders

Bacterial

- Wide variety of bacteria causing metritis, pyometra and mastitis
- In guinea pigs consider Bordetella (see *Respiratory Disorders*), Erysipelas, *Streptococcus equi equisimilis* (mastitis/metritis)as well as other infections (*E. coli, Klebsiella, Proteus, Staphylococci,* and other streptococci)
- Preputial gland abscess (chinchillas).

Neoplasia

- Ovarian teratoma
- Ovarian cystadenoma
- Leiomyoma (often concurrent with cystic ovarian disease)
- Mammary tumours (fibroadenomas, fibrocarcinomas).

Other non-infectious problems

- Balanoposthitis. Often secondary to foreign body, e.g. hair ring, bedding particles)
- Mastitis secondary to bites or abrasions from bedding/cage furniture
- Cystic ovarian disease (Nielsen et al 2003)
- Cystic endometrial hyperplasia, endometritis, mucometra (often concurrent with cystic ovarian disease)
- Pregnancy toxaemia (see 'Ketosis', in *Systemic Disorders*).

Findings on clinical examination

- Vaginal discharge from metritis, pyosalpinx, abortion, stillbirths (guinea pigs with bordetellosis, erysipelas, *S. e. equisimilis*)
- Abdominal enlargement (cystic ovarian disease)
- Hyperaemic or even blackened vulva with discharge (metritis) (chinchillas)
- Paraphimosis
- Mastitis
- Slight increase in size and firm texture (localized disease)
- Marked swelling, pain, discolouration, fever, anorexia, depression, weight loss, litter abandonment, high mortality rate (systemic disease)
- Other clinical signs, e.g. pneumonia (systemic disease)
- High temperature
- Non-pruritic alopecia (cystic ovarian disease)
- Large, palpable masses in the abdomen (cystic ovarian disease, neoplasia).

Investigations

1. Radiography
2. Routine haematology and biochemistry
   a. Leucopaenia suggests endotoxin production (with mastitis)
3. Culture and sensitivity
4. Cytology
5. Endoscopy
   a. Endoscopic laparotomy
6. Ultrasonography
   a. Cystic structures visible, often bilateral but asymmetrical. Can be several centimetres in diameter (cystic ovaries esp. guinea pigs)
7. Biopsy.

Management

- Supportive treatment, such as fluid therapy and assisted feeding.

Treatment/specific therapy

- Metritis
  - Vaginal/uterine irrigation with warm saline and antibiotic solution
  - Oxytocin at 1 IU/guinea pig s.c., i.m.
  - Antibiosis
  - Ovario-hysterectomy
- Preputial gland abscess
  - Lance and flush. Use appropriate antibiosis
- Balanoposthitis
  - Remove any foreign bodies, hair, etc.
  - Clean daily with dilute chlorhexidine solution
  - Antibiosis
- Paraphimosis

- As for balanoposthitis
- Attend to other underlying conditions, e.g. urethral calculi, fur ring (chinchillas)
  - If fur ring, gently extrude penis and remove accumulated fur; wash down with dilute chlorhexidine solution.
- Mastitis
  - Broad-spectrum antibiosis, e.g. co-trimoxazole at 30 mg/kg b.i.d. p.o. or enrofloxacin at 5 mg/kg s.i.d. p.o. or s.c.
  - Fluid therapy
  - Wean or foster any young as soon as possible
- Cystic ovarian disease
  - Ovario-hysterectomy (treatment of choice)
  - HCG 1000 IU weekly for 1–3 weeks
  - Draw fluid off by paracentesis
- Neoplasia
  - Surgery.

Reproductive disorders

Viral

- Caviid herpesvirus type 1 (cytomegalovirus CMV) (guinea pigs)
- Caviid herpesvirus type 2 (Epstein–Barr-like virus) (guinea pigs)
- Caviid herpesvirus type 3 (guinea pigs).

Bacterial

- A variety of bacterial infections, including mycoplasmosis, can lead to reproductive failures, abortions and stillbirths
- Puerperal septicaemia.

Protozoal

- *Toxoplasma gondii.*

Parasitic

- *Trixacarus caviae* infestation (abortion in extreme cases) (see *Skin Disorders*).

Nutritional

- Hypovitaminosis C (see *Nutritional Disorders*)
- Hypocalcaemia (eclampsia).

Neoplasia

Other non-infectious problems

- Diabetes mellitus (see *Pancreatic Disorders*)
- Ketosis
- Retained fetus
- Fetal mummification
- Dystocia
  - Fetal malpresentation

- Fetal oversize
- Uterine inertia
- Agalactia.

Findings on clinical examination

- Abortion (caviid herpesviruses, toxoplasmosis)
- Vulvar haemorrhage (vaginitis, pyometra, toxoplasmosis)
- Anorexia
- Depression
- Muscle spasms, seizures in pregnant or lactating female guinea pigs (eclampsia)
- Young may be palpable in abdominal cavity
- Failure to breed.

Investigations

1. Radiography
2. Routine haematology and biochemistry
   a. Blood calcium (guinea pig: 2.0–3.03 mmol/L; chinchilla 2.5–3.75 mmol/L)
   b. Anaemia, hypoglycemia, hyperkalaemia, hyponatraemia, hypochloraemia and hyperlipidaemia (ketosis)
3. Serology for toxoplasmosis
4. Culture and sensitivity
5. Cytology
6. Endoscopy
7. Ultrasonography
8. Biopsy
9. Postmortem
   a. Hepatic lipidosis, enlarged adrenal glands, empty stomach/gut (ketosis)
   b. Hepatic lipidosis.

Management

- Fluid therapy
- Keep warm.

Treatment/specific therapy

- Caviid herpesviruses. Infection is transplacental, sexually transmitted and possibly via urine and saliva. CHV type 2 can be transmitted via fomites
- Toxoplasmosis
  - Co-trimoxazole at 30 mg/kg b.i.d. p.o. for at least 3 weeks or alternatively try a combination therapy consisting of:
    - Co-trimoxazole at 30 mg/kg b.i.d. p.o.
    - Pyrimethamine at 0.5 mg/kg b.i.d. p.o.
    - Folic acid at 3.0–5.0 s.i.d.
- Eclampsia

- Usually peri- or postparturient females affected
- Calcium gluconate i.v. or i.p. at 94–140 mg/kg
- Supplement pregnant females guinea pigs with calcium
- Early weaning of young
- Gut stasis and gastric dilation and hind-limb paralysis in lactating chinchillas often the result of hypocalcaemia; usually seen in lactating chinchillas at 2–3 weeks postpartum. Calcium gluconate i.v. or i.p. at 94–140 mg/kg (see *Systemic Disorders*)
- Retained fetus; mummified fetus and dystocia
  - If birth takes longer than 4 h (chinchilla), may require intervention
  - Radiography
  - If radiographs appear normal, attempt calcium at 0.5 mL of 20% calcium solution followed by oxytocin 1 IU/guinea pig
  - If no improvement, consider caesarean section
- Puerperal septicemia
  - Antibiotics
  - Fluid therapy
  - Uterine irrigation
- Agalactia
  - Usually due to an underlying problem so investigate for this
  - Oxytocin at 1 IU/guinea pig to encourage milk let down
  - Foster or hand rear kits
- Dystocia
  - Radiography
  - If uterine inertia, try oxytocin 1 IU/guinea pig, otherwise consider caesarean section.

References

Azuma Y, Maehara K, Tokunaga T et al 1999 Systemic effects of the occlusal destruction in guinea pigs. In Vivo 13(6):519–524

Beck W 2007 Ectoparasites, endoparasites, and heartworm control in small mammals. Comp Cont Edu Vet 29(5A):3–8

Castro M I, Alex S, Young R A et al 1986 Total and free serum thyroid hormone concentrations in fetal and adult pregnant and non-pregnant guinea pigs. Endocrinology 118:533–537

Crossley D A 2001 Dental disease in chinchillas in the UK. J Small Anim Pract 42(1):12–19

Fujieda K, Goff A K, Pugeat M et al 1982 Regulation of the pituitary-adrenal axis and corticosteroidhyphen;binding globulin-cortisol interaction in the guinea pig. Endocrinology 111:1944–1950

Hammer M, Klopfleisch R, Teifke J P et al 2005 Cavernous or capillary haemangioma in two unrelated guinea pigs. Vet Rec 157:352–353

Huerkamp M J, Murray K A, Orosz S E 1996 Guinea pigs. In: Laber-Laird K, Swindle M, Flecknell P (eds) Handbook of rodent and rabbit medicine. Pergamon, Oxford

Keeble E 2001 Endocrine diseases in small mammals. In Practice 23(10):570–585

Kenagy G J, Veloso C, Bozinovic F 1999 Daily rhythms of food intake and feces reingestion in the degu, an herbivorous Chilean rodent: optimizing digestion through coprophagy. Physiol Biochem Zool 72(1):78–86

Kimoto A 1993 Change in trigeminal mesencephalic neurons after teeth extraction in guinea pig [Abstract, in Japanese] Kokubyo Gakkai Zasshi 60(1):199–212

Linde A, Summerfield N J, Johnston M et al 2004 Echocardiography in the chinchilla. J Vet Intern Med 18:772–774

Linek M, Bourdeau P 2005 Alopecia in two guinea pigs due to hypopodes of Acarus farris (Acaridae:Astigmata) Vet Rec 157:58–60

Meingassner J G, Burtscher H 1977 Double infection of the brain with Frenkelia species and Toxoplasma gondii in Chinchilla laniger. Veterinary Pathology 14(2):146–153

Najecki D, Tate B 1999 Husbandry and management of the degu. Lab Animal 28(3):54–62

Nielsen T D, Holt S, Ruelokke M L et al 2003 Ovarian cysts in guinea pigs: influence of age and reproductive status on prevalence and size. J Small Anim Pract 44:257–260

Richardson V C G 2003 Diseases of small domestic rodents, 2nd edn. Blackwell, Oxford

Singh B R, Alam J, Hansda D 2005 Alopecia induced salmonellosis in guinea pigs. Vet Rec 156:516–518

Strake J G, Davis L A, LaRegina M et al 1996 Chinchillas. In: Laber-Laird K, Swindle M, Flecknell P (eds) Handbook of rodent and rabbit medicine. Pergamon, Oxford, p 172

Van Gestel J F E, Engelen M A C M 2004 Comparative efficacy of lufenuron and itraconazole in a guinea pig model of cutaneous Microsporum canis. Free Comm Abst. Session 1: Fungal and Bacterial diseases. Vet Dermatol 15(Suppl 1):20–40

Wasson K, Criley J M, Clabaugh M B et al 2000 Therapeutic efficacy of oral lactobacillus preparation for antibiotic-associated enteritis in guinea pigs. Contemp Top Lab Anim Sci 39(1):32–38

Zeugswetter F, Fenske M, Hassan J et al 2007 Cushing's syndrome in a guinea pig. Vet Rec 160:878–880

CHAPTER

4

Small rodents

Small rodents are popular both as children's (and adult) pets, but also as show animals. Rats in particular have a very enthusiastic following. Those species that are likely to be encountered in the veterinary surgery are:

- Mice (*Mus musculus*)
- Rats (*Rattus norvegicus*)
- Mongolian gerbil (*Meriones unguiculatus*)
- Hamsters
  - Syrian (golden) *Mesocricetus auratus*
  - Russian hamster (*Phodopus sungorus*)
  - Roborovski's hamster (*Phodopus roborovskii*)
  - Chinese hamster (*Cricetulus griseus*).

Table 4.1 Small rodents: Key facts

		Mouse	Rat	Gerbil	Syrian hamster	Russian hamster	Chinese hamster
Average life span (years)		2–3	3–4	2–3	2–3	9–15 (months)	2
Weight (g)	Male	20–40	250–1000+	117	85–130	30–35	30–35
	Female			100	95–150		
Body temperature (°C)		37.5	38	38	36–37.4		
Respiratory rate (breaths/min)		100–250	70–150	90–140	75		
Heart rate (beats/min)		500–600	300–450	200–360	300–600		
Gestation (days)		19–21	21–23	24–26	15–16	18–20	20–21
Age at weaning (days)		21–28	21–28	21–24	21–28	21–28	21
Sexual maturity (weeks)		5–8	6–8	10–12	6–8	6–8	7–14

• Hamsters species differ in their standard husbandry. Syrian hamsters are solitary and will fight if kept together. *Phodopus spp* are highly sociable and fare best in small groups, and, indeed, live longer if kept that way. The Chinese hamster falls between the two and is best kept in pairs.

Consultation and handling

Small rodents are prey animals and may become stressed by the presence of potential predators such as cats, dogs and unfamiliar people; this includes auditory and olfactory signals, so where possible they should be housed separately from such animals, and hands should be well cleaned to remove other species' odours before handling.

Many small rodents move quickly and unpredictably and care should be taken to prevent unwanted escapes or potentially disastrous leaps to the floor. Gently wrapping in a towel will often help with the handling and control of an excitable rodent. A sure way to annoy a pet rat (and alienate its owner) is to attempt to grasp it by the scruff of the neck. Most are used to being gently handled and are unlikely to bite. If in doubt, use a towel. Do not attempt to pick a hamster straight from its bed; they are territorial of this and are likely to bite. Instead, gently tease or tip it out. Recalcitrant hamsters are more easily scruffed and, although this will help with an examination of the teeth, it may upset the rodent.

Hamsters are permissive hibernators and may attempt hibernation if temperatures fall consistently below 4.5°C. Poor food availability, altered photoperiod and other factors may also induce hibernation, although this varies between individuals. Hibernation is not continuous but is interrupted every 2–3 days by bouts of normal activity including foraging. During hibernation, hamsters remain sensitive to tactile stimulation and can be gently aroused. Exposure to normal room temperatures (18–22°C) and lighting (12–14 h) are unlikely to trigger hibernation. Many owners misinterpret clinical signs of illness (lack of movement and lethargy, anorexia) with hibernation, often delaying presentation to the veterinary surgeon.

Nursing care

See *Nursing Care* in *Rabbits* for general principles.

Small rodents by virtue of their size and the high risk of predation are forced to obtain most of their water from preformed (food) and metabolic sources. Dehydration can be a real issue, especially at higher environmental temperatures (Table 4.2).

Fluids can be given s.c., i.p. or i.o. However, for small rodents, the intravenous route (Fig. 4.1) for fluid administration is largely impractical, but Table 4.3 gives suggested sites.

Jugular catheterization can be attempted in all species but it is difficult and may result in respiratory embarrassment. Many of these sites may also require anaesthesia and surgical cut down, which may not be appropriate for the welfare of the patient. In hypovolaemic patients vascular access may be impossible. It is better to consider either i.p. or i.o. administration.

Table 4.2 Small rodents: Nursing care

Species	Weight (g)	Maintenance daily water intake (mL/ kg per day)	Approximate volumes for fluid replacement therapy (mL/kg body weight)		
			Subcutaneous	Intraperitoneal	Shock
Syrian hamster	85–130 (M) 95–150 (F)	100	30	30	65–80
Gerbil	45–130 (M) 50–85 (F)	Allow 3–4 mL/day	20–40	40–60	60–85
Rat	267–520 (M) 250–325 (F)	0.8–1.1	25	25	50–70
Mouse	20–40 (M) 25–63 (F)	1.5	30–60	60	70–80

Hypothermia

Much endogenous body heat is generated by gut and muscle activity; sick, inactive or anaesthetized rodents are prone to hypothermia (Jepson 2004). Use a heat source, e.g. electric heat mat, plus insulation such as silver foil over the feet, pinnae and tail (reduces heat lost by conduction) and bubble wrap (reduces heat lost by

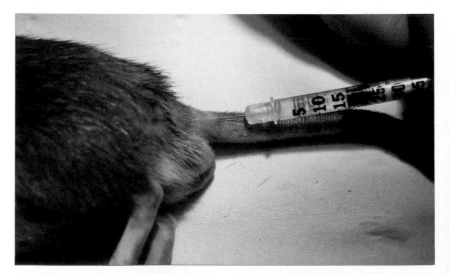

Fig. 4.1. Intravenous fluids given through the lateral tail vein.

Table 4.3 Small rodents: Sites for fluid administration

Intravenous (rat and mouse)	Lateral tail vein (helps if warm!) (Fig. 4.1)
Intravenous (hamster)	Very difficult: lateral tarsal vein, anterior cephalic vein and lingual vein
Intravenous (gerbil)	Lateral tail vein or saphenous vein
Intraperitoneal (all three species)	Hold the patient vertically downward and inject into the lower left quadrant
Intraosseous (all three species)	Under GA to insert either an intraosseous catheter or a hypodermic needle into the marrow of either the femur (via the greater trochanter) or tibia (through the tibial crest). Fluids, colloids and even blood can be i.o. if necessary.

convection). Maintain in warm air, e.g. incubator, or use a commercial medial warm air generator.

Nutritional status

Many small rodents are presented as emergencies after a prolonged period of ill-health that will have affected their food intake. These animals are often hypoglycaemic – testing with a commercial glucometer on a small sample of blood – and i.v. or i.p. glucose can be given to these cases once identified.

Analgesia

Table 4.4 Small rodents: Analgesic doses

Analgesic	Dose			
	Rat	Mouse	Hamster	Gerbil
Buprenorphine	0.05–1.0 mg/kg s.c., i.p. every 6–12 h	0.05–1.0 mg/kg s.c., i.p. b.i.d. every 12 h	0.1 mg/kg s.c. every 6–12 h	0.1 mg/kg s.c. every 6–12 h
Butorphanol	0.2–2.0 mg/kg s.c. every 2–4 h	1.0–2.0 mg/kg s.c. every 2–4 h		
Carprofen	1.0–5.0 mg/kg s.c. or p.o. s.i.d. or b.i.d.	1.0–5.0 mg/kg s.c. or p.o. s.i.d. or b.i.d.		
Ketoprofen	2.0–5.0 mg/kg s.c., i.m. every 12–24 h	2.0–5.0 mg/kg s.c., i.m. every 12–24 h		

Continued

Table 4.4   Small rodents: Analgesic doses—cont'd

Analgesic	Dose			
	Rat	Mouse	Hamster	Gerbil
Meloxicam	0.5–2.0 mg/kg s.c., p.o. s.i.d.	1.0–2.0 mg/kg s.c., p.o. s.i.d.		
Morphine	2.0–5.0 mg/kg s.c., i.m. every 4 h	2.0–5.0 mg/kg s.c., i.m. every 4 h		
Pethidine	10–20 mg/kg i.m., s.c., i.p. q.i.d.	10–20 mg/kg i.m., s.c., i.p. q.i.d.	10–20 mg/kg i.m., s.c., i.p. q.i.d.	10–20 mg/kg i.m., s.c., i.p. q.i.d.
Nalbuphine	4.0–8.0 mg/kg s.c. every 2–4 h	4.0–8.0 mg/kg s.c. every 2–4 h		

Anaesthesia

Small rodents may have subclinical respiratory infections.

It is important to keep small rodents warm as they have a large surface area compared with volume, which results in significant heat loss during surgery. This also applies during anaesthesia – hypothermia acts as a general depressant and is also immunosuppressive. Merely applying insulation such as bubble wrap is often insufficient – inactive, anaesthetized rodents are not generating heat and you may be insulating it from a higher ambient temperature. Place these animals on to a heat mat, on to which is placed an absorptive towel or other material to both protect the mat from becoming wet, and reduce the slight risk of localized burns.

Use reflective foil over hairless areas where heat loss can occur, e.g. tails, feet, pinnae on mice and rats.

There is no need to starve – prolonged fasting can lead to hypoglycaemia.

Pre-medication

1. Pre-medication is rarely used, but does permit easier, smoother anaesthetic induction; this should be balanced against increased recovery times where short operations are performed.
2. Suitable pre-medications include:
   a. Acepromazine at 0.5–5.0 mg/kg i.m. or i.p.
   b. Diazepam at 2.5–5.0 mg/kg i.m. or i.p.
   c. Midazolam: 2.5–5.0 mg/kg i.m. or i.p.
3. *Pre-medicate 45–60 min before* gaseous anaesthesia.
4. Mask down or use induction chamber with isoflurane. Induction is usually quick due to high respiratory rates.

Parenteral anaesthesia

1. Always weigh accurately.
2. Always supply oxygen by face mask.
3. Many rodents fail to lose withdrawal reflex and may respond to surgical stimuli, therefore may need to use low concentration of inhalation anaesthetic or infiltrate with local anaesthetic.
4. There is a range of published anaesthetic regimes. The author has found the following of use:
   a. Ketamine 50–100 mg/kg plus Xylazine 2.0–10 mg/kg i.p.
   b. Ketamine 50–100 mg/kg plus 0.25–1.0 mg/kg medetomidine i.p.

Cardiopulmonary resuscitation

For respiratory arrest

1. Administer 100% oxygen.
2. Assist ventilation – compress thorax at around 60×/min.
3. Doxapram sublingual or at 10 mg/kg i.v. or i.p. – *Note*: this will increase the animal's oxygen demand.
4. If appropriate, give atipamezole.

For cardiac arrest

1. As for respiratory arrest.
But also:
2. Compress thorax at around 90×/min.
3. If asystole – give adrenaline at 0.1 mg/kg of 1:10 000.
4. If ventricular fibrillation – lidocaine (lignocaine) at 1–2 mg/kg.

Skin disorders

Syrian hamsters have large, bilaterally symmetrical hip glands; these are scent glands used for marking burrow walls and in males they can be particularly pronounced in both size and the amount of sebaceous secretion they produce. These are frequently mistaken as skin lesions. Dwarf hamsters and gerbils possess ventral scent glands visible on the abdomen.

Pruritus

- Ectoparasites (Fig. 4.2)
- Otitis externa (ear mites)
- Pyoderma (see also *Abscessation* below)
- Diet-associated dermatitis (mouse, see *Dietary*)
- Allergic dermatitis
  - Swollen feet, palpebral swelling, ocular discharge and sneezing (hamsters)

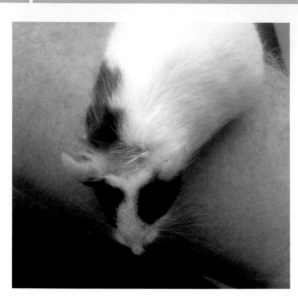

Fig. 4.2. Trauma from *Myobia musculi* infestation in a mouse.

- Contact allergy to nickel (mouse). Typically see inflammation on nose, feet and tail
- Nasal dermatitis (gerbil).

Alopecia

- Ectoparasites (see below)
- Dermatophytosis (rat, mouse) (often asymptomatic)
  - *Trichophyton spp* and *Microsporon spp*
- Barbering (usually done by dominant individual in group)
- Muzzle alopecia. Secondary to repetitive rubbing of muzzle against bars during cage-bar chewing
- *Staphylococcus aureus* dermatitis (gerbil). Localized alopecia and erythema around the external nares
- Nasal dermatitis (gerbil). Alopecia and pruritic reddened scabs appear first around the external nares, mainly on the upper lip. May spread over the head and to the forepaws
- Wood shaving and sawdust bedding made from treated wood
- Low protein diet (<16%) (hamster)
- Hormonal alopecia (see *Endocrine Disorders*)
- Cystic ovaries (see *Reproductive Disorders*)
- Satinization in hamsters. Individuals homozygous for the satin gene may have only a thin coating of hair.

Scaling and crusting

- Ectoparasites (*Radfordia* (rats), *Demodex*, *Notoedres* (hamsters)
- Dermatophytosis (rat, mouse) (often asymptomatic)
- Build up of wax and debris in the ear canals (ear mites, otitis externa).

Erosions and ulceration

- *Notoedres* (hamsters)
- On the dorsum of mice (ectoparasitic: *Myobia musculi* and *Mycoptes musculinus*). Resultant self-inflicted trauma can be severe. Black-coated strains of mice may be more prone to hypersensitivity reactions to these mites (Csiza & McMartin 1976, cited in Girling 2007)
- Bite wounds
- Sores and ulcers on the medial aspect of the legs of hamsters – abrasions secondary to wire wheel.

Nodules and non-healing wounds

- Ectromelia virus (mousepox); orthopox virus
- Rat poxvirus (orthopox virus)
- Hamster polyomavirus (HaPV, Papova virus)
- Self-inflicted trauma
- Abscessation. Often resulting from bites; can be from pyoderma or bacteraemic spread. *Staphylococcus aureus* is a common isolate, but others include *Streptococcus spp, Pasteurella spp* and in the mouse, *Actinobacillus spp* and *Corynebacterium spp* as well
- Rats with *Corynebacterium kutscheri* may have slightly enlarged cervical lymph nodes in addition to mild-to-severe respiratory disease
- *Streptobacillus moniliformis* is a rare oral commensal in rats that can cause abscessation in rats following rats and rat-bite (Haverill) fever in man.

Changes in pigmentation

- Rash (Ectromelia virus in the mouse); nickel contact allergy (mouse)
- Seborrhea (esp. older adult male rats).

Ectoparasites

- Rats
  - Mites: *Radfordia ensifera* (fur mite), *Myobia musculi* (fur mite), *Sarcoptes scabei, Demodex nanus, Ornithonyssus bacoti* (tropical rat mite)
  - Ear mites: *Notoedres muris* – may infest the pinnae, face, tail and extremities
  - Lice: *Polyplax spinulosa* (sucking louse)
  - Fleas *Ctenocephalides felis, Xenopsylla spp, Leptosylla spp, Nosopsyllus spp*
- Mouse
  - Mites: *Myobia musculi* (fur mite), *Mycoptes musculinus* (fur mite), *Radfordia affinis* (fur mite); *Sarcoptes scabei* (rare), *Psorergates simplex spp* (follicular mite – rare)
  - Ear mites: *Notoedres muris*
  - Lice: *Polyplax serrata* (sucking lice), *P. spinulosa*
  - Fleas: *Ctenocephalides felis*
- Hamster
  - *Demodex criceti* and *D. aurati*. Infestation more common than disease
  - *Sarcoptes scabei*
  - *Ctenocephalides felis*
  - Ear mites: *Notoedres notoedres* and *N. cati* (but can have a more generalized distribution including the face, genitalia, limbs and tail
  - *Ornithonyssus bacoti* (tropical rat mite) (Fox et al 2004)

- Gerbil
  - Mites: *Demodex meroni, Liponyssoides sanguineus* (esp. Egyptian gerbils, *Meriones libycus*). Rarely *Sarcoptes scabei* and *Notoedres muris*
  - Storage mites (*Acarus farris*) on cereal based foods may occasionally cause irritation.

Neoplasia

- Squamous cell carcinoma
- Mammary adenocarcinomas (mouse) (see *Reproductive Disorders*)
- Melanoma
- Haemangiosarcomas
- Trichoepitheliomas (in hamsters may be related to HaPV infection).

Necrosis of extremities

- Shortening of extremities secondary to necrosis (mouse: Ectromelia virus)
- Ringtail (annular constrictions of the tail) (rats).

Other

- Anaemia, debilitation (*Ornithonyssus bacoti* (tropical rat mite, heavy infestations of lice)
- *Note* lice (*Polyplax spp*) can be vectors for *Encephalitozoon cuniculi, Eperythrozoon coccoides* and *Haemobartonella muris*
- Fleas (*Xenopsylla spp* and *Nosopsyllus spp*) can be vectors for *Yersinia pestis* (plague), *Rickettsia typhus* and act as intermediate hosts for *Hymenolepis spp* (see *Gastrointestinal Tract Disorders*).

Findings on clinical examination

- Areas of alopecia
- Swellings, often firm consistency even if abscess. Displacement of normal outline of coat may indicate swelling
- Cuts and abrasions
- Extreme pruritus
- Systemic signs
- Overgrown claws
- Pododermatitis – swelling and abscessation of the soles of the feet, especially the hind feet
- Areas of inflammation and excoriation around the nares in gerbils (nasal dermatitis, Staphylococcal dermatitis)
- Hair loss and sores on legs of hamsters (repetitive trauma from wire wheel)
- Hair loss on one side of mouth (persistent bar gnawing)
- Seborrhoea
- Multiple small lumps around neck in hamsters (with subsequent ulceration), weight loss; mortalities (can be up to 15–20%) (HaPV).

Investigations

1. Microscopy: examine fur pluck, acetate strips or skin scrapes to affected area and examine for ectoparasites

2. Examine teeth. Rodents with dental disease may have difficulty grooming normally
3. Radiography
   a. Pododermatitis – often underlying osteoarthritis
4. Routine haematology and biochemistry
   a. Eosinophilia (ectoparasitism)
5. Serology for ectromelia virus
6. Bacteriology and mycology: hair pluck or swab lesions for routine culture and sensitivity
7. Cytology
8. Gram stain
   a. Fine-needle aspirate followed by staining with rapid Romanowsky stains
9. Biopsy obvious lesions
10. Ultraviolet (Wood's) lamp – positive for *Microsporium canis* only (not all strains fluoresce). Also porphyrins fluoresce (nasal dermatitis in gerbils)
11. Endocrine analysis: Thyroxine (see *Endocrine Disorders*), oestradiol
12. If barbering suspected, examine hair under microscope to see if chewed; separate from other animals; supply extra hay.

Management

1. Pododermatitis
   a. Soft bedding
   b. Covering antibiosis
   c. Regular cleansing
   d. Application of topical amorphous hydrogel dressings, e.g. IntraSite Gel (Smith and Nephew Healthcare Ltd) encourage secondary healing
   e. Attend to any underlying osteoarthritis with NSAIDs, e.g. meloxicam.

Treatment/specific therapy

- Poxviruses (including Ectromelia virus)
  - No treatment; supportive only. Consider euthanasia. Rat poxvirus is a potential zoonosis
- Hamster polyomavirus (HaPV, Papova virus)
  - No treatment
  - Transmitted via the urine
  - Cull affected and in-contact animals.
- *Corynebacterium kutscheri* (pseudotuberculosis)
  - Appropriate antibiosis. Prevalence is variable
- Dermatophytosis
  - Griseofulvin at 25 mg/kg once daily for 30–60 days
  - Miconazole/chlorhexidine (Malaseb, Leo) shampoo – bath once daily
  - Itraconazole 5 mg/kg s.i.d. p.o. for 30 days
  - Improve ventilation
- Ectoparasites
  - Ivermectin at 0.2 mg/kg or as topical (450 µg/tube) 'spot on' (Xeno450, Genitrix) weekly for 3–4 weeks
  - Dust with pyrethrin powder

- For cases of severe self-inflicted trauma then NSAIDs plus prophylactic toe clipping may be necessary to reduce excoriation, plus antibiotics to control secondary infections
- *Notoedres* in Syrian hamsters (Beco et al 2001)
  - Ivermectin at 400 µg/kg s.c. every 7 days for a minimum of 8 weeks
  - Moxidectin at 400 µg/kg p.o. every 7 days for a minimum of 8 weeks
- *Demodex* mites
  - Amitraz as wash at 100 mg/L applied topically every 7 days until resolution
  - Ivermectin as for *Notoedres*
  - Some mice may fail to respond to treatment; it is thought that some of these individuals may have inherent, genetic immune deficits whilst others may develop a hypersensitivity to mite antigen that is difficult to control
- Storage mites
  - Topical fipronil spray applied with a cotton bud
  - Dispose of affected foods and clean storage containers
- *Ornithonyssus bacoti* is a potential zoonosis (Beck & Pfister 2004)
- Ringtail
  - Surgical removal of affected part. Linked to low humidity (RH <40%) so increase to 50–70%.
- Allergic dermatitis
  - Separate from all potential allergens, and where appropriate seek alternatives, including beddings, certain foods (see below), metallic objects (including caging), environmental triggers such as cigarette smoke
  - For suspected dietary allergies an elimination protocol can be developed – remove all high risk triggers, e.g. sunflower seeds, peanuts, coloured dog biscuits and replace with cooked rice, maize flakes and fruits (including dried) (Richardson 2003)
- Diet-associated dermatitis
  - Change food to more appropriate material (see *Dietary*)
- NSAIDs to control pruritus
- Abscessation
  - Systemic antibiosis
  - Bath wounds and apply topical antibiosis
  - May require surgical removal
- Neoplasia
  - Surgical removal
  - Where surgery is considered non-viable, accessible cutaneous tumours can be treated by injecting cisplatin directly into the tissue mass on a weekly basis as a debulking exercise
- Staphylococcal dermatitis
  - Topical and systemic antibiosis
  - Environmental modification: high humidity, fighting, and trauma are thought to predispose
- Nasal dermatitis
  - May be linked to focal hyperplasia of the Harderian glands and increased lachrymal secretion
  - Environmental modification; may be associated with trauma from burrowing into certain beddings; provision of sand may improve the condition
  - Topical ophthalmic treatment may be beneficial

- Sores on legs from wire wheel
  - Treat with topical preparations and switch to a solid backed and rimmed wheel
- Seborrhoea
  - Treat symptomatically with appropriate shampoos.

Respiratory tract disorders

Viral

- Paramyxovirus
- Sendai virus (rats and mice; forms part of rat pneumonia complex)
- Sialodacryoadenitis (SDAV) (coronavirus) (rats) (see also *Gastrointestinal Tract* and *Ophthalmic Disorders*)
- Mouse hepatitis virus (MHV) (mouse) (see also *Gastrointestinal Tract Disorders*).

Bacterial

- *Pasteurella pneumotropica*
- Mycoplasmosis esp. M. pulmonis (rats and mice; forms part of rat pneumonia complex)
- Cilia associated respiratory bacillus (CAR) (part of rat pneumonia complex)
- *Streptococcus pneumoniae* (rats) (see also *Cardiovascular and Haematological Disorders*)
- *Corynebacterium kutscheri* (pseudotuberculosis). Often subclinical (rats and mice)
- Listeriosis (bushy-tailed jirds, *Sekeetamys calurus*); acute pneumonitis (see also *Gastrointestinal Tract Disorders*).

Fungal

Neoplasia

- Alveologenic carcinoma
- Pulmonary metastases from other neoplasia especially uterine adenocarcinomas.

Other non-infectious problems

- Allergic disorders, e.g. to fine sawdust
- Heart disease (see *Cardiovascular and Haematological Disorders*)
- High environmental ammonia levels.

Findings on clinical examination

- Upper respiratory signs, such as sneezing, porphyrin staining around the eyes (Fig. 4.3)
- Swollen neck and eyes; ophthalmic lesions (SDAV in rats)
- Respiratory distress – can be severe
- Cyanosis of mucous membranes, feet, nares and tails (rats and mice)
- Tachypnoea. Estimates for the normal respiratory rates of small mammals can be achieved with the following formula: Respiratory rate = $53.5 \times wt^{-0.26}$, where wt = body weight in kg.
- Dyspnoea
- Marked lung sounds

149

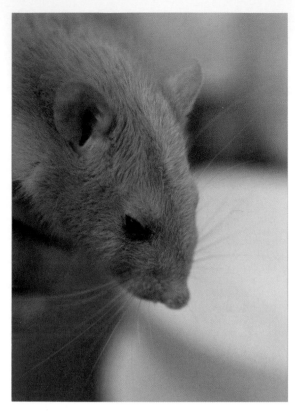

Fig. 4.3. Porphyrin-stained tears in a rat.

- Rhinitis + nasal discharge
- Torticollis, circling and other neurological disorders (see *Neurological Disorders*)
- Weight loss, anorexia
- Pyrexia.

Investigations

1. Differentiate porphyrin staining from blood by either using blood 'dipstick' tests or UV light (porphyrins fluoresce)
2. Radiography
   a. Pneumonia
3. Routine haematology and biochemistry
4. PCR for *M. pulmonis*. Sendai virus, CAR, SDAV, MHV
5. Culture and sensitivity (including from tracheal wash)
6. Cytology form tracheal wash
7. Pleural tap and cytology

8. Culture and sensitivity
9. Mycoplasma culture
10. Cytology
   a. Gram staining of discharges or effusions
11. Endoscopy
12. Ultrasonography.

Management

• A clean, well-ventilated, but not draughty, air space is necessary.
• Some of the smaller module-based rodent housing has poor ventilation which can produce areas of high humidity and high ammonia levels. Both of these can predispose to respiratory disease.

Treatment/specific therapy

• Viral infections
  • Control of secondary infections
  • For ADAV, MHV and Sendai virus, attempt removal from breeding colonies by euthanizing all unweaned and weanling young and preventing breeding for 8 weeks. This allows immunocompetent adults to seroconvert and eradicate these viruses
• Bacterial disease including mycoplasmosis
  • Appropriate antibiosis
  • *M. pulmonis* infections may be exacerbated by concurrent SDAV
• Rat pneumonia complex
  • Broad-spectrum antibiotics
  • NSAIDs, e.g. meloxicam
  • Mucolytics such as bromhexine and N-acetyl-cysteine may be useful
  • Improved environmental conditions, i.e. sanitation and ventilation
  • Often cure is impractical; control of the condition is often the case
• Allergic disease
  • Often only one in a group affected
  • Consider NSAIDs or antihistamines as a control
  • Avoid suspected antigens.

Gastrointestinal tract disorders

Disorders of the oral cavity

In small rodents, the cheek teeth either grow very slowly or not at all so dental disease involving these is rare. Gnawing in rodents involves a significant rostrocaudal movement of the lower jaw relative to the upper, therefore the lower incisors are naturally long. True indicators of incisor malocclusion include uneven wear, sloping of the cutting edges, fractured teeth, altered pigmentation, obvious pathological overgrowth.

The hemi-mandibular junction is flexible and it is normal for the lower incisors to be able to deviate from each other during manipulation.

Permanent dental formula of a rodent

$$I : \frac{1}{1} , C : \frac{0}{0} , PM : \frac{0}{0} , M : \frac{3}{3}$$

Dental disorders

- Incisor malocclusion; secondary to fractures, developmental problems, hereditary predisposition
- In some cage bar-chewing rodents the cutting edges of the incisors may show a slope to one side associated with uneven wear due to repetitive gnawing on vertical bars
- Some rodents with grossly overgrown incisors may present with weight loss secondary to extreme incisor malocclusion that results in an inability to physically close the mouth for mastication
- Dental caries can be common in rodents fed treats high in sugar and other carbohydrates, or acidic foods
- Burr back overgrown incisors. Avoid rotation of tooth during this process to reduce risk of trauma
- Provide something to gnaw on, e.g. safe wood or dog biscuit
- Incisor extraction. Significant risk of mandibular fracture
- Tooth root abscessation
  - Surgical debridement and covering antibiosis.

Cheek pouches

Very well developed in hamsters and some other rodents, e.g. chipmunks.
- Cheek pouch impaction
  - Food accumulation; may begin to autolyse and secondary infection ensues. Empty under general anaesthetic
- Cheek pouch eversion/prolapse/neoplasia (Fig. 4.4)
  - Some cases may respond to gently replacement
  - Requires surgical resection.

Foreign bodies

- The rodent may display an apparent malocclusion, hypersalivation, discomfort around the mouth. Require removal possibly under GA.

Differential diagnoses for gastrointestinal disorders

Coprophagy is commonly practiced by many small rodents. Hamsters have a stomach divided into two compartments: an aglandular forestomach (which allows some pre-gastric fermentation to occur, especially of ingested faeces) and the true glandular stomach.

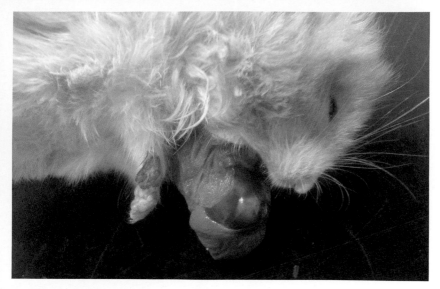

Fig. 4.4. Prolapsed cheek pouch secondary to neoplasia.

Viral

* Sialodacryoadenitis (SDAV) (coronavirus) (rats: see also *Respiratory Tract* and *Ophthalmic Disorders*)
* Mouse hepatitis virus (MHV) (coronavirus) (mouse: see also *Respiratory Tract Disorders*)
* Rotavirus (mouse)
* Reovirus (mouse).

Bacterial

* *Citrobacter freundii* (mouse)
* *Clostridium piliforme* (Tyzzer's disease) all rodents especially gerbils
* *Salmonellosis* esp. *S. enteriditis* and *S. typhimurium*
* Listeriosis (bushy-tailed jirds, *Sekeetamys calurus*), disease was characterized by acute deaths without clinical signs
* Proliferative ileitis or 'wet-tail' in hamsters
* *Lawsonia intracellularis*
* *Campylobacter spp*
* *E. coli*
* *Yersina pseudotuberculosis*
* *Pasteurella* (enteritis in hamsters).

Protozoal

* Rat
  * *Cryptosporidium parvum*
  * *Eimeria spp* (rare)
  * *Giardia muris*
  * *Spironucleus muris*

- Mouse
  - *Cryptosporidium muris, C. parvum*
  - *Eimeria spp:* common in wild mice (*E. falciformis, E. musculi, E. schueffneri, E. krijgsmanni, E. keilini, E. hindlei*)
  - *Giardia muris*
  - *Trichomonas muris*
  - *Spironucleus muris*
  - *Entamoeba muris*
- Hamster
  - *Cryptosporidium spp* (see 'Proliferative ileitis' in *Treatment/specific therapy*)
  - *Giardia spp*
  - *Balantidium coli* and *B. caviae*
  - *Spironucleus muris*
  - *Tritrichomonas muris. Balantidium*
  - *Entamoeba muris.*

Parasitic

- Rat
  - Nematodes: *Aspiculuris tetraptera, Syphacia muris (pinworms), Trichosomoides crassicauda*
  - Cestodes: *Hymenolepis nana* and *diminuta*
- Mouse
  - Nematodes: *Aspiculuris tetraptera, Syphacia obvelata, Trichuris muris*
  - Cestodes: *Hymenolepis nana, H. diminuta* and *H. microstoma*
- Gerbil
  - Nematodes: *Syphacia muris* and *S. obvelata* (pinworms), *Dentostomella translucida* (oxyurid)
  - Cestodes: *Hymenolepis nana*
- Hamster
  - Nematodes: *Syphacia obvelata* (pinworms) and *Aspiculuris tetraptera*
  - Cestodes: *Hymenolepis nana.*

Nutritional

- Sudden change in dietary composition, e.g. influx of vegetable material.

Neoplasia

- Intestinal polyps
- Forestomach papillomas
- Intestinal adenocarcinoma.

Other non-infectious problems

- Antibiotic-induced enterotoxicosis (often secondary to *Clostridium difficile*)
- Intussusception
- Rectal prolapse
- Gut stasis/impaction.

Findings on clinical examination

- Diarrhoea, soiling around the perineum
- Non-specific signs of ill-health, e.g. hunched posture, ruffled coat

- Weight loss
- Rectal prolapse (*C. freundii* in mice)
- Death
- Cervical thickening (swollen salivary glands, lymph nodes), ocular swelling (swollen lachrymal glands) and ocular discharge (SDAV in rats)
- Central nervous signs, e.g. head tilt, ataxia (indicate neurological involvement, e.g. with *Clostridium piliforme*
- Testicular enlargement suggestive of salmonellosis in gerbils (Laber-Laird 1996)
- Proliferative ileitis (wet-tail) in hamsters
- Acute: acute enteritis with profuse and often haemorrhagic, diarrhoea
- Subacute: stunting, dehydration and diarrhoea, palpable abdominal viscus, mortalities
- Chronic: few overt, clinical signs; palpable ileal lesions, sudden death. This may explain some outbreaks without contact with other hamsters.

Investigations

1. Faecal examination
   a. Microscopy of wet prep; floatation
1. *Aspiculuris* ova are symmetrical; *Syphacia* asymmetrical (slightly banana-shaped). *Syphacia* deposits eggs around anus so use acetate strip test for *Syphacia* while *Aspiculuris* does not
2. *H. diminuta* and *H. microstoma* ova have polar filaments. *H. nana* and *H diminutia* eggs have three pairs of hooks
3. *Spironucleus muris* – look for cysts in faeces (shaped like Easter eggs); trophozoites in small intestine (wet mounts, histology). Usually subclinical
2. Radiography
   a. Intestinal obstruction (parasites, neoplasia, foreign bodies)
   b. Ileus (obstruction, compromise of gut motility, dietary-induced gut disorder)
3. Routine haematology and biochemistry
4. PCR for *C. piliforme*, SDAV, MHV
5. Culture and sensitivity
6. Ultrasonography
7. Endoscopy
8. Biopsy
   a. 'Wet-tail' without ileal hyperplasia may be caused by *E. coli*
9. Postmortem
   a. Gross thickening of colon and rectum (*C. freundii* in mice)
   b. Yellowish foci in the liver and myocardium (*Cl. piliformis*)
   c. Multiple microabscessation, especially liver and spleen (*Yersinia*).

Management

- Fluid therapy
- In cases of severe disruption of the gut environment and its commensal flora, consider supplementation with vitamin B compounds
- Probiotics may be of benefit.

Treatment/specific therapy

- Bacterial diseases including *C. freundii*
  - Appropriate antibiosis
  - Address any stress factors, e.g. environmental temperatures and over-crowding
- *Clostridium piliformis* (Tyzzer's disease)
  - Appropriate antibiosis and supportive care
- *Yersinia*
  - Appropriate antibiosis
  - Strict sanitation
  - Prevent access of wild rodents and birds to pet rodent food/living areas
- Proliferative ileitis (wet-tail) in hamsters
  - Fluid therapy plus good nursing care (see *Nursing Care*)
  - Appropriate antibiosis
    - Enrofloxacin at 5 mg/kg p.o., s.c. or as 10 mg/100 mL fresh drinking water daily
    - Erythromycin at 100 mg/L fresh (distilled or de-ionized) drinking water
    - Oxytetracycline at 400 mg/L fresh drinking water
  - *Cryptosporidium*: no effective treatment. Consider potentiated sulphonamides or nitazoxanide
  - Strict sanitation
- Protozoa
  - Sulphadimidine at 0.2% in drinking water for 7–10 days
  - Metronidazole at 2.5 mg/mL in drinking water
- Nematodes
  - Ivermectin at 0.2 mg/kg or as topical (450 µg/tube)spot on (Xeno450, Genitrix) weekly for 3–4 weeks
  - Topical emodepside plus praziquantel preparations (Profender, Bayer) at 0.004 mL/30 g body weight (Mehlhorn et al 2005a)
  - Topical imidacloprid and moxidectin compound (Advocate Cat, Bayer) reduced *T. muris* burdens by up to 95% at a concentration of 128 mg imidacloprid and 32 mg moxidectin/kg body weight (Melhorn et al 2005b)
- Cestodes including *Hymenolepis spp*
  - Praziquantel at 5.0–10 mg/kg p.o., s.c. Repeat after 10 days
  - *Note* that all species have intermediate arthropod hosts, but *H. nana* can have a direct life cycle. Zoonotic hazard, especially with *H. nana*, as no intermediate host required
- Sudden dietary changes
  - Switch to dried food only
  - If pronounced diarrhoea consider fluid therapy (see *Nursing Care*)
  - Do not use antibiotics unless specifically indicated as these may retard the re-establishment of the normal gut flora
- Antibiotic-induced enterotoxicosis
  - As for 'Sudden dietary changes', above
  - Cease antibiotic administration
  - Supplementation with probiotics *may* be useful
  - Vitamin B supplementation
- Intussusception
  - Especially seen in hamsters
  - Euthanasia or surgical correction

- Rectal prolapse
  - May be secondary to diarrhoea or intussusception
  - Surgical correction
  - Supportive nursing
- Gut stasis/impaction
  - May be linked to systemic disease, dry foods and foreign bodies (e.g. bedding fibres)
  - Laxatives and gut motility enhancers, e.g. metoclopramide at 0.2–1.0 mg/kg may be of benefit
  - Surgical removal of foreign bodies.

Nutritional disorders

- Diet-associated dermatitis (mouse). Possibly linked to high sunflower and nut diet (Richardson 2003)
- Hypovitaminosis E in hamsters (see *Musculoskeletal Disorders* and *Reproductive Disorders*).

Findings on clinical examination

- Pruritus in mice (diet-associated dermatitis).

Treatment/specific therapy

- Diet associated dermatitis
  - NSAIDs, e.g. meloxicam
  - Place on simpler diet or proprietary pelleted mouse food.

Hepatic disorders

A gall bladder is present in the mouse, gerbil and hamster, but absent in the rat.

Bacterial
- Listeriosis (gerbils)
- Salmonellosis.

Neoplasia
- Hepatic carcinoma.

Other non-infectious disorders
- Amyloidosis (see *Systemic Disorders*).

Findings on clinical examination

- Vague signs of ill-health
- Diarrhoea
- Weight loss

- Jaundice
- Polydipsia/polyuria
- Poor blood clotting (hepatic lipidosis)
- Hepatomegaly.

Investigations

1. Radiography
2. Routine haematology and biochemistry
3. Culture and sensitivity
4. Endoscopy
5. Biopsy
6. Ultrasonography.

Management

- Fluid therapy
- Milk thistle (*Silybum marianum*) is hepatoprotectant; dose at 4–15 mg/kg b.i.d. or t.i.d.
- Lactulose at 0.5 mL/kg b.i.d. p.o.

Treatment/specific therapy

1. Bacterial infections
   a. Guarded prognosis
   b. Antibiosis.

Pancreatic disorders

Diabetes mellitus (see *Endocrine Disorders*).

Cardiovascular and haematological disorders

Cardiac disease is considered very common in Syrian hamsters, such that heart failure may represent a common ageing-related cause of mortality (Schmidt & Reavill 2007). Rodent heart rates are fast. As a guide the normal heart rate of a rodent can be reasonably estimated with the following formula: Heart rate = $241 \times wt^{-0.25}$ where wt = body weight in kg.

Viral

- Encephalomyocarditis virus (hamsters)
- Hamster leukaemia virus.

Bacterial

- *Streptococcus pneumoniae* (rats) (see also *Respiratory Tract disorders*)
- *Bacillus piliformis* (Tyzzer's disease)
- *Erysipelas rhusiopathiae* (see *Systemic Disorders*)

- Septicaemia (phlebotomothrombosis), e.g. with *Salmonella spp*
- Myocarditis (suppurative).

Fungal

Protozoal

- *Haemobartonella muris* (rat)
- *Eperythrozoon coccoides* (mouse).

Parasitic

Dietary

Neoplasia

- Lymphocytic leukaemia.

Other non-infectious problems

- Cardiomyopathy (Syrian hamsters)
- Autosomal recessive in the BIO 14.6 strain
- Inherited DCM in BIO TO-2 strain
- Congenital cardiac and aortic anomalies (Syrian hamsters)
- Atrial thromboses (Syrian hamsters)
- Calcifying vasculopathy (Syrian hamsters)
- Myocardial fibrosis (acute and chronic)
- Polyarteritis nodosus (rat) – can cause aneurysms, thrombus formation and stenosis of blood vessels leading to multiple organ disruption or failure
- Anaemia secondary to other causes, e.g. haemorrhage, haemolytic anaemias, anaemia of chronic disease, neoplasia, chronic renal disease.

Findings on clinical examination

- Anaemia
- Exercise intolerance
- Heart abnormalities, e.g. dysrhythmias, abnormal heart sounds
- Exaggerated breathing postures (air hunger) and other respiratory signs
- Pulmonary oedema
- Cyanosed extremities
- Splenomegaly, hepatomegaly
- Lymphadenopathy
- Sudden death (may be due to rupture of aneurysms formed in polyarteritis nodosus).

Investigations

1. Radiography
   a. Pericardial effusions (*Streptococcus pneumoniae*)
2. Routine haematology and biochemistry
3. Culture and sensitivity
   a. Gram stain effusions (*Streptococcus pneumoniae*)

4. Endoscopy
5. Ultrasonography
6. ECG.

Management

● Supportive treatment including vitamin B12 for anaemia.

Treatment/specific therapy

● Cardiomyopathies
  ● Benazepril at <0.1 mg/kg p.o. s.i.d.
  ● Furosemide 0.3–4 mg/kg p.o., s.c., i.m., i.v. s.i.d., b.i.d.
● Intraerythrocytic protozoa
  ● *H. muris* and *E. coccoides* transmitted by *Polyplax* lice (see *Skin Disorders*) so control by treatment for these
● Hamster leukaemia virus
  ● No effective treatment.

Systemic disorders

See also *Endocrine Disorders*.

Viral

● Ectromelia virus (mouse pox) (orthopox virus)
● Lymphocytic choriomeningitis virus (LCMV) (arenavirus)
● Hamster polyomavirus (HaPV, Papova virus) (see also *Skin Disorders*).

Bacterial

● Salmonellosis esp. *S. enteritidis*
● *Streptobacillus moniliformis*
● *Erysipelas rhusiopathiae* (rare) (see also *Cardiovascular and Haematological Disorders*).

Neoplasia

● Lymphoma (in hamsters can be related to HaPV).

Other non-infectious problems

● Dental disease (see *Gastrointestinal Tract Disorders*)
● Amyloidosis
● Dystrophic calcification
● Polyarteritis nodosus (rat) – can cause aneurysms, thrombus formation and stenosis of blood vessels leading to multiple organ disruption or failure
● Pregnancy toxaemia in hamsters
● Polycystic disease in hamsters
● Hypothermia.

Findings on clinical examination

- Extreme weight loss
- Hunched posture, staring, ruffled fur
- Loss of interest in surroundings
- Overgrowth of incisors causing masticatory difficulties
- Sudden death
- Arthritis, limb abnormalities, distal limb necrosis (mice: *Streptobacillosis*, Ectromelia virus and see *Skin Disorders*)
- Stunting of mice, renal disease (LCMV)
- Sudden death
- Multiple small lumps around the neck area in hamsters (HaPV) (see *Skin Disorders*)
- Polyarthritis, myocarditis and endocarditis (*Erysipelas*)
- Subnormal body temperature (using rectal thermometer and/or remote thermal sensing).

Investigations

1. Radiography
2. Routine haematology and biochemistry
3. Serology for LCMV
4. Culture and sensitivity
5. Endoscopy
6. Biopsy
7. Ultrasonography
8. Postmortem
   a. Multifocal necrosis of liver, lymphoid tissue, intestine, spleen, integument, and other organs (mouse; Ectromelia virus)
   b. One to many cysts in a one or more organs. Cysts contain an amber fluid (hamster: polycystic kidney disease)
   c. Polyarthritis, myocarditis, endocarditis (*Erysipelas*).

Management

- Supportive care including fluid therapy, covering antibiosis where applicable.

Treatment/specific therapy

- LCMV. Potentially fatal zoonosis so consider euthanasia
- Salmonellosis. Can consider treatment with appropriate antibiosis, but is potential zoonosis
- *Streptobacillosis*. Appropriate antibiosis. Asymptomatically carried by rats in the oral cavity; is potentially zoonotic as 'rat bite fever'
- Erysipelas
  - Appropriate antibiosis
- Pregnancy toxaemia

- Similar to ketosis seen in guinea pigs (see 'Ketosis', in *Guinea Pigs, Chinchillas and Degus*)
- Polycystic disease
  - Hereditary disorders. Rare in hamsters below 1 year of age
  - No treatment
- Hypothermia
  - See *Nursing Care.*

Musculoskeletal disorders

Viral

- Lymphocytic choriomeningitis virus (LCMV).

Nutritional

- Hypovitaminosis E (see also *Reproductive Disorders*).

Neoplasia

Other non-infectious problems

- Limb bone fractures
- Spinal trauma
- Myopathies in hamsters
- Progressive hind-limb paralysis in hamsters
- Kinked tail in mice (inherited)
- See also *Neurological Disorders.*

Findings on clinical examination

- Muscle weakness and paralysis
- Reproductive problems in hamsters (hypovitaminosis E).

Investigations

1. Radiography
2. Routine haematology and biochemistry
3. Culture and sensitivity
4. Endoscopy
5. Biopsy
6. Ultrasonography.

Treatment/specific therapy

- LCMV. Potentially fatal zoonosis so consider euthanasia
- Hypovitaminosis E
  - Supplement with dietary vitamin E

- Fractures
  - Closed fractures can be treated conservatively with cage rest and analgesia
  - Internal fixation may be possible in some cases using a hypodermic needle as an intramedullary pin; external fixation and supportive dressings are likely to be chewed and damaged
  - Open fractures may require amputation
- Myopathies in hamsters
  - Often strain specific
  - Affected hamsters have shortened life spans
  - Not all muscle groups are affected equally – the limb adductor muscles are the first and most severely affected
- Progressive hind-limb paralysis in Syrian hamsters
  - Sex-linked, occurs in males; BIO 12.14 strain. A degenerative peripheral neuropathy.

Neurological disorders

Viral

- Murine encephalitis virus (MEV) (rare) (mouse, rat)
- Rabies (very rare; wild rodents).

Bacterial

- Mycoplasma pulmonis (rat, mouse) (see *Respiratory Tract Disorders*)
- Streptococcus pneumoniae (rat, mouse) (see *Respiratory Tract Disorders*)
- *Clostridium piliforme* (see *Gastrointestinal Tract Disorders*), esp. gerbil.

Protozoal

- *Encephalitozoon cuniculi* (rats).

Neoplasia

- Pituitary hyperplasia/adenomas in rats (see *Endocrine Disorders*)

Other non-infectious problems

- Trauma
- Radiculoneuropathy (spinal nerve root degeneration)
- Seizures – inherited predisposition in gerbils. Possibly linked to a deficiency of glutamine synthetase
- Streptomycin administration in gerbils (causes neuromuscular blockade, paralysis and death).
- See also *Musculoskeletal Disorders*.

Findings on clinical examination

- Torticollis (including otitis media/interna)
- Circling (including otitis media/interna)
- Weakness
- Flaccid paralysis of hind legs
- Seizures. In gerbils can last for up to 5 min.

Investigations

1. Radiography
2. Routine haematology and biochemistry
3. Serology for MEV, *E. cuniculi*, rabies (very rare)
4. Culture and sensitivity
5. Endoscopy
6. Biopsy
7. Ultrasonography.

Management

- Supportive care including hand feeding and attending to sores and abrasions.

Treatment/specific therapy

- Viral disorders
  - Rare; if diagnosed consider euthanasia
- Rabies – euthanasia
- Otitis media
  - Treat with appropriate antibiotics both topical and systemic. Ensure eardrum is intact before treatment
- Otitis interna
  - Appropriate systemic antibiosis depending upon aetiology
  - If bulla osteotomy required, swab for culture and sensitivity
- *E. cuniculi*
  - Co-trimoxazole at 30 mg/kg b.i.d. p.o. for at least 3 weeks
  - Albendazole at 10 mg/kg p.o. for 6 weeks
  - Fenbendazole at 10 mg/kg p.o. for 1 month
- Radiculoneuropathy. Consider euthanasia. Small 'carts' have been used to support the back-end of rats with similar disorders thereby allowing some voluntary movement. The ethics of this should be considered carefully
- Seizures
  - Phenobarbitone at 10–20 mg/kg b.i.d.
  - Diphenylhydantoin at 25–50 mg/kg b.i.d.

Ophthalmic disorders

In rats, mice and gerbils the Harderian gland can produce tears rich in porphyrins when the rodent has a concurrent illness. These porphyrins can stain the fur around the eyes and external nares a reddish-brown colour – this can be mistaken by owners for haemorrhage; differentiate either by exposing to UV light (porphyrins fluoresce) or by testing on a urine dipstick (Fig. 4.3).

Viral

- Sialodacryoadenitis (SDAV) (coronavirus) (rats).

Bacterial

• Uveitis.

Parasitic

• Rhabditis *orbitalis* (rare).

Neoplasia

Other non-infectious problems

• Allergies
• Prolapse (especially Syrian hamsters)
• Glaucoma (possibly inherited in Campbell's Russian hamsters)
• Keratitis sicca
• Microphthalmia/anophthalmia (recessive disorder in black-eyed white, white-bellied and dominant-spot Syrian hamsters, see Richardson 2003)
• Diabetes mellitus (Russian and Chinese hamsters).

Findings on clinical examination

• Porphyrin secretion around the eyes (SDAV in rats)
• Suborbital swelling (SDAV in rats)
• Keratitis
• Uveitis
• Cataracts (see *Endocrine Disorders*)
• Corneal ulceration
• Deaths in weanling rats (SDAV in rats)
• Upper respiratory tract signs and swollen neck/salivary glands (SDAV in rats; see *Gastrointestinal* and *Respiratory Tract Disorders*)
• Swollen globe (glaucoma). May prolapse and/or ulcerate
• Nematodes present on the cornea (*Rhabditis orbitalis*).

Investigations

1. Routine ophthalmic examination
2. Radiography
3. Routine haematology and biochemistry
4. Culture and sensitivity
5. Endoscopy
6. Biopsy
7. Ultrasonography
8. Tonometry
   a. Rat: 13.9 ± 4.2 mmHg (Lewis rats)
   b. Mice: 13.7 ± 0.8 mmHg (C3H strain); 12.3 ± 0.5 mmHg (B6 strain); 9.4 ± 0.5 (A/J); 7.7 ± 0.5 mmHg (BALBc).

Treatment/specific therapy

• Uveitis
  • Topical ophthalmic steroid or NSAID preparations

- Topical ophthalmic antibiotic preparations plus systemic antibiosis if appropriate
  - Enucleation if severe
- Prolapse/ulceration
  - Tarsorrhaphy
- Glaucoma
  - Enucleation (hereditary form)
  - Otherwise treat as for uveitis
- Keratitis sicca
  - Topical cyclosporin A ointment
  - Covering antibiosis
- *Rhabditis orbitalis*
  - Ivermectin at 400 µg/kg; repeat weekly as necessary.

Endocrine disorders

Neoplasia

- Thyroid neoplasia
  - C-cell tumours (rats)
  - Follicular cell adenomas (mice)
- Hyperadrenocortism (Cushing's disease)
  - Adrenocortical adenoma/carcinoma
  - Pituitary adenoma
- Insulinomas.

Other non-infectious problems

- Hypothyroidism
- Diabetes mellitus (inherited in Russian and Chinese hamsters)
- Iatrogenic hyperadrenocortism (glucocorticoid therapy).

Findings on clinical examination

- Bilateral symmetrical alopecia of flanks
- Weight loss
- Ataxia, head tilt and other CNS signs (pituitary hyperplasia/adenomas)
- Thin skin (hyperadrenocortism)
- Alopecia, hyperpigmentation, cold intolerance, thick skin and lethargy (hypothyroidism in hamsters)
- Hyperpigmentation
- Polydipsia, polyuria, polyphagia (hyperadrenocortism, diabetes mellitus)
- Cataracts, weight loss (diabetes mellitus)
- Secondary infections and parasitic infestations (diabetes mellitus)
- Intermittent weakness, collapse, seizures (insulinoma)
- Pseudopregnancy, mammary gland hyperplasia/neoplasia (pituitary hyperplasia/adenomas in rats) (see also *Reproductive Disorders*).

Investigations

1. Radiography
2. Routine haematology and biochemistry
   a. Diabetes mellitus (Table 4.5)
   b. Hyperadrenocortism (Table 4.6)
   Note that hamsters may secrete both cortisol and corticosterone so diagnosis on cortisol levels alone may be inaccurate
   c. Hypothyroidism (Table 4.7)
3. Culture and sensitivity
4. Urinalysis
   a. Ketonuria occasionally seen in diabetic hamsters
5. Endoscopy
6. Biopsy
7. Ultrasonography
   a. Enlarged adrenal gland(s).

Table 4.5 Small rodents: Diabetes mellitus

Species	Blood glucose: normal range (mmol/L)	Blood glucose: diabetic (mmol/L)
Syrian hamster	3.6–7.0	>16
Gerbil	2.8–7.5	
Rat	4.7–7.3	
Mouse	3.3–12.7	

Table 4.6 Small rodents: Hyperadrenocortism

Species	Blood cortisol		ALP (iu/L)	
	Normal range (nmol/L)	Hyperadrenocortism (mmol/L)	Normal range	Hyperadreno-cortism
Syrian hamster	13.8–27.6	<110.4	8–18	>40
Rat			39–216	
Mouse			28–94	

Table 4.7 Small rodents: Serum thyroxine levels

Species	T4$_{(total)}$ nM/L	T3$_{(total)}$ nM/L	T4$_{(free)}$ pM/L	T3$_{(free)}$ pM/L
Syrian hamster	46.3	0.7		
Mouse	39.7–61.0	1.3–1.7		
Rat	43.8–80.0	0.8–1.2	15.0–36.0	1.7–16.0

After Hulbert (2000).

Treatment/specific therapy

- Diabetes mellitus
  - Provide a high-fibre, low-fat diet
  - Oral hypoglycaemic agents such as glibenclamide may prove useful in hamsters
  - In rats, Keeble (2001) reports that twice-daily treatment with a medium duration insulin product at 1.0 IU/kg can give stabilization, combined with twice daily urinary glucose monitoring
  - In hamsters, neutral protamine Hagedorn (NPH) insulin may be useful, but titration and subsequent dosage may prove difficult long term at home
  - In gerbils diabetes mellitus is associated with obesity and high sunflower intake.
- Insulinoma
  - Surgical resection
  - Glucocorticoid therapy may give palliative results for a period of time
- Hyperadrenocortism
  - Pituitary hyperplasia/adenomas in rats
    - Toremifene at 12 mg/kg p.o. s.i.d.
    - Early ovario-hysterectomy may prevent adenoma formation
  - Surgical adrenalectomy
  - Hamsters (Keeble 2001)
    - Metyrapone 8 mg p.o. s.i.d. for 4 weeks
    - Mitotane 5 mg p.o. s.i.d. for 4 weeks
    - Trilostane
  - Palliative and supportive treatment
- Hypothyroidism
  - Supplement with thyroxine, e.g. levothyroxine at 10 µg/kg daily in divided doses
- Thyroid neoplasia in rats
  - Usually involves C-cells and, therefore, does not produce typical thyroid disease-associated signs.

Urinary disorders

Viral

- Lymphocytic choriomeningitis virus (LCMV) (arenavirus) (mouse, hamster).

Bacterial

- Cystitis
- Leptospirosis (wild rodents) (usually asymptomatic but is significant zoonosis).

Parasitic

- *Trichosomoides crassicauda* (bladder thread worm)
- *Encephalitozoon cuniculi* (rats).

Neoplasia

- Can be related to *T. crassicauda* infestations in the rat.

Other non-infectious problems

- Glomerulosclerosis, with an interstitial fibrosis (rats)
- Glomerulonephritis
- Amyloidosis
- Urolithiasis (esp. hamsters).

Findings on clinical examination

- Non-specific signs of ill-health, e.g. hunched posture, ruffled coat, reduced appetite
- Weight loss
- Polydipsia, polyuria
- Ascites
- Fibrous osteodystrophy
- Dysuria
- Haematuria
- Preputial haemorrhage
- Uroliths may be palpable in the penile urethra of males (esp. hamsters)
- Hair-like nematode visible in rat urine (*Trichosomoides crassicauda*).

Investigations

1. Urinalysis (Table 4.8)
2. Radiography
3. Calculi (may accompany *T. crassicauda* infestations in the rat)
4. Routine haematology and biochemistry
   a. Rats with glomerulosclerosis, biochemistry findings may show elevated urea (normal 2.2–8.3 mmol/L) and creatinine (normal 17.7–70.7 μmol/L)
   b. Eosinophilia (*Trichosomoides crassicauda*)
5. Serology for LCMV
6. Culture and sensitivity
7. Endoscopy
8. Ultrasonography
9. Biopsy.

Management

- Supportive care especially fluid therapy
- Feed more natural diet; rats fed more refined foods tend to develop chronic renal disease earlier (Fallon 1996).

Treatment/specific therapy

- LCMV. Potentially fatal zoonosis so consider euthanasia
- *Trichosomoides crassicauda*
  - Combination therapy (Bowman et al 2004) of:
    - Ivermectin at 0.2 mg/kg s.c. weekly for 3 weeks
    - Fenbendazole at 20 mg/kg p.o. s.i.d. for 5 days
  - Thorough and repeated cage sanitation

Table 4.8 Small rodents: Typical urinalysis values

Value	Rat	Syrian hamster
Urine volume	5.5 mL/100 g per day	Around 7.0 mL/day total
Crystals		Triple phosphate and calcium carbonate crystals (in some cricetids allantoin is excreted)
Protein	<0.5 g/L. *Note* by 12–14 months old, up to 50% of rats will have a proteinuria >2.0 g/L	0–3 g/L; >30 g/L reported for renal disease
Urine gravity		1.014–1.060
pH		≈8.5
WBCs	Few	
Parasites	*Trichosomoides crassicauda* (bladder thread worm). Bioperculated, light brown, larvated ova in urine. May be accompanied by urinary WBCs	

- Urolithiasis
  - Cystotomy and/or urethrotomy
  - Hamsters especially prone as naturally produce triple phosphate and calcium carbonate crystals in their urine.

Reproductive disorders

The mammary tissue in small rodents, especially rats and mice, can be quite extensive and may extend laterally up the neck, flanks and perineum.

Viral

- Mouse mammary tumour viruses (MMTV) (retroviruses)
- Lymphocytic choriomeningitis virus (LCMV) (hamster, mouse) – see *Systemic Disorders*.

Bacterial

- *Mycoplasma pulmonis* (endometritis, pyometra) (rats) (see *Respiratory Tract Disorders*)
- *Staphylococcus aureus* (preputial gland abscess (mouse, rat)
- *Streptococcus spp; Streptococcal* mastitis in hamsters
- *Pasteurella pneumotropica* (preputial gland abscess, pyometra (mouse, rat, hamster)
- Salmonellosis (cause of testicular hyperplasia in gerbils – see *Gastrointestinal Tract Disorders*)
- Mastitis.

Nutritional

- Hypovitaminosis E in hamsters.

Neoplasia

- Uterine neoplasia (Fig. 4.5)
- Preputial gland neoplasia
- Mammary gland adenocarcinomas and carcinomas (especially mice). May be triggered by MMTV
- Mammary gland fibroadenomas (especially rats). These can grow extremely large and suffer significant abrasions
- Ovarian neoplasia
- Interstitial cell tumours and other testicular neoplasia
- Pituitary hyperplasia/adenoma (rat) (see *Endocrine Disorders*).

Other non-infectious problems

- Uterine prolapse (mouse) (rare)
- Ovarian follicular cysts (cystic ovaries)
- Pseudopregnancy
- Physiological post-oestrus vaginal discharge (hamster). This is clear and should not be mistaken for a vaginitis
- Pregnancy toxaemia (see *Systemic Disorders*).

Findings on clinical examination

- Swollen viscus palpable in females (uterine neoplasia, pyometra, pregnancy)
- Swollen abdomen (pregnancy, phantom pregnancy, abdominal mass, ascites)
- Symmetrical alopecia (cystic ovaries)
- Bilateral swelling around penis (preputial gland abscess, mouse, rat)
- Unilateral swelling next to penis (preputial gland neoplasia)
- Single or multiple swellings of mammary tissue. *Note* that in rats and mice the distribution of mammary tissue can be extensive, spreading some way up the flank, neck and perineal area
- Mastitis

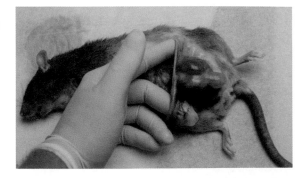

Fig. 4.5. Postmortem showing uterine neoplasm in a rat.

- Pseudopregnancy, mammary gland hyperplasia/neoplasia, CNS signs, hyperadrenocortism (pituitary hyperplasia/adenomas in rats) (see also *Endocrine Disorders*)
- Male sterility, abnormal gestation, muscular weakness and paralysis in hamsters (hypovitaminosis E)
- Testicular enlargement
  - If unilateral consider neoplasia. This appearance may be exacerbated as the other testicle may also reduce in size. Occasionally a hard mass may be palpable in an otherwise normal testicle
  - Bilateral in gerbils – salmonellosis.

Investigations

1. Radiography
   a. Enlarged uterus (pyometra, neoplasia)
2. Ovarian cysts
3. Routine haematology and biochemistry
4. Serology for LCMV (hamster)
5. Culture and sensitivity
6. Endoscopy
7. Biopsy
8. Ultrasonography
   a. Ovarian cysts.

Treatment/specific therapy

- Bacterial diseases
  - Appropriate antibiosis
  - Bacterial infections, e.g. pyometra may follow an outbreak of respiratory disease
- LCMV may induce pyometra
- Preputial gland abscess
  - Lance, flush and drain. Appropriate antibiosis
- Preputial gland neoplasm; surgical removal
- Mammary gland neoplasia
  - Surgical resection
  - Early ovario-hysterectomy may reduce incidence of mammary neoplasia in rats
- Other neoplasia; surgical removal where practical
- Uterine prolapse
  - Replace uterus and apply suture to retain. Poor prognosis. May require ovario-hysterectomy
- Mastitis
  - Systemic antibiosis
  - May require debriding and application of antibiotics or medications to enhance healing, e.g. topical amorphous hydrogel dressings to encourage secondary healing such as IntraSite Gel (Smith and Nephew Healthcare Ltd.)
- Pseudopregnancy
  - In hamsters, lasts 7–13 days. Usually resolves spontaneously
- Ovarian cysts
  - Ovario-hysterectomy (treatment of choice)

- Draw fluid off by paracentesis
- Attempt HCG at 1000 IU/kg weekly for 1–3 weeks
- Hypovitaminosis E in hamsters
  - Supplement with vitamin E.

References

Beck W, Pfister K 2004 Mites as newly emerging disease pathogens in rodents and human beings. Free Comm Abst Vet Dermatol 15(Suppl 1):20–40

Beco L, Petite A, Olivry T 2001 Comparison of subcutaneous ivermectin and oral moxidectin for the treatment of notoedric acariasis in hamsters. Vet Rec 149:324–327

Bowman M R, Pare J A, Pinckney R D 2004 Trichosomoides crassicauda infection in a pet hooded rat. Vet Rec 154:374–375

Fallon M T 1996 Rats and mice. In: Laber-Laird K, Swindle M, Flecknell P (eds) Handbook of rodent and rabbit medicine. Pergamon, Oxford, p 28

Fox M T, Baker A S, Farquhar R et al 2004 First record of Ornithonyssus bacoti from a domestic pet in the United Kingdom. Vet Rec 154:437–438

Girling S 2007 Common parasitic skin problems of rodents. Vet Rev July:36–41

Hulbert A J 2000 Thyroid hormones and their effects: a new perspective. Biol Rev 75:519–631

Jepson L 2004 Management of small rodent emergencies. BSAVA Congress. Scientific Proceedings 373–376

Keeble E 2001 Endocrine diseases in small mammals. In Practice 570–585

Laber-Laird K 1996 Gerbils. In: Laber-Laird K, Swindle M, Flecknell P (eds) Handbook of rodent and rabbit medicine. Pergamon, Oxford, p 48

Mehlhorn H, Schmahl G, Frese M et al 2005a Effects of a combination of emodepside and praziquantel on parasites of reptiles and rodents. Parasitol Res 97:S64–S69

Melhorn H, Schmahl G, Mevissen 2005b Efficacy of a combination of imidacloprid and moxidectin against parasites of reptiles and rodents: case reports. Parasitol Res 97:S97–S101

Richardson V C G 2003 Diseases of small domestic rodents, 2nd edn. Blackwell, Oxford

Schmidt R E, Reavill D R 2007 Cardiovascular disease in hamsters: review and retrospective study. J Exot Pet Med 16(1):49–51

5

Parrots and related species

Members of the parrot family are the commonest avian pet and, therefore, the most likely to be presented to the veterinarian. Table 5.1 shows the most commonly encountered species.

Consultation and handling

Psychologically, most pet birds are little different from their wild ancestors – the veterinary surgeon constitutes a potential predator so the bird is likely to exhibit a flight or fight response when handled. Exceptions to this are hand-reared parrots (or imprinted raptors and owls). However, in extremis, birds vary in their susceptibility to stress, and while some, such as the larger psittacines, can be handled relatively safely, others, such as canaries, carry a greater risk.

A great many captive-bred, hand-reared birds can be superficially examined while perched on the owner or on a freestanding perch, thereby minimizing stress. If care and patience is undertaken, then auscultation of the lungs and air sacs, plus some assessment of body condition can be achieved in this way.

It is important to weigh parrots at every consultation (Fig. 5.1); tame birds can be accurately weighed using a small perch designed to fit on to standard weighing scales.

Aggressive birds, or birds unused to handling, may require to be 'towelled' in order to examine them. Use a large towel that will cover most of the bird. Drop or place it over the bird such that the head is covered and the bird cannot see your hands. With one hand, grab the bird's head or neck from behind so that there is control of the beak, and use the other hand to gather up the rest of the bird into the towel. Do not in any way compress the sternum, as this will seriously compromise the bird's breathing.

Birds will attempt to mask signs of illness and so may not exhibit clinical signs until a disease course is quite advanced. It is important to observe the bird from a distance for several minutes prior to handling, as a relaxed bird is more likely to show signs of ill-health.

Table 5.1 Parrots and related species: Key facts

	African grey parrot	Blue-fronted Amazon parrot	Blue and gold macaw	Moluccan cockatoo	Peach-faced lovebird	Cockatiel	Budgerigar
Average life span (years)	50–70	40–50+	50–80+	50+	10+	10–20+	4–13
Weight (g)	300–400	320–460	950–1175	640–1025	50–61	80–90	45–50 (60 g+ for large show budgerigars)
Sexing	DNA or surgical sexing	DNA or surgical sexing	DNA or surgical sexing	DNA or surgical sexing. Also males have black irides, females have reddish brown	DNA sexing	The small, ventral (true) tail feathers (not the overlying longer remiges) are barred in females (hard to assess in Lutinos). The red-orange colour of the cheek patches are more pronounced in males. Resemble females but the tail is shorter and the cere is pinkish rather than grey	Cere is blue and smooth in males; brown and rough in females. Young blue mutation females may have a pastel-blue cere
Estimating age	Young <5 months have dark grey irides, adults have yellow	In very young birds the irides are black or dark brown; adults have yellowish irides	Young birds have dark brown irides	Younger are a duller colour with less yellow and blue on the head	Young birds have dark/black saddle marks on the mandible and maxilla		Young birds (<6 weeks) have barred feathering on the forehead
Normal clutch size	3–4	3–4	2–3	2	3–8	4–7	3–8
Incubation (days)	28	30	28	30 days	21–24	17–23	17–20 (begins with the second egg)

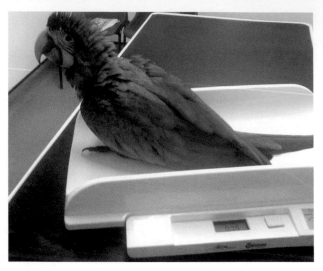

Fig. 5.1. Weighing a young harlequin macaw (hybrid blue and gold X green-wing).

Important non-specific clinical signs in parrots

- Heavy lidded/dark periorbital colouring
- Fluffed up/feather plucking
- Abnormal or absent feeding/drinking behaviour
- Polydipsia/polyuria
- Lethargy
- Abnormal activity
- Change from normal perching activity or on floor of cage
- Abnormal profile
- Abnormal breathing action
- Abnormal vocalization
- Tail-bobbing. A sign of dyspnoea. Respiratory rates of psittacines are high, but a recovery time exceeding 3 min would be considered abnormal
- Regurgitation.

From Malley (1996).

Avian emergencies

1. It is best to attempt an initial assessment *before* handling a stressed or extremely ill bird, as this may allow you to take some diagnostic shortcuts thereby reducing handling time.
2. Remove the bird to as quiet and darkened area as possible so as to reduce stress, preferably into a heated chamber such as an incubator, and supply oxygen as close to the bird's head as possible.

3. Allow the bird a few minutes to relax in this warm, high oxygen environment before continuing with the examination.
4. If it is imperative to handle the bird, *warn the owner first* that although you must do this, there is a chance of losing the bird. If necessary ask the owner to sign a consent form.
5. Handle the bird either with your hands or with a towel. Never use gloves or gauntlets. With larger psittacines, if necessary have an assistant grip the head firmly from behind if you are concerned about being bitten. Do not grip around or otherwise compress the sternum as this will compromise respiration.
6. Consider inducing anaesthesia by masking the bird down with isoflurane or sevoflurane for a more detailed examination. For those birds with respiratory or cardiovascular compromise, the relative risks and benefits of anaesthesia need to be considered.

Nursing care

Thermoregulation

Avian core body temperature often exceeds 40.5°C and birds have a large surface area relative to body mass, which means that they must expend a great deal of energy in thermal homeostasis. Feathers act as an insulative layer but do not grow back as readily as mammalian fur, so as few as possible should be removed, should surgery be indicated.

Heat loss and, therefore, energy conservation can be reduced by placing the bird close to a heat source – vivarium heat mats are ideal for this. Place a towel or similar over the mat to prevent burns and protect the mat from fluids. Young chicks are unable to thermoregulate, so must be maintained in an incubator.

Fluid therapy

Birds are primarily uricotelic which, as in reptiles, predisposes them to gout-related problems. Blood volume is between 4.4 and 8.3 mL/100 g body weight in chickens. In some species, it can be as high as 14 mL/100 g.

Dehydration

1. Most critically ill birds should assumed to be 5–10% dehydrated.
2. Increased skin turgor over the foot or upper eyelid, collapse or poor filling of the ulnar vein, sunken or glazed eyes, dry and tacky mucus membranes, tachycardia, depression and red or wrinkled skin in psittacine neonates all indicate dehydration.
3. The daily maintenance water requirement for psittacine birds is around 50 mL/kg per day, with that of passerines and young birds being much higher.
4. A 500 g (0.5 kg) bird with 10% (0.1) dehydration, therefore, requires (0.5 × 0.1) litres = 0.05 L = 50 mL fluid. As in other species, which fluids are given depends upon the reason for giving fluids. Half of the fluid deficit should be replaced within the first 12–24 h. The remaining 50% is divided over the following 48 h, to be given alongside the daily maintenance.

Fluid administration

- *Per cloaca.* Water can be absorbed from the cloaca (and naturally from material refluxed into the colon) so this can be used as route for rehydrating with small volumes where there is a risk of aspiration pneumonia (Table 5.2).
- *Oral fluids* are usually given by crop tube. Not suitable for birds which are regurgitating, recumbent or fitting.
- *Intravenous.* Birds can tolerate fluid replacement rates of up to 10 mL/kg given in a bolus, if given slowly over 5–7 min. Sites include the right jugular vein, brachial vein (Fig. 5.2) and the medial metatarsal vein. Intravenous catheters are difficult to maintain in birds so bolus administration is preferred. Isotonic solutions should be administered slowly at a rate of 10–15 mL/kg. A 'shock' dose of 90 mL/kg can be used if large volumes are needed rapidly. Suggested individual bolus volumes are listed in Table 5.3.

Table 5.2 Parrots and related species: Cloacal administration

Species	Suggested volumes for cloacal administration (mL)
Budgerigar	0.5
Cockatiel	1
Amazon	4
Macaw	6–7

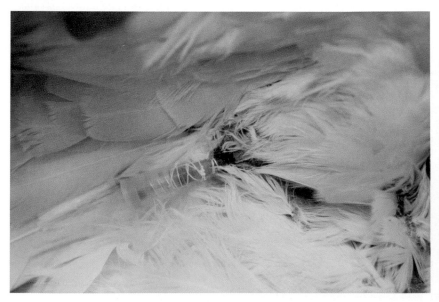

Fig. 5.2. Placement of an intravenous catheter into the brachial vein of a cockatoo. Use a collar if to be kept in place for several days.

Table 5.3 Parrots and related species: Suggested individual bolus volumes

Species	Bolus volume (mL)
Budgerigar	1–2
Cockatiel	2–3
Conure	4–6
Amazon	8–10
Macaw	15–25

- *Subcutaneous fluids* can be given into the interscapular area (not caudal neck to avoid the cervico-cephalic air sac) or the inguinal region. Small volume (5–10 mL/kg) should be given at each site and absorption may be poor.
- *Intraosseous.* Distal ulna and proximal tibiotarsus. Strict asepsis + anaesthesia. All types of fluid including blood transfusions. Do not use very acidic, alkaline or hypertonic solutions i.o. without diluting them first.

Choice of parenteral fluids

- Crystalloids. Only 25% of a crystalloid solution remains in the peripheral vasculature 30 min after administration. Hartman's solution contains lactate that is converted to bicarbonate by the liver and so may help correct acidosis but is contraindicated with hypernatraemia.
- Hypertonic saline at 3–7.5% will help to correct circulatory collapse by triggering fluid shifts from the interstitial space into the circulation, followed quickly by isotonic solutions to prevent tissue dehydration. Do not use hypertonic solutions if cranial haemorrhages are suspected.
- Colloids. Bolus administration of hetastarch at 10–15 mL/kg i.v. t.i.d. for up to four treatments may be safe and effective for hypoproteinaemia.
- Oxyglobin can be given at a dose rate of up to 15 mL/kg i.v. or i.o.
- Whole blood. Birds are tolerant of anaemia but a transfusion should be considered if the PCV falls below 15.0 L/L. Use blood from the same or similar species; blood groups, etc., have been only poorly investigated.

Nutritional supplementation

If the bird is eating normally then supply its usual diet. For short-term management, recovery diets commercially available for dogs and cats (non-milk based) may be crop tubed for carnivorous, insectivorous or omnivorous birds. Dextrose can be given orally, by subcutaneous injection up to 2.5% or i.v. It is a metabolic acidifying agent and may be contraindicated in cases of metabolic acidosis. Note that most birds are diurnal and will not feed in the dark. For parrots, hand-rearing formula can be used.

Wing clipping of pet parrots

A badly clipped bird is not only at increased risk of damage to itself, but such clipping may predispose to feather picking and self-mutilation. Wing clipping can be controversial but the major justification for wing clipping is that by doing so it facilitates the necessary interaction between a pet parrot and the other family members, allowing the bird to become involved with, and behave as, part of the family (or 'flock') rather than it be confined to its cage. However, the ideal would be that the bird is left fully flighted and controlled verbally using commands such as 'step up', 'step down', 'leave' and 'no'.

Wing clipping

1. Both wings should be clipped, allowing the bird to maintain its balance.
2. It is the primary flight feathers that allow lift and it is these that should be trimmed such that the cut end is tucked beneath the coverts.
3. Developing 'pin' feathers should not be cut as these will haemorrhage; instead leave alone and leave a feather along side it or on either side for support to prevent accidental damage.

Microchipping

1. Microchips are placed into the left pectoral musculature.
2. Occasionally haemorrhage may occur but usually digital pressure is sufficient for haemostasis.
3. Microchips inserted subcutaneously, although potentially less traumatic, are readily palpable and subject to removal and fraud.

Analgesia

Table 5.4 Parrots and related species: Analgesic doses

Analgesic	Dose
Butorphanol	0.5–4.0 mg/kg i.m. every 2–4 h
Carprofen	1.0–4.0 mg/kg s.c. p.o. b.i.d.
Ketoprofen	1.0–5.0 mg/kg i.m. b.i.d. or t.i.d.
Meloxicam	0.1–0.5 mg/kg s.c., p.o. s.i.d.
Morphine	0.1–3.0 mg/kg i.v.

Anaesthesia

From a practical point of view, induction and maintenance with gaseous anaesthesia is of choice. Atropine can be given as pre-medication at 0.05–0.1 mg/kg s.c. This reduces mucus and counters bradycardia from vagal stimulation during surgery.

Gaseous anaesthetic protocol

1. Hold the bird's head into a mask or place into an induction chamber. Isoflurane offers a rapid induction and recovery (as does sevoflurane).
2. Intubate (uncuffed endotracheal tube) whenever possible.
3. During anaesthesia, regularly positive-pressure ventilates to reduce risk of CO_2 build up in the abdominal air sacs.
4. Main sources of heat loss are the extremities (especially the feet), and the air sacs. Wrap the feet with silver foil and maintain the bird on an external heat source.
5. If using halothane, start at low concentrations (0.5–1.0%) and gradually increase to 3.0–4.0%. Induction at high concentrations can lead to dangerously high levels of halothane present in posterior air sacs. Attempts to resuscitate bird by flushing through with oxygen or manual ventilation will only force this reservoir of halothane through the lungs further increasing blood concentrations.

Parenteral anaesthesia

1. Always weigh the bird accurately before using parenteral anaesthesia, and always intubate and maintain on oxygen whenever possible.
2. A range of anaesthetic protocols are available from the literature. The ones the author has used include:
   a. Ketamine at 5–30 mg/kg i.v. or i.m. No analgesic effect. Avoid birds with potential liver/kidney complications
   b. Ketamine 5 mg/kg + xylazine 0.25–1.0 mg/kg i.v. or i.m.
   c. Ketamine 5–20 mg/kg + midazolam 0.25 mg/kg i.v. or i.m. This gives good sedation, muscle relaxation and recovery
   d. Ketamine 3–6 mg/kg + medetomidine 150–300 µg/kg i.v. or i.m.
   e. Both medetomidine and xylazine can be reversed with atipamezole at 5× medetomidine dose.

Air sac perfusion anaesthesia

Avian respiratory anatomy means that the trachea can be 'bypassed' by insertion of a suitable cannula into one of the caudal air sacs (abdominal or caudal thoracic) for delivery of oxygen and anaesthetic gasses. This technique is suitable for oral or tracheal obstructions or if surgery is required at or around oral cavity. Glottal or tracheal foreign bodies or other obstructions will usually give their presence away by producing a whistling sound during the respiratory cycle. These birds are extremely liable to sudden death. The main priority is to establish a patent airway as quickly as possible, therefore the need to anaesthetize and insert an air sac tube.

Air sac perfusion anaesthesia technique

1. Use soft tube with holes in walls.
2. 4 mm diameter tube for 350 g bird, increasing pro rata.
3. A left lateral approach is used with the left leg extended cranially and a small incision made behind the last rib and ventral to the flexor cruis medialis muscle (Fig. 5.3).
4. A small pair of haemostats can then be used to enter the coelom in a craniomedial direction, which will provide access to the caudal thoracic air sac.
5. A tube is then secured in place with a suture and attached to the anaesthetic machine. *Note* that a higher airflow rate (> 50% above normal) will be required to maintain anaesthesia this way.
6. Can be left *in situ* for 1–3 weeks.

Recovery

- Keep quiet
- Wrap wings gently in towel/paper toweling to reduce injury from flapping
- Keep warm, preferably mid-20s°C
- Recovery must be fast from anaesthetic – birds under 100 g should be eating within 30 min.

Cardiopulmonary resuscitation

1. Can use doxapram at 5–7 mg/kg i.m. or sublingually.
2. Intubate if not already done so.
3. Intermittent positive pressure ventilation once every 5 s.
4. If in cardiac arrest, begin rapid chest compressions.
5. Give epinephrine at 0.5–1.0 mL/kg of 1:1000 i.t., i.c., i.o., i.p.

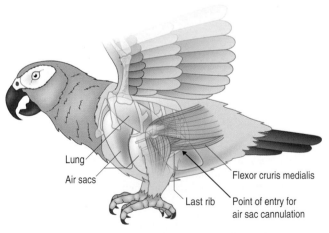

Lung
Air sacs
Flexor cruris medialis
Last rib
Point of entry for air sac cannulation

Fig. 5.3. Anatomical markers for the placement of an air sac tube.

Skin disorders

Avian skin is very thin with the epidermis only up to 10 cells thick in feathered areas. There are few cutaneous glands:

1. Uropygial gland. Not present in all species, e.g. Amazon parrots and *Pionus* parrots. When present, it lies dorsally near the tip of the tail. There can be up to 18 orifices depending upon species. Usually bare except for a tuft of down feathers known as uropygial wick. Secretes a lipoid sebaceous secretion – sebum – that is water repellent. It also helps to keep plumage supple and smooth, contains vitamin D_3 precursors, has antibacterial and antifungal properties and enhances feather colouration. However, most sebum is produced from epidermal cells that contain keratin-bound phospholipids that coats the skin and feathers.
2. Small wax secreting glands are present in the external wall of the auditory meatus.
3. There are mucus secreting vent glands.
4. There are no sweat glands.

Commensal bacterial numbers on the skin of birds are considered to be lower than those found on mammals. Yeasts are infrequent commensals. *Malassezia* not isolated from normal or self-mutilating birds (Preziosi et al 2006); in the same study, *Candida albicans* was isolated but significance was unclear.

Feathers serve a number of functions including insulation, protection from trauma, accessories to flight, species recognition patterns and display. There are several types and sub-groups of feathers.

Feather types

1. Contour feathers are divided into:
   a. Flight feathers
      i. Remiges (carried on the wing)
         (1) Primary – borne on the manus
         (2) Secondary – borne on the antibrachium
      ii. Retrices (carried on the tail).
   b. Body feathers
   c. Coverts – cover the bases of the retrices or remiges
   d. Ear coverts – screen the external opening of the ear and improve hearing.
2. Other feathers include down feathers, filoplumes, bristles, semi-plumes. Various intermediate forms of feather will be encountered. Powder feathers usually structured like down feathers, occasionally semi-plumes and contours shed a fine white powder of keratin on to contour feathers to provide waterproofing. Particularly obvious in African grey parrots and cockatoos.

Signs of skin disease

Pruritus

* Flies
   * Hippoboscids (flat flies/louse flies) occasionally encountered especially with aviary birds. Can transmit haemoparasites such as *Haemoproteus* and *Leukocytozoon*, as well as transfer mites and lice between individuals
* Lice. Can reach significant numbers on debilitated birds

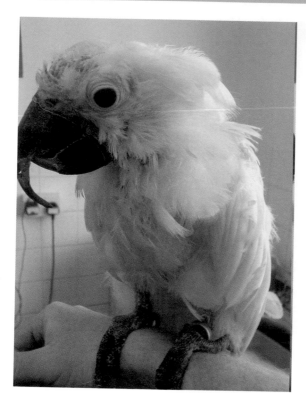

Fig. 5.5. Psittacine beak and feather disease (PBFD) in a sulphur crested cockatoo.

Nodules and non-healing wounds

- Avian pox virus (skin pox)
  - Wart-like lesions of the skin. Yellowish nodules form on the beak, eyelids and other areas of the skin that disintegrate and discharge a serosanguineous fluid. The areas then scab over. When present on the feet, lesions may occlude distal vasculature resulting in tissue necrosis of the lower extremities. *Note* can occur as a diphtheritic form or a septicaemic form
- Staphylococcus may occasionally be encountered as a cause of dermatitis. More often it is isolated as a secondary invader in bumblefoot
- Candidiasis has been seen as focal raised lesions as well as more generalized ulcerations. Head lesions reported in Eclectus parrots, Amazons and cockatiels. *Aspergillus* lesions, *Trichosporon asahii* and dermatophytosis are both occasionally encountered
- Feather cysts. Secondary to follicle damage; the developing feather is unable to emerge and forms a large, cyst-like structure
- Cryptococcosis (Berrocal 2004)
- Mycobacteria (Ferrer et al 1997)
- 'Bumblefoot' – typically chronic infection and abscessation of the feet, especially the plantar surfaces. Often due to *Staphylococci* or *Streptococci*.

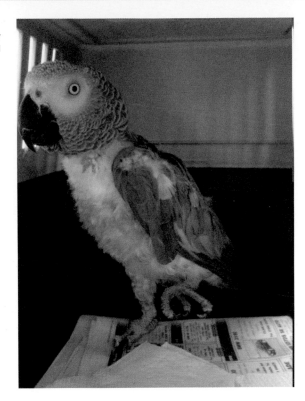

Fig. 5.6. Abnormal red pigmentation in an African grey parrot with psittacine beak and feather disease (PBFD).

Changes in pigmentation

- Erysipelothrix infections may cause an erythema of the skin. In an acute infection with sudden death.

Chronic ulcerative dermatitis (CUD)

- Usually associated with chronic conditions such as mycobacteriosis, tumours, abscesses or xanthomas. Poor nutrition may also contribute. Four main presentations are:
  a. Prepatagial CUD. Wing web area. Possibly linked to *Giardia* or hypovitaminosis E. Usually very pruritic and painful. Patagium may also be affected. Commonly seen in chronic self-mutilating African greys (Fig. 5.7)
  b. Proventer CUD. Keel area – common in African greys and large Amazons. Secondary to trauma following hard landings. Bruises or splits forming ulcers
  c. Postventer CUD. Between cloaca and tail. Possibly similar aetiology to proventer CUD. Poor nutrition also implicated

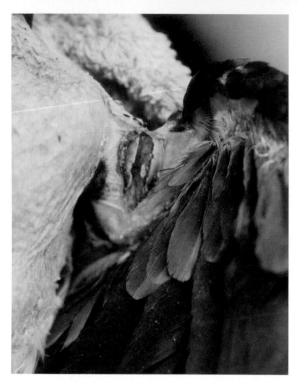

Fig. 5.7. Prepatagial chronic ulcerative dermatitis in an African grey parrot.

    d. Squamous cell carcinoma (Klaphake et al 2006).
- Ectoparasites (see 'Pruritus', above).

Alopecia

- Pruritic (self-mutilation) versus non-pruritic. PBFD is provisionally differentiated from self-inflicted trauma in single birds as feathers on head also affected; normally bird cannot reach these to self-damage.

Neoplasia

- Lipomas (Fig. 5.8), fibrosarcomas, liposarcomas and squamous cell carcinomas are some of the commoner skin neoplasms reported from birds. Xanthomas common especially in budgerigars. These are non-neoplastic yellowish nodules or plaques caused by an accumulation of cholesterol and fats. Can be ulcerative. Often found over an area of pathology such as a lipoma.

Allergies

- There is a strong suggestion that allergies may be the cause of skin disease in some cases, especially old world psittacines.

Fig. 5.8. Lipoma in a budgerigar.

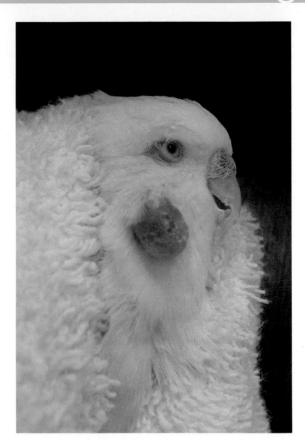

Findings on clinical examination

- Observe bird in cage or at rest on owner. Assess if it show signs of typical sick bird – ruffled, fluffed up feathers, sleepiness, and tail 'pumping'. Is it pruritic?
- Assess the surroundings. Are faeces normal? Stress or sudden influx of fruit may trigger very loose faeces
- Handle the bird:
  - Examine nares, beak, eyes and buccal cavity including choana. Look particularly for signs of vitamin A deficiency (see *Nutritional Disorders*)
  - Examine skin – note signs of inflammation, hyperkeratosis, ulceration, and trauma
- Assess feather quality:
  - Stress lines – lines visible on the vanes of the feather that denote areas of poor quality of the barbs. Thought to be linked to release of endogenous corticosteroid

- Frayed, dirty or matted. Inappropriate sized caging may cause repeated damaged to the retrices of those birds with long tails such as parakeets and macaws
- Abnormal feather colouration may result from nutritional deficiencies, hepatopathies or PBFD
- Examination for parasites:
  - Pluck one or two feathers for examination under a light microscope for ectoparasites and feather pulp examination
- Examine uropygial (preen) gland, cloaca and feet
- Auscultate heart, lungs, air sacs
- Palpate abdomen
- Anaesthesia may be required for anaesthesia with birds difficult to handle safely (Fig. 5.9).

Investigations

1. Routine haematology and biochemistry
   a. Zinc and lead levels may be appropriate to investigate low-grade heavy metal poisoning. Collect samples for zinc in either heparin or plain tube (without gel as this may contain zinc). Although blood levels can be indicative of zinc toxicity there is no absolute correlation between blood zinc levels and clinical signs. As a general rule, if zinc levels are >32.0–50.0 μmol/L and there are consistent clinical signs (see *Neurological Disorders* and *Gastrointestinal Tract Disorders*), then zinc toxicity should be suspected. Significant zinc levels are often accompanied by an absolute or relative monocytosis

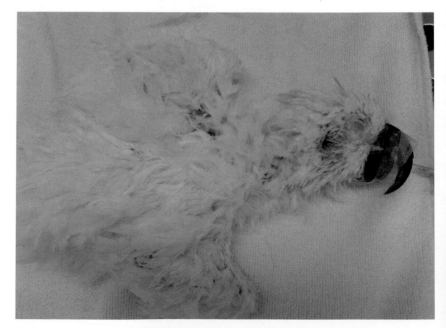

Fig. 5.9. Anaesthesia of a cockatoo for further skin investigation.

2. Aseptic collection of samples for bacteriology/mycology
3. Cytology
4. Radiography. A standing view using horizontal beam is useful for detecting metallic foreign bodies in the conscious bird, otherwise lateral and VD views, under GA, are required for meaningful radiography
5. Endoscopy
6. Serology for PBFD, polyomavirus, *Aspergillus* antigen and *Chlamydophila* antigen should be taken if thought necessary
7. Fresh faecal samples for parasitic examination – look for *Giardia*, nematode eggs, etc. Smears can be dried and stained
8. Bulk faecal samples (collected over 3–5 days) can be submitted for *Chlamydophila* PCR
9. Diagnostic imaging including radiography and endoscopy
10. Biopsy
    a. *Note* eosinophilic dermatitis linked to *Trichosporon asahii* infection.

Management

- Optimize diet – consider converting on to pelleted foods; use of multivitamin supplements; reducing seed intake and increasing fruit consumption where appropriate
- Where there is significant feather loss, consider supplementary heating to counter loss of insulation
- Covering broad-spectrum antibiotics may be useful if there are obvious skin lesions
- If pruritic consider analgesia – meloxicam (Metacam oral suspension) at 1 drop/500 g body weight twice daily. Do not use steroids
- Collars
  - Collars are inherently very stressful to parrots – they interfere with normal feeding (many parrots transfer their food to their mouth with a foot), flight, climbing and crop function. They are heavy relative to the weight of the bird and generally alienate the bird from its immediate surroundings. They also do not address any underlying cause or pathology and if these are not addressed then feather plucking/self-mutilation may resume when the collar is removed
  - Therefore, collars should be used judiciously and on a case-by-case basis
  - If possible hospitalize the parrot for 24–48 h to enable the bird to get used to the collar, as well as allowing any minor adjustments and reassessments to be made
  - A collar should be removed only after the bird has been clinically well for a reasonable period of time, as it is likely that, as in other species, abnormal or triggering sensations will persist for some time following the clinical resolution of lesions. Early removal often results in repeat damage.

Treatment/specific therapy

- Ectoparasites
  - Ticks: treat with ivermectin or fipronil. Remove ticks manually where possible
  - Red mite and other species
    - Ivermectin at 0.2 mg/kg p.o., s.c. or i.m.

- Does the bird self-mutilate when owner present or absent. If seen, how does bird behave whilst self-mutilating? Does it appear pruritic, vocalize or scream or even interrupt a favoured activity in order to self-mutilate?
- Try to find out what the bird's normal demeanor is. Is the bird normally relaxed, fearful, aggressive?
- How has the self-mutilation progressed? Where did the bird start plucking and how did it progress?
- How does the owner respond? In some psychological cases the noisy excitable response of the owner can become a reward for this behaviour!

Environmental

Lighting

- Photoperiod. Many of the birds kept as pets are equatorial in origin and so are physiologically attuned for a 12 h day/night cycle.
- Intensity. The majority of psittacines are open scrub (budgerigars) or high canopy (parrots) species that are exposed to high-intensity sunlight. This would include UV light that may act as a natural anti-parasiticide, bacteriocide and fungicide.
- Spectrum. UV lighting in particular may be important with vitamin D3 synthesis from precursors excreted by the uropygial gland. In mammals vitamin D is important for normal skin function and this may also be the case in birds.

Diet

- Seed-based diets are inappropriate for sole, long-term maintenance of many psittacines. Fat and hence energy levels are too high, protein levels relatively low and of poor quality. They are also low in vitamin levels.
- Attempt to wean on to newer pelleted diets. This can be difficult to do, plus anecdotally there seem to be occasional behavioral reactions to colourings used. Otherwise some basic research may be needed to ascertain suitable foods.

Water

- Amazons, African greys and many others are from humid, tropical rainforest areas. A daily dowsing with water and consequent necessary preening may encourage normal feather and skin integrity. Daily spraying with luke-warm water, or access to a bath is appreciated by many birds.

Environmental toxins

- Zinc, often from galvanized caging or cheap metallic toys. Blood levels can be indicative of zinc toxicity, but as with lead, there is no absolute correlation between blood zinc levels and clinical signs. As a general rule if zinc levels are >32.0–50.0 µmol/L and there are consistent clinical signs (see *Neurological Disorders* and *Gastrointestinal Tract Disorders*) then zinc toxicity should be suspected. Significant levels often accompanied by an absolute or relative monocytosis. Feather plucking can be associated with chronic low-grade zinc toxicity; gut problems may be seen as can cause gut stasis. In acute poisonings can damage liver and kidneys causing vomiting, polyuria, haematuria. Consider radiography to look for metallic foreign bodies in the gizzard. Other heavy metals such as lead, copper and iron may cause similar signs.

Treatment for zinc toxicity

- Sodium calcium edetate at 35 mg/kg bid for 5 days, stop for 3–4 days then repeat. Continue until zinc levels fall
- Dimercaptosuccinic acid (DMSA) at 30 mg/kg p.o. b.i.d. for 10 days or 5 days per week for 3–5 weeks
- Penicillamine at 55 mg/kg p.o. b.i.d. for 7–14 days.

- Tobacco smoke. May predispose to brittle feather production, as may an excessively dry atmosphere
- Toys. Psittacines are gregarious creatures. Most live as a pair within a flock and are constantly interacting with their flock members. All single psittacines should have a toy 'friend' that they can feed, huddle up to, beat up, and generally completely dominate. Other toys should be rotated or changed with great frequency. Particularly useful toys are:
  - Wooden objects, as these can be systematically destroyed, exercising the beak and claws and occupying valuable time
  - Toys into which food can be placed and with which the parrot must work to obtain its food.

Findings on clinical examination

- Note if the condition is symmetrical. Self-mutilation due to psychological causes is often not symmetrical in early stages.
- Handle the bird:
  - Examine nares, beak, eyes and buccal cavity including choana. Look particularly for signs of vitamin A deficiency.
  - Examine skin – note signs of inflammation, hyperkeratosis, ulceration, trauma and seborrhea.
- Assess feather quality:
  - Stress lines – lines visible on the vanes of the feather that denote areas of poor quality of the barbs. These may indicate that a significant stressor has happened to the bird at a crucial point in the development of that feather. This may have been a disease or nutritional deficiency.
  - Frayed, dirty or matted. Inappropriate sized caging may cause repeated damage to the retrices of those birds with long tails such as parakeets and macaws.
  - Abnormal colouration may result from nutritional deficiencies, hepatopathies or PBFD.
- Parasites:
  - Pluck one or two feathers for examination under a light microscope for ectoparasites and feather pulp examination.
- Feather scoring. This allows a structured approach to defining and monitoring the extent of the self-mutilation. A final score is arrived at and noted, allowing an objective view of improvement or deterioration to be assessed. Feather scoring may prove difficult with a recalcitrant bird and should a GA be needed, e.g. for radiography – this would provide an ideal opportunity to assess this. (The feather scoring system in Figure 5.10 is from Meehan et al 2003a.)

BODY AND LEGS	Score	Chest and flank	Back	Legs
All or most feathers removed, down removed and skin exposed, evidence of skin or tissue injury	0			
All or most feathers removed, down removed and skin exposed, no evidence of skin or tissue injury	0.25			
All or most feathers removed, some down removed, patches of skin exposed	0.5			
All or most feathers removed, down exposed and intact *or* Feathers removed from more than half the area, some down removed, patches of skin exposed	0.75			
Feathers removed from less than half the area, some down removed and skin exposed	1.0			
Feathers removed from more than half the area, down exposed and intact	1.25			
Feathers removed from less than half the area, down exposed and intact	1.5			
Feathers intact with fraying and breakage	1.75			
Feathers intact with little or no fraying and breakage	2.0			
WINGS				
All or most primaries, secondaries and coverts removed, down removed, skin exposed, evidence of skin or tissue injury			0	
All or most primaries, secondaries and coverts removed, down removed, skin exposed, no evidence of injury			0.5	
More than half of coverts removed, down exposed and intact *or* more than half of primaries and secondaries removed, down exposed and intact			1.0	
Fewer than half of coverts removed, down exposed and intact *or* fewer than half of primaries and secondaries removed, down exposed and intact or primaries and secondaries intact with significant breakage and fraying			1.5	
Feathers intact with little or no fraying or breakage			2.0	
TAIL				
All or most tail feathers removed or broken			0	
Some tail feathers removed or broken *or* Significant fraying of tail feathers			1.0	
Feathers intact with little or no fraying or breakage			2.0	

Fig. 5.10. Feather scoring system.

Investigations

1. A general blood screen is highly recommended. Especially interested in WBC count and differential, liver and kidney biochemistry and zinc
2. Blood samples for PBFD or polyomavirus PCR
3. Chlamydophila serology
4. Fresh faecal samples for parasitic examination – look for *Giardia*, nematode eggs etc.
5. Bulk faecal samples (collected over 3–5 days) can be submitted for *Chlamydophila* PCR
6. Diagnostic imaging including radiography and endoscopy
7. Aseptic collection of samples for bacteriology/mycology
8. Biopsy.

Pathological causes of self-mutilation

Refer to *Skin Disorders,* above.
  Otherwise significant conditions include:
- *Chlamydophilosis*
- *Staphylococcus* has been linked to feather-picking in a budgerigar and feather loss in an unspecified psittacine (Hermans et al 2000)
- *Aspergillus*
- Proventricular dilatation disease (PDD)
- Other diseases including hepatopathies, renal disease etc.
- Endocrinological
  - Hypothyroidism. Rare (see *Endocrine Disorders*)
  - Sex hormone disturbances. Self-mutilation can be associated with seasonal changes or sexual activity. May pick at leggings. It is normal in many species to remove a patch of feathers ventrally at nesting time to form the brood patch whereby eggs can be kept warm. Consider measuring serum oestrogen or androstenedione levels. Possible sex predisposition towards females.

Psychological causes of self-mutilation

- Frequently over-diagnosed. Should only be considered when other aetiologies reasonably eliminated
- True cause not yet elucidated. Adverse environmental stimuli likely to be involved in many cases (see Garner et al 2005); may in some cases be linked to commercial bird-rearing techniques and practices that nestling parrots are exposed to at a time of neurological development with high psychological sensitivity and receptivity
- Suggested manifestations include:
  - Attention seeking. Abnormal behaviour is reinforced by the owner paying attention when bird self-mutilates
  - Displacement behaviour. In the wild stressful situations can be avoided by flying off. In captivity this may not be an option and so fear/aggression may be channelled into exaggerated 'normal' behaviour such as preening
  - Boredom, including the concept of time budgets. In the wild, a parrot will spend a significant amount of time flying to and from roosts and food sources,

interacting with flock mates, avoiding predators and so on. In captivity this time void can be filled by extending other normal behavioural repertoires that it can undertake such as eating (esp. Amazon parrots) or preening
• Separation anxiety. The high intelligence of parrots suggests that this could be quite common
• Obsessive compulsive disorders. Akin to stereotypic disorders – bird will stop favoured activity just to pluck.

Psychotropic drugs

These should not be considered a first line of action; their use should be considered once a physical or environmental problem has been reasonably ruled out or addressed. Suggested medications include:
1. Amitriptyline at 1.0–5.0 mg/kg p.o. b.i.d.
2. Doxepin at 0.6 mg/kg i.m. or i.v. s.i.d. or 2 drops of 5.0 mg/kg solution per 30 mL drinking water
3. Fluoxetine at 0.4 mg/kg p.o. s.i.d.
4. Haloperidol at 0.1–0.4 mg/kg p.o. s.i.d.
   a. Alternatively, dilute 3.0 mg into 1 L of fresh drinking water, offered fresh daily; increase the dose progressively by double dosing every 2 weeks until a dose of 12.0 mg/L is achieved
   b. Continue treatment for at least 3–4 months before gradually withdrawing over a period of time
   c. May induce Parkinson-like tremors which disappear when drug is withdrawn
   d. Haloperidol works reasonably well with self-mutilating birds; behaviour of the bird is likely to alter for the better long before feather improvements are seen.

Management

1. Correct diet. Ideally change to pelleted foods. At the very least, begin supplementation with multivitamin and/or calcium (if appropriate)
2. Address any environmental issues such as photoperiod, irritants such as smoking and so on
3. Remove any metallic objects from the cage
4. Consider environmental enrichment techniques (more/different toys; companion of same species if no risk of infection), etc. If left alone for long periods, consider leaving radio or TV on. Birds naturally inhabit noisy environments – silence usually means there is a predator about. Environmental enrichment (including provision of a conspecific companion) has been found to be beneficial in birds displaying both self-mutilation (van Hoek & King 1997) and stereotypies (Meehan et al 2003b, Meehan et al 2004)
5. If pruritic consider analgesia – meloxicam (Metacam oral suspension) at drop/500 g body weight twice daily
6. Attend to any obvious wounds. Application of topical amorphous hydrogel dressings, e.g. IntraSite Gel (Smith and Nephew Healthcare Ltd.) encourage secondary healing
7. Where there is significant feather loss, consider supplementary heating to counter loss of insulation

8. Undertake specific treatment regimes as results of tests dictate
9. Avoid the use of collars unless absolutely necessary. May stress bird and interfere with normal behaviour including feeding and crop function
10. Basic training – 'Step up', 'Step down', 'No', and 'Stay' – can be useful in both interacting with the bird in a controlled manner and filling in valuable time. The ideal is to establish a *parent:child* or *leader:follower* relationship rather than a *partner:partner* one
11. Do not forget the owner. They are likely to be embarrassed at the state of the bird and feel guilty if they have been feeding their bird on the wrong food, or if some other managemental deficit is identified, but you need them on board for what is liable to be a prolonged haul. They must be encouraged not to lose heart, as improvement may take some time.

Upper respiratory tract disorders

Nasal tract

Cere colour in budgerigars is a secondary sexual characteristic; in most sexually mature males it is a smooth, bright blue structure, while in most females it has a rougher texture, and is brown in colour. Young female light blue birds may have a pastel blue cere leading to incorrect sexing; these darken to a more normal female-type cere with maturity. Gonadal tumours may secrete inappropriate sex hormones that can lead to a change in cere colour of adult birds.

Rhinitis

Viral

- Paramyxovirus (see *Lower Respiratory Tract Disorders*, below)
- Influenza A (orthomyxovirus) (see *Lower Respiratory Tract Disorders*, below).

Bacterial

- Chlamydophilosis
- Mycoplasmosis
- Other bacteria.

Fungal

- *Aspergillus*
- *Candida* (see Treatment in *Lower Respiratory Tract Disorders*, below).

Dietary

- Hypovitaminosis A (see *Nutritional Disorders*).

Neoplasia

Other non-infectious problems

- Choanal atresia
- Allergies
- Rhinoliths. Require surgical removal followed by antibiotic cover. Often linked to hypovitaminosis A (Fig. 5.11).

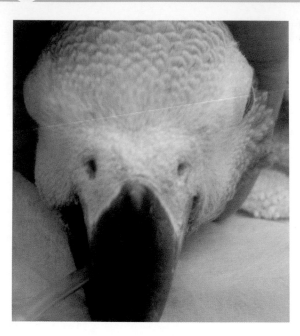

Fig. 5.11. Blocked nares in an African grey parrot.

Investigations

1. Radiography
2. Rhinogram
3. Routine haematology and biochemistry
4. Culture and sensitivity
5. Endoscopy of choana
6. Biopsy.

Sinusitis

- Typically presents as swelling of the infra-orbital sinus
- For possible aetiologies, see both *Rhinitis* and *Lower Respiratory Tract Disorders*, below
- Bacterial
- *Mycobacterium spp*
- Mycoplasmal
- Fungal
- Papillomas
- Sunken eye sinusitis. Collapse of the outer delineating skin due to negative pressure in the infraorbital sinus, which results from blockage of normal connecting diverticuli. Should return to normal when sinus problem resolved
- Neoplasia
- Teratoma (Diaz-Figueroa et al 2005)
- Thymoma (Diaz-Figueroa et al 2004).

Treatment

- Appropriate antibiosis
- Flushing of the infra-orbital sinus; followed by culture and sensitivity plus cytology as appropriate
- Surgical removal of inspissated material.

Lower respiratory tract disorders

Viral

- Paramyxovirus
- Avian pox virus (diphtheritic form)
- Amazon tracheitis virus (herpesvirus)
- Orthoreovirus
- Influenza A (orthomyxovirus)
- Adenovirus (interstitial pneumonia)
- Proventricular dilatation disease (secondary aspiration and inhalation pneumonia).

Bacterial

- *Mycoplasma spp*
- Chlamydophilosis. Primarily *C. psittaci* but other serotypes occasionally encountered.
- *E. coli*
- *Pseudomonas spp*
- *Bordetella avium*
- *Mycobacterium avium*
- Others.

Fungal

- *Aspergillosis*
- *Cryptococcosis.*

Protozoal

- *Sarcocystis falculata* (*Coccidia*).

Parasitic

- Tracheal mites *Sternostoma tracheacolum* (in small parakeets and cockatiels)
- Air sac worms, e.g. filariid nematodes
- *Cyathostoma* and *Syngamus spp* (rare).

Dietary

- Hypovitaminosis A
- Squamous metaplasia of the respiratory tract predisposes to respiratory infections.

Neoplasia

- Glottal neoplasia
- Haemangiosarcoma (Hanley et al 2005)
- Hepatic neoplasia or other coelomic mass

Other non-infectious problems

- Tracheal foreign body. Seed husk a common finding in cockatiels
- Polytetrafluoroethane (PTFE) toxicity from overheating of Teflon®
- Inhalation of other fumes from fires
- Abdominal disease, e.g. neoplasia, haemocoelom, yolk serositis
- Hypothyroidism (goitre) in budgerigars on a seed only diet
- Air sac rupture (usually pathological)
- Cigarette smoke
- Creosote
- Anaemia
- Allergic, asthma-like conditions
- Chronic pulmonary interstitial fibrosis (CPIF), especially in older Amazon parrots (Zandvliet et al 2001). Pre-existing pulmonary damage or allergies may contribute to the aetiology of CPIF.

Findings on clinical examination

- Dyspnoea and tachypnea. Can be very severe
- Open-mouth breathing
- Change in voice. May cease 'talking'
- Sneezing
- Head swinging and neck stretching. Forward-leaning and extended neck strongly suggests tracheal obstruction
- Coughing occasionally encountered but is uncommon. Beware parrots that imitate their owner's cough
- Tail pumping
- Increased recovery time/exercise intolerance
- Increased inspiratory sounds often associated with upper respiratory tract disease
- Increased expiratory sounds often associated with lower respiratory tract disease
- Abdomen may be distended (fluid, neoplasia, haemorrhage)
- Subcutaneous air-filled swelling; may vary in size (ruptured air sac)
- Yellow urates and peracute death common with *Sarcocystis*. Old world parrots are especially susceptible.

Investigations

1. Radiography
   a. Ventro-dorsal view is best for detecting abnormalities of the lungs and air sacs
   b. Distension of abdominal air sacs indicate upper respiratory obstruction, e.g. tracheal fungal granuloma or seed husk
2. Fluoroscopy
3. Routine haematology and biochemistry
   a. Very high heterophil count ($15-40 \times 10^9$/L) indicative of aspergillosis
   b. High PCV – 0.55–0.74 L/L in chronic pulmonary interstitial hyperplasia. Also often have a respiratory acidosis with a pH of 7.16–7.3 ($n = 7.35 \pm 0.08$), hypoxaemia: pO_2 of 33.69–52.77 ($n = 49.46 \pm 7.62$)

and hypercapnia: pCO_2 of 48.77–80.08 ($n = 37.92 \pm 4.23$) (figures from Zandvliet et al 2001).
   c. High AST and CK often with sarcocystis.
4. Serology for sarcocystis, *Aspergillus* and *Chlamydophila*. Ideally investigate with repeat sampling to assess rising titre, but screening tests may also be useful

Table 5.5   Parrots and related species: *Chlamydophila* serology

Result of *Chlamydophila* serology	Interpretation
Negative (no antibodies to *C. psittaci*)	May not have sero-converted. Retest in 7–10 days in acutely ill birds
Weak positive	Suspicious, but interpretation may depend upon species tested and test used. May also reflect previous exposure
Strong positive	Highly indicative of infection, especially if accompanied by consistent clinical signs

5. Haemagglutination inhibition tests and ELISAs may be of benefit in detecting influenza A
6. Culture and sensitivity
   a. Tracheal lavage. Needs GA
7. Cytology
8. Endoscopic biopsy
9. Endoscopy
   a. Endoscopic examination of trachea and syrinx
   b. Air sacs and lungs (high-risk procedure)
10. Transillumination of trachea in small psittacines may reveal mites or nematodes (rare)
   a. Mite or nematode eggs may be detected in faeces or sputum microscopic examination
11. Faecal samples
   a. *Chlamydophila* PCR.
   b. Modified Ziehl–Neelsen staining of faecal samples or PCR for mycobacteriosis.

Management

1. Reduce stress as much as possible. Placing bird in a darkened room may help
2. Covering broad-spectrum antibiosis. May be given by nebulization
3. Provide oxygen support
4. Nutritional support
5. Placement of a tube into a caudal air sac to allow normal breathing in cases of tracheal blockage
6. Bronchodilators, e.g. aminophylline 4.0 mg/kg p.o. or i.m. b.i.d.
7. Mucolytics, e.g. bromhexine at 3.0–6.0 mg/kg i.m. or 6.5 mg/L fresh drinking water daily.

Treatment/specific therapy

- Foreign body
  - Remove if possible. May require endoscopy or tracheotomy
- Emphysema
  - Physical tapping and draining of air from emphysematous lesions. May need to be repeated. If necessary, place a stent if fails to resolve quickly
- Viral diseases
  - Provide supportive treatment and covering antibiosis
  - Amazon tracheitis virus. Acyclovir at 10–40 mg/kg i.v. or s.c. t.i.d.
  - Influenza – provide covering antibiosis. Potentially a zoonosis and reverse zoonosis so avoid contact with infected people
  - Paramyxovirus – supportive treatment. Paramyxovirus A (Newcastle disease) is notifiable in the UK
- Chlamydophilosis
  - Enrofloxacin at 5.0 mg/kg i.m. s.i.d. or 0.5 mL into 100 mL drinking water fresh daily
  - Doxycycline
    - Doxycycline hyclate intravenous human preparation given 60–100 mg/kg i.m. every 5–7 days for 45 days.
    - Doxycycline hyclate as an in-water powdered medication. Use de-ionized water. However, Flammer et al (2003) found that drinking water with 400 mg of doxycycline/L over a 14-day period failed to maintain therapeutic plasma doxycycline concentrations
    - In the same study, hulled seed coated with sunflower oil and doxycycline powder to a concentration of 300 mg of doxycycline hyclate/kg maintained therapeutic plasma doxycycline concentrations for 42 days without notable adverse effects
      Note birds may be intermittent excreters so at least three consecutive negative samples should be achieved before ceasing treatment
- Bacteria – appropriate antibiosis
- Mycobacteriosis
  - Potential zoonosis. Consider euthanasia
  - Two suggested treatment regimes (Rupiper et al 2000) are:
    - Ethambutol (200 mg), isoniazid (200 mg) and rifampin (300 mg) all crushed together and mixed with 10 mL of a simple syrup. This is administered s.i.d. according to Table 5.6

Table 5.6 Parrots and related species: Volumes required for suggested treatment regime of *Mycobacteriosis*

Bird weight (g)	Volume of mixture (mL)
<100	0.1
100–250	0.2
250–500	0.3
500–1000	0.4

- Combination therapy of:
  - Ethambutol (10 mg/kg p.o. b.i.d.)
  - Streptomycin (30 mg/kg i.m. b.i.d.)
  - Rifampin (15 mg/kg p.o. b.i.d.)
- Fungal diseases: specific antifungal regimes for *Aspergillus* and *Candida*
  - Clotrimazole (incl. nebulization)
  - Itraconazole at 5 mg/kg s.i.d. p.o. *Note* that this is potentially toxic to African grey parrots in particular
  - Miconazole (Daktarin Oral Gel, Jansssen-Cilag) at 0.1 mL per 500 g body weight
  - Terbinafine at 15 mg/kg once daily
    Note that *Aspergillus* can be a serious sequel to prolonged/inappropriate steroid use (Verstappen et al 2005)
- Air sac worms: ivermectin at 200 μg/kg. Repeat after 2 weeks
  - *Cyathostoma* and *Syngamus spp.* Indirect life cycle using earthworms, slugs and snails. Treat with fenbendazole at 50 mg/kg p.o. as a one off dose
- Haemocoelom – PCR for polyomavirus. Provide supportive care, but unlikely to survive
- Hypothyroidism in budgerigars: usually supplementation with iodine or commercially available iodine-impregnated seeds such as Trill® (Pedigree Petfoods) will resolve the problem
- PTFE poisoning. If still alive (most birds die very quickly) remove from source of toxicity. NSAIDs may be useful in the control of the pulmonary inflammation that is caused
- Fume inhalation. In addition to general therapy, consider NSAIDs, e.g. meloxicam (Metacam oral suspension) at 1 drop/500 g body weight twice daily. Steroids can be counter-productive in some cases
- Suspected allergic conditions may respond to steroids (beware iatrogenic effects) and bronchodilators (see *Management*, above). These may be given by nebulization. Alternatively try oral meloxicam.

Gastrointestinal tract disorders

The beak

> #### Beak trimming
> 1. The beak is a highly sensitive organ and should be regarded as such.
> 2. In some birds just the maxilla overgrows, in others both the maxilla and mandible need attention, usually due to an underlying malocclusion.
> 3. With large parrots in particular, radiograph the skull to ascertain the extent of the underly maxillary bone before shortening the beak.
> 4. Burring and reshaping of the beak with dental burrs while under GA is preferable a traumatic to the bird than clipping the beak with nail clippers (Fig. 5.12).

Neoplasia

- Squamous cell carcinoma, basal cell carcinoma and Girling 2004).

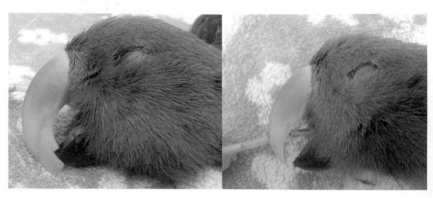

Fig. 5.12. Before and after re-shaping of the beak of an Eclectus parrot, using a dental burr.

Other non-infectious problems
- Maxillary or mandibular fracture
- Lateral deviation of the maxilla (scissor beak). Can be linked to repetitive bar chewing at the same spot.

Findings on clinical examination

- Damaged area of beak. Often marked haemorrhage (fracture)
- Overgrowth of the maxilla or mandible; may be asymmetric.

Investigations

- Radiography.

Management

1. Severe fractures are unlikely to heal. Remove distal part and if the bird is able to use remains of beak to prehend food, then allow to heal
2. Mild fractures may respond to pinning and cerclage wire plus application of supportive dental acrylics
   Provide covering antibiosis.

nt/specific therapy

nalities resulting from fractures will need repeated attention to burr
mal keratin growth that frequently results
young chicks in which the beak has not calcified, repeated
ing may work. If the beak is too calcified then an acrylic
on the mandible to try and force the maxilla back into

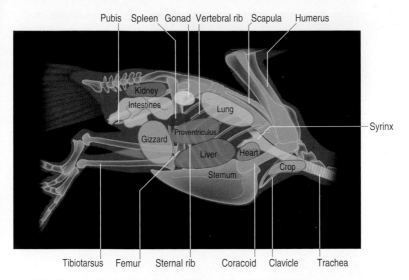

Pubis Spleen Gonad Vertebral rib Scapula Humerus

Kidney
Intestines
Lung
Gizzard
Proventriculus
Liver
Heart
Syrinx
Sternum
Crop

Tibiotarsus Femur Sternal rib Coracoid Clavicle Trachea

Fig. 5.14. Diagram of radiographic anatomy of a psittacine (lateral view).

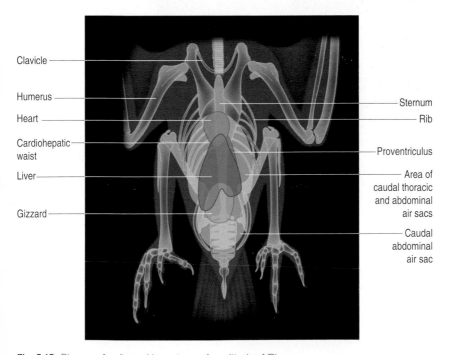

Clavicle
Humerus
Heart
Cardiohepatic waist
Liver
Gizzard

Sternum
Rib
Proventriculus
Area of caudal thoracic and abdominal air sacs
Caudal abdominal air sac

Fig. 5.15. Diagram of radiographic anatomy of a psittacine (VD).

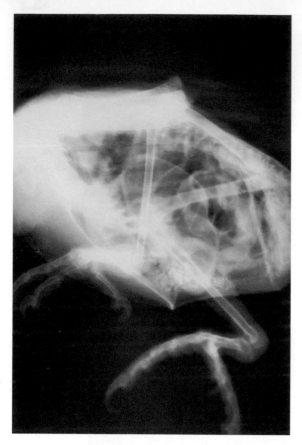

Fig. 5.16. Radiograph of a young African grey parrot with ileus.

- Contrast radiography of old, discharging tongue lesions to investigate presence of possible foreign body
- Ileus may indicate an enteritis, heavy metal toxicity or PDD (Fig. 5.16)
- Endoscopy
  - Creamy-yellow lesions in the crop and/or oesophagus suggest trichomoniasis. Take grab biopsy and look at wet prep under microscope
- Ultrasonography
- Fluoroscopy.

Management

1. Supportive treatment including fluids (see *Nursing Care*)
2. For proventriculitis, consider:
   a. Metoclopramide at 0.2–0.5 mg/kg i.m. or p.o.
   b. Cimetidine at 5 mg/kg b.i.d. p.o.
   c. Gavage with activated charcoal.

Treatment/specific therapy

- Trichomonas
  - Metronidazole at 50 mg/kg orally every 12 h for three occasions; alternatively 30 mg/kg b.i.d. for 5–7 days (Girling 2004)
- Candida
  - Nystatin at 300 000 iu/kg p.o. b.i.d. for 10 days
  - Amphotericin B at 1 mL/kg orally b.i.d.
- Sour crop – flush with warmed saline. May need to be done under GA; consider intubation and packing of the choana prior to flushing
- Megabacteriosis (*Macrorhabdus ornithogaster*)
  - Amphotericin B at 1 mL/kg orally of 100 mg/mL suspension b.i.d.; for budgerigars 0.5 mg/bird b.i.d. until organism is eliminated
  - Ketoconazole at 10 mg/kg b.i.d.
- Laceration of the tongue may require suturing
- Foreign body: removal either via the oral cavity or surgery (ingluviotomy). If flushing out crop, do so under GA, intubated with head held down and choana packed to reduce risk of aspiration
- Zinc or other heavy metal toxicity
  - Sodium calcium edetate at 35 mg/kg b.i.d. for 5 days, stop for 3–4 days then repeat. Continue until zinc levels fall
  - Dimercaptosuccinic acid (DMSA) at 30 mg/kg p.o. b.i.d. for 10 days or 5 days a week for 3–5 weeks
  - Penicillamine at 55 mg/kg p.o. b.i.d. for 7–14 days
- PDD (see *Gastrointestinal Tract Disorders*)
- Crop fistula in hand-reared psittacines. These may require surgical debridement and closure (two layered). Aetiology is due to being fed on food that is too hot
- Crop stasis due to dilute preparation: increasing the concentration of the food mix to 20–30% dry matter will often rectify this problem
- Ingluvoliths – removal via the oral route or break down into smaller particles using warmed saline (Girling 2004)
- Goitre
  - Supplement with iodine. A stock solution of 2.0 mL of strong Lugol's iodine solution in 30 mL water is prepared; one drop of this is added to 250 mL drinking water daily for treatment and 2–3 times weekly for prevention.

Assessment of droppings

Normally, there are both faecal and urinary portions to a bird dropping. The faecal part should be dark and well formed; the urinary part should contain white crystals of uric acid plus a small amount of liquid urine. However, faecal consistency reflects diet and, therefore, varies according to species, from small, hard droppings in budgerigars to liquid 'squirts; in lorikeets. Therefore, birds presented with diarrhoea should have their faeces closely examined to differentiate genuine loss of faecal consistency from polyuria.

Assessment of avian droppings

Faecal portion

- The faecal portion may be small or absent if:
  - Bird is anorexic
  - Cloacoliths or other obstructions are present
- May be poorly formed – genuine diarrhoea (Fig. 5.17)
- May be abnormally coloured:
  - Blood may be present
  - Certain highly pigmented fruits may do this
- May contain abnormalities such as:
  - Undigested seeds
  - Worm eggs or protozoal cysts (on microscopic examination).

Urinary portion

- May be dry if:
  - Bird is on an all seed diet, e.g. budgerigar
- May have a high water content if:
  - Bird is on a high water-content diet, e.g. fruit or vegetables
  - The bird is polydipsic
  - If the bird is polyuric, always collect a sample and check for glucose, blood and protein
- May be abnormally coloured:
  - Light to dark green may indicate liver disease due to high biliverdin levels
  - Greenish to a bronze colour may indicate liver disease, but can also occur after trauma.

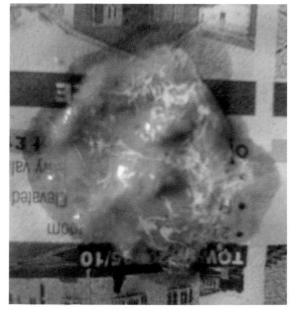

Fig. 5.17. Genuine diarrhoea in a parrot – *note* the loss of faecal consistency.

Always collect a fresh sample.
- Microscopic examination of a wet preparation will often pick up protozoa and worm eggs
- Faecal flotation for protozoal oocyst counts
- Gram stain: the normal gut flora of psittacines should be predominantly G +ve. A Gram stain should highlight changes in the bacterial flora including yeast overgrowths
- Swab for bacterial culture and sensitivity if appropriate.

Differential diagnosis for gastrointestinal disorders

Viral

- Proventricular dilatation disease (PDD) (putative paramyxovirus, Grund et al 2002). Formerly known as macaw wasting disease; can affect a variety of psittacines
- Paramyxovirus
- Chronic paramyxovirus infection can cause cloacal dilatation
- Papillomatosis (a possible herpesvirus)
- Orthoreovirus and orthoreovirus-like agent (budgerigars)
- Pacheco's disease
- Polyomavirus
- Rotavirus
- Picornavirus
- Adenovirus.

Bacterial

- Hepatitis, proventriculitis, enteritis due to:
- *E. coli*
- *Klebsiella spp*
- *Pseudomonas spp*
- Salmonellosis
- *Yersinia pseudotuberculosis*
- Chlamydophilosis (psittacosis)
- *Mycobacterium avium* (avian tuberculosis).
- Clostridia
- *Clostridium colinum* and *Cl perfringens* in lories (Pizarro et al 2005)
- Megacolon secondary to *Clostridium tertium*.

Fungal

- Candida
- Megabacteriosis (*Macrorhabdus ornithogaster*)
- Mucormycosis
- Protozoal
- *Giardia*
- *Spironucleus* (Philbey et al 2002).

Parasitic

- Uncommon in psittacines but ground-feeding Australian parakeets are particularly at risk
- Nematodes:
  - Ascarids (esp. *Ascaris platyceri* and *Ascaridia hermaphrodita*) and *Porrocaecum spp*

- *Capillaria*
- *Thelazia* and *Oxyspirura spp*
- Spiruroids: Proventricular worms, e.g. *Geopetitia, Dispharynx, Habronema* and *Tetrameres spp*
- Cestodes, e.g. *Raillietina spp.*

Dietary

- Dietary indiscretion

Neoplasia

- Gastric carcinoma
- Gastric adenoma
- Papilloma (papillomatosis – see *Viral*, above).

Other non-infectious problems

- Calcinosis circumscripta (deep granuloma in tongue)
- Proventricular ulceration
- Proventricular impaction
- Foreign body
- Sloughed koilin due to ventriculitis
- Dysplastic koilin
- Intussusception
- Cloacal prolapse
- Megacloaca
- Cloacal impaction.

Findings on clinical examination

- Weight loss
- Vague signs of ill-health, e.g. cessation of talking
- Passing undigested seeds in faeces (PDD)
- Melaena (ulceration, severe enteritis)
- Haemorrhagic faeces (Pacheco's disease)
- Neurological signs (PDD, paramyxovirus)
- Vent soiled with accumulated faeces
  - Budgerigars – usually due to obesity (cannot clean themselves) or herniation of abdominal musculature
  - Central American parrots, e.g. Amazons, macaws and hawk-headed parrots: likely to be papillomatosis. This affects the cloaca, but also the oral cavity and proximal gastrointestinal tract
- Yellow-green diarrhoea; wasting and deaths (spironucleosis)
- Wide range of clinical signs including GIT and respiratory may be seen with systemic bacterial infections such as *Salmonella* and *Yersinia*. Occasionally neurological may be seen with *Salmonella*
- Green diarrhoea, dyspnoea and sneezing (*Chlamydophilosis*)
- Weight loss (*Mycobacterium avium*). May also exhibit slow-growing masses
- Cloacal tissue visibly protruding from vent (cloacal prolapse)
- Physiological enlargement of the cloaca in reproductively active Vasa parrots (*Coracopis vasa*) and lesser Vasa parrot (*C. nigra*)
- Sudden death (*Clostridial* infection). May be linked to stress triggers
- Sudden, mass deaths in budgerigars (orthoreovirus-like agents).

Investigations

1. Routine haematology and biochemistry
2. Samples for culture and sensitivity
   a. Faecal examination
   b. Gram stain
   c. Modified Ziehl–Neelsen staining for mycobacteriosis
   d. Wet preparation/flotation for worm eggs/protozoa (Fig. 5.18)
   e. Abundant motile trophozoites (*Spironucleus*)
3. Proventricular wash for proventricular worm eggs
4. Fine needle aspirate/staining/cytology of any abnormal masses (including staining for mycobacteria)
5. Radiography (including contrast studies)
   a. Dilated crop, proventriculus, gizzard and gut (PDD, severe enteritis)
   b. Contrast studies for PDD, proventricular ulceration, foreign bod
   c. Dilated cloaca (megacloaca)
6. Fluoroscopy
7. Chlamydophila PCR; ideally take three samples from each bird: conjunctiva, choana and faeces. Serology for *Chlamydophilosis*
8. Mycobacterium avium PCR on faeces/suspect material
9. PCR for Pacheco's disease and polyomavirus
10. Orthoretroviral infection: isolation of orthoreovirus from faeces, biopsy samples, ascitic fluid or respiratory secretions. ELISA and virus neutralizing tests
11. Endoscopy
12. Ultrasonography
13. Biopsy
    a. Full thickness crop wall including large blood vessel for PPD will allow diagnosis in 75% of cases (Gregory et al 1996). Biopsy of proventriculus is a more difficult operation and carries a higher risk
14. Postmortem of affected birds
    a. *Yersinia*: a degree of hepatomegaly; patchy discolouration of the liver and in more advanced cases, miliary lesions in liver, kidneys and spleen

Fig. 5.18. Diagram showing some eggs of intestinal parasites of psittacines. (Not drawn to scale.)

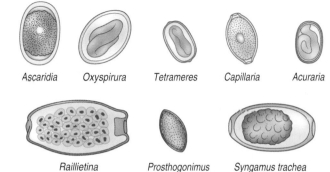

Ascaridia   Oxyspirura   Tetrameres   Capillaria   Acuraria

Raillietina   Prosthogonimus   Syngamus trachea

Management

1. Supportive management including covering antibiosis
2. Fluid therapy.

Treatment/specific therapy

* Pacheco's disease – see *Hepatic Disorders*
* Orthoreoviral infection: supportive treatment: new world species often respond well but old world species carry a poorer prognosis
* Other viral diseases
  * Symptomatic and supportive treatment only
* Parasites
  * Birds in outside aviaries should be wormed twice yearly (avoid breeding season) or have faecal screens every 6 months. All new birds should be wormed during quarantine
  * Suitable treatments include fenbendazole at 50 mg/kg as a once only dose, or water-soluble avermectins, e.g. moxidectin 0.1% added to drinking water at 20 mg/L for 48 h. *Note* fenbendazole may be toxic to cockatiels (Lloyd 2003)
  * *Capillaria.* Infection is direct, but intermediate stages can be carried by earthworms so remove faecal material regularly and prevent access to soil. Treat with fenbendazole at 50 mg/kg by crop tube; this may need repeating every 2 weeks until the bird is clear
  * *Ascaridia* and *Porrocaecum spp.* The life cycle is direct, although earthworms may act as transport hosts
  * *Thelazia* and *Oxyspirura spp.* Carried by intermediate arthropod host
  * Proventricular worms, e.g. *Geopetitia, Dispharynx, Habronema* and *Tetrameres spp.* Indirect life cycle using insect intermediate hosts
  * Cestodes: single dose of praziquantel at 8–10 mg/kg p.o.
* *Giardia*
  * Metronidazole at 20 mg/kg p.o. b.i.d.
* Spironucleus
  * Metronidazole as above
  * Dimetridazole failed to work (Philbey 2002)
* Candida and mucormycosis
  * Nystatin at 300 000 iu/kg p.o. b.i.d. for 10 days
  * Amphotericin B at 1 mL/kg orally b.i.d.
* Proventricular dilatation disease. Poor response to treatment but some individuals recover. Treatment should include:
  * Broad-spectrum antibiosis, e.g. enrofloxacin at 5–20 mg/kg s.i.d., co-trimoxazole at 30 mg/kg b.i.d.
  * Motility modifiers, e.g. cisapride at 1.0 mg/kg b.i.d. p.o.; metoclopramide 0.5 mg/kg p.o., i.m., i.v.
  * Cox 2 inhibitors such as Celebrex (Pfizer) at 10 mg/kg s.i.d. appear to be beneficial in some cases
  * Meloxicam (Metacam oral suspension) at 1 drop/500 g body weight twice daily
  * Keep in-contact birds in strict isolation
  * Institute good hygiene, ventilation and other good management
  * Immediate and thorough investigation of any sick or dead birds

- Probably an isolation period of 2–3 years without any fresh incidence of PDD is needed before declaring an aviary free of the disease (Doneley et al 2007)
- Obesity in budgerigars: consider supplementing with L-carnitine (1000 mg/kg food)
- Abdominal herniation in budgerigars will often require surgery to remove excess abdominal musculature
- Papillomatosis. Surgical removal of papillomas from cloaca and oral cavity if causing problems. Infected birds often subsequently develop neoplasia of the pancreas, and bile duct carcinoma has been report in affected Amazon parrots
- Salmonella: antibiotics based upon culture and sensitivity
  - Autogenous vaccination can clear carriers (Harcourt-Brown 1986). Two doses are given 2 weeks apart and each dose consists of 1.0 mL orally and 0.5 mL s.c.
- Other bacterial infections: appropriate antibiosis
- *Yersinia*: prevent access of wild birds and rodents to aviaries and food stocks
- Clostridial infections: metronidazole at 20 mg/kg p.o. b.i.d.
- *Macrorhabdus ornithogaster* – see under *Vomiting/regurgitation/dysphagia*
- *Mycobacterium avium*. Potential zoonosis so recommend euthanasia. For suggested treatment protocols, see under *Lower Respiratory Tract Disorders*
- Chlamydophilosis (see *Lower Respiratory Tract Disorders*)
- Proventricular ulceration
  - Cimetidine at 5 mg/kg p.o. b.i.d.
  - Address underlying factors including possible secondary bacterial and fungal ulceration
- Proventricular impaction
  - Flush with warm saline either via mouth or via ingluviotomy incision
  - If fails may need to undertake a proventriculotomy
- Cloacal prolapse – requires cloacopexy
  - A purse-string suture may provide temporary alleviation of the condition, but cloacopexy should give more permanent results
  - Investigate the possibility of underlying predisposing factors, e.g. cloactitis, etc.
- Megacloaca – cloacal reductive surgery (Graham et al 2004)
- Cloacal impaction. Requires manual removal, usually under an anaesthetic
  - Covering antibiotics; investigate and deal with underlying factors.

Nutrition

The diet of most psittacine birds is very poor compared with their comparable diet in the wild. Nutritional problems arise by two means:
1. Provision of inappropriate food
2. Selectivity of the bird (Werquin et al 2005).
These apply especially to a sunflower-seed-based diet.

Nutritional disorders

- Incorrect protein levels
  - In cockatiels, the optimum protein levels for growth and weaning is around 20% crude protein, but:
    - 5% causes severe stunting followed by 100% mortality
    - 10–15% leads to stunting and some mortality
    - 25% gives good weight gain but also behavioural problems such as aggression
    - 35% gives paradoxical poor growth and aggression

- Hypervitaminosis A: excessively high levels of vitamin A have been associated with cataract formation and bone abnormalities. High levels of carotenoids can cause a yellowing discolouration of skin and fat
- Hypovitaminosis A: hyperkeratosis and squamous metaplasia of epithelia, including the pharynx, respiratory tract and occasionally renal tubules. Often there are sterile white plaques visible in oral mucosa, and blunting or loss of the choanal papillae. Rhinitis (and occasionally rhinoliths) and blepharitis are common. Sneezing may occur, and there is a predisposition towards respiratory infections. In severe cases, metaplasia of the renale tubules can result in visceral gout
- Hypervitaminosis D_3: can result in calcification of viscera, especially the kidneys, triggering a visceral gout
- Metabolic bone disease. This is often a hypovitaminosis D_3 combined with a hypocalcaemia and hyperphosphataemia. In particular, African grey Parrots appear to have difficulty in mobilizing skeletal calcium reserves. Such birds often present with a hypocalcaemic tetany – wings fluttering violently in apparent 'fits'. Such birds often have high parathormone levels, low 25-hydroxycholecalciferol levels as well as low serum ionized and non-ionized calcium levels

Clinical signs of metabolic bone disease is birds

- General weakness (Fig. 5.19)
- Pathological fractures and/or bending of bones
- Rickets
- Paralysis
- Tetany
- Dystocia
- Low clutch size, thin or soft shelled eggs and low hatchability. (Egg laying hens may have an episode of acute hypocalcemia that can result in partial paresis and perhaps egg binding.)
- Polydipsia/polyuria occasionally seen due too increased phosphorus turnover triggering a diuresis
- Birds, especially the young, with bone and joint deformities might be deficient in both calcium and vitamin D_3.

- Hypovitaminosis E: affected birds may become lethargic and show coordination and equilibrium problems. Complete paralysis can occur. Other signs include white muscle disease. If the gizzard is affected, then undigested seed may be passed. Splayed legs and oedema of the neck, wings and breast may be seen. Reproductive problems can be encountered including infertility and low hatchability due to weakness in the pipping muscle of the chick
- Hypovitaminosis K can occur with coccidiostats and long-term antibiosis that destroys the normal gut flora. Failure to produce vitamin K leads to blood clotting problems, which can present as excessive haemorrhage
- Riboflavin (vitamin B2). However, adult hens deficient in B2 develop fatty livers, elongated flight feathers, have low egg production and low hatchability. In chicks the signs are weakness and diarrhoea, inward curling toes and depigmented feathers (achromatosis) in cockatiels

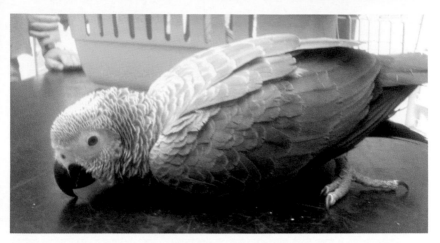

Fig. 5.19. Hypocalcaemia in an African grey parrot – *note* the three-point stance using the beak to aid support.

- Pantothenic acid: cockatiels raised on a pantothenic acid deficient diet fail to grow contour feathers on the chest and back and die at three weeks of age. Others signs include dermatitis on the face and feet, decreased growth, decreased feathering and incoordination
- Biotin. Deficiencies can occur due to ingested mycotoxins in the diet affecting biotin uptake. Signs as for pantothenic acid
- Folic acid. Genuine deficiencies can occur with long-term antibiosis. Signs include anemia, immunosuppression, poor egg production, low hatchability and stunting of chicks, often accompanied by deformation of upper beaks
- Vitamin B12: deficiencies are rare, but include anaemia, poor feathering, reduced growth, reduced food intake, nervous disorders, gizzard erosions and fatty accumulations in the heart, liver and kidneys
- Choline. Deficiencies include poor growth of young birds, fatty liver syndrome in adults and calcification of soft tissues. Cockatiels on a low choline diet exhibited unpigmented wing and tail feathers, but no calcification
- Iodine. In budgerigars linked to goitre formation (see *Differential Diagnoses for Vomiting/Regurgitation/Dysphagia*)
- Hypocalcaemia: often combined with hypovitaminosis D3 (see 'Metabolic bone disease', above)
- Obesity. Common in Amazon parrots, Galah cockatoos, cockatiels and budgerigars. Subcutaneous fat deposits may be visible and there is infiltration of internal organs with fatty tissue. May give rise to atherosclerosis and sequelae, e.g. cerebrovascular accidents
- Hepatic lipidosis: obesity; lethargy, depression, and anorexia. Neurological signs may be seen, consistent with hepatic encephalopathy. Urates may be yellow or green
- Atherosclerosis (see *Cardiovascular and Haematological Disorders*)
- Haemochromatosis (iron storage disease). Hepatomegaly. Rare.

Investigations

1. Haematology and biochemistry
   a. Hepatic lipidosis may show an increased LDH, AST, triglycerides and bile acids
   b. Blood levels for calcium (including ionized calcium), phosphorus
   c. Vitamin D_3 (blood 25-hydroxycholecalciferol levels >50 nmol/L)
   d. Vitamin A levels (retinol 0.471 ± 0.209 µg/mL) (Torregrossa et al 2005)
   e. Vitamin E levels (α-tocopherol 13.5 ± 6.60 µg/mL)
2. Radiography
   a. Hepatomegaly (hepatic lipidosis, neoplasia)
   b. Hypervitaminosis D_3: calcification of the kidneys
   c. Skeletal abnormalities: pathological fractures, healed fractures, bone deformities, osteomalacia (metabolic bone disease)
3. Liver biopsy
4. Dietary analysis.

Management

1. Dietary imbalances often predispose to secondary pathogen invasion, so covering antibiosis should be considered. Aim to switch to a more healthy diet which, depending upon the species, should consist of:
   a. Exchanging seed mix for a good proprietary pelleted food, e.g. Harrison's Bird food
   b. Enhancing the diet by increasing the consumption of coloured vegetable such as sweet peppers and non-citrus fruits
   c. Using appropriate vitamin and mineral supplements
   d. Sprouting seeds helps to convert some of the fat into carbohydrate
   e. Altering diets can be time consuming. Many parrots are seriously neophobic and are reluctant to eat novel substances
2. Milk thistle (*Silybum marianum*) is hepatoprotectant. Dose at 4–15 mg/kg b.i.d. or t.i.d. (Wade 2004)
3. Provide exposure to UVB light – especially important for African grey parrots.

Treatment/specific therapy

* Hepatic lipidosis
  * Poor prognosis
  * Provision of interosseous fluids (Hartmann's), diet high in nutrients (include fructose, biotin, choline, and lactulose) and broad spectrum antibiotic therapy may be useful
  * Consider L-carnitine (see 'Obesity', below)
* Hypovitaminosis A
  * Injectable vitamin A at 5000 IU/kg daily for 2 weeks, then adopt maintenance rate of 5000 IU p.o. or feed coloured vegetables such as carrots and peppers
* Metabolic bone disease
  * Supplement with vitamin D_3 at 5000 IU/kg daily, but also calcium as well
  * Provide access to full spectrum lighting with an ultraviolet B component, e.g. sunshine or commercially available lighting to allow natural endogenous vitamin D_3 production

- Hypervitaminosis D_3
  - In some cases, clinical signs regress when D_3 levels were returned to normal. Macaws particularly seem to be susceptible to high vitamin D_3 levels, and it is recommended that vitamin D_3 levels should not be higher than 2000 IU/kg of a parrots diet (with a gross energy diet range of 3200–4200 kcal/kg)
- Vitamin E
  - Works synergistically with selenium, and can be given combined (Vitesel, Norbrook) at 0.01 mL/kg i.m. every 7–14 days
- Other hypovitaminoses: supplement with appropriate vitamin preparations. Complete revision of diet recommended
- Iodine: supplement with iodine (see *Differential Diagnosis for Vomiting/Regurgitation/Dysphagia*)
- Haemochromatosis. Select low iron diet. May be linked to chronic inflammatory conditions
- Obesity. In budgerigars, L-carnitine at 1000 mg/kg food has been effective in inducing weight loss along with shrinkage of lipomas
- Hypocalcaemia
  - Calcium gluconate 10% at 100–200 mg/kg (1.0–2.0 mL/kg) i.m. s.i.d. or 50–100 mg/kg by slow i.v.

Hepatic disorders

Note that psittacines lack a gall bladder.

Viral

- Pacheco's disease (herpesvirus)
- Polyomavirus
- Adenovirus.

Bacterial

- Bacterial hepatitis
- Chlamydophilosis
- *Yersinia pseudotuberculosis*
- Mycobacteriosis.

Fungal

- Aflatoxicosis.

Nutritional

- Haemochromatosis
- Hepatic lipidosis.

Neoplasia

- Hepatic tumours
- Lymphoma (likely linked to retrovirus infection) (see *Cardiovascular and Haematological Disorders*).

Other non-infectious problems

- Cirrhosis
- Steroid hepatopathy (iatrogenic)
- Amyloidosis.

Findings on clinical examination

- Unwell bird, fluffed up appearance
- Anorexia
- Polydipsia/polyuria
- Very green or yellow appearance of faeces
- Ascites (secondary to portal hypertension)
- Respiratory signs (ascites/chlamydophilosis)
- Multifocal follicular and feather pulp haemorrhages (polyomavirus).

Investigations

1. Radiography
   a. Hepatomegaly (Pacheco's disease, neoplasia, haemochromatosis)
   b. Ascites
2. Routine haematology and biochemistry
   a. Liver enzymes raised. AST is not liver specific, but raised AST plus bile acid levels indicate liver disease; raised AST + CK suggests muscle injury. In end-stage liver disease, plasma liver enzymes levels may be normal or low
3. Culture and sensitivity
4. Coelomic tap (culture and sensitivity, cytology)
5. Faecal or cloacal swab for Pacheco's disease PCR
6. Endoscopy
   a. Hepatomegaly, splenomegaly, renal enlargement
7. Ultrasonography
   a. Hepatomegaly (Pacheco's disease)
8. Biopsy.

Management

1. Supportive therapy including fluids
2. Lactulose at 0.5 mL/kg b.i.d.
3. Milk thistle (*Silybum marianum*) is hepatoprotectant. Dose at 4–15 mg/kg b.i.d. or t.i.d. (Wade 2004).

Treatment/specific therapy

- Pacheco's disease is usually rapidly fatal. Try acyclovir at 80 mg/kg p.o. t.i.d. for 7–10 days or 40 mg/kg i.v. or s.c. t.i.d. (cited in Girling 2003)
- Haemochromatosis (see 'Dietary')
- Hepatic lipidosis (see 'Dietary').

Splenic disorders

- Chlamydophilosis (see *Lower Respiratory Tract Disorders*)
- Lymphoma (see *Cardiovascular and Haematological Disorders*).

Cardiovascular and haematological disorders

Where possible, auscultate tame birds while at rest on a perch or the owner, as stressed birds exhibit such high heart rates that meaningful auscultation is difficult. Any abnormal heart rate or rhythm is likely to be associated with heart disease or a more systemic illness.

Viral

- Polyoma virus (hydropericardium)
- PDD (myocarditis).

Bacterial

- Valvular endocarditis. Can be thrombotic
- Bacterial infiltration
- Pericarditis
- Chronic systemic lung disease.

Fungal

- Pericarditis
- Chronic systemic lung disease.

Protozoal

- *Haemoproteus*
- *Leucocytozoon*
- *Akiba spp*
- *Plasmodium*.

Nutritional

- Fat accumulation (lipomatosis cordis)
- Atherosclerosis (esp. Amazons and African greys).

Neoplasia

- Lymphoma/lymphosarcoma.

Other non-infectious problems

- Chronic pulmonary interstitial fibrosis, especially in older Amazon parrots (Zandvliet et al 2001). Very commonly causes a right ventricular enlargement (see *Respiratory Tract Disorders*)
- Right ventricular enlargement also from other causes of systemic lung disease, e.g. chronic mycosis
- Pericardial effusion with or without ascites
- Ventricular hypertrophy or dilatation
- Myxomatous degeneration of atrioventricular valve (Oglesbee & Lehmkuhl 2001)
- Calcification of the blood vessels
- Lack of exercise (plus poor diet)
- Avocado toxicity (hydropericardium)
- Urate deposits in the aorta
- Congenital.

Findings on clinical examination

- Exercise intolerance
- Apparent respiratory signs
- Auscultation: dysrhythmias and altered heart sounds, e.g. murmurs
- Vomiting and wasting (leucocytozoon)
- Concomitant signs such as ascites, pulmonary disease, air sacculitis
- Neurological signs (typically cerebrovascular accidents secondary to atherosclerosis).

Investigations

1. Radiography
   a. Normal radiographic heart parameters
   b. Liver enlargement

Table 5.7 Parrots and related species: Normal radiographic heart parameters

Ratio of cardiac silhouette width to:	(%)
Sternum length (measured on the bird)	35–41
Width of thorax (measured on VD radiograph)	51–61
Width of coracoid (measured on VD radiograph)	545–672

From Straub et al (2002).

2. Routine haematology and biochemistry
   a. Blood cholesterol levels are a major risk factor for atherosclerosis

Table 5.8 Parrots and related species: Blood cholesterol levels

Species	Cholesterol (mmol/L)		Triglycerides (mmol/L)	
	Bavelaar et al[a]	Polo et al[b]	Bavelaar et al[a]	Polo et al[b]
Palm cockatoo	–	3.6 ± 0.5 (2.8–4.2)	–	1.2 ± 0.5 (0.8–1.9)
Long-billed cockatoo	5.65–6.33	–	0.79–1.78	–
Amazon (yellow-headed Amazon)	7.46–9.65	7.1 ± 2.5 (4.3–10.9)	1.7–2.86	1.6 ± 0.4 (1.1–2.1)
Blue and gold macaw	4.2–4.77	4.2 ± 0.9 (3.1–6.7)	0.35–0.52	1.2 ± 0.7 (0.4–2.5)
Scarlet macaw	5.0–5.3	4.1 ± 1.1 (2.3–6.4)	0.38–0.66	1.0 ± 0.3 (0.5–1.6)
Red fan parrot	4.09–4.54		0.35–0.38	–
African grey parrot	–	8.38 ± 2.57 (5.31–18.62)[c]	–	–

[a]Values from Bavelaar et al (2005).
[b]Values from Polo et al (1998).
[c]Bavelaar & Beynen (2003).

Table 5.9 Parrots and related species: Normal lead II ECGs

Variable	Hyacinth macaw	Green wing macaw	African grey parrot
Body weight (g)	1331 ± 149	1214 ± 173	–
Heart rate (beats/min)	283 ± 65	280 ± 97	–
Electrical axis (˚)	−101 (81–109)	−98 (86–131)	–
P, duration (s)	0.02 (0.015–0.025)	0.018 (0.015–0.025)	0.012–0.018
P, amplitude (mV)	0.3 (0.19–0.4)	0.2 (0.075–0.3)	0.25–0.55
QRS duration (s)	0.02 (0.015–0.025)	0.02 (0.013–0.025)	0.010–0.016
QRS, amplitude (mV)	0.65 (0.35–1.0)	0.5 (0.35–0.85)	–
R, amplitude (mV)	0.045 (0.04–0.08)	0.05 (0.02–0.2)	0.0–0.2
T, duration (s)	0.05 (0.035–0.075)	0.045 (0.035–0.05)	–
T, amplitude (mV)	0.3 (0.1–0.7)	0.25 (0.1–0.45)	0.18–0.60
PR interval (s)	0.055 (0.05–0.075)	0.05 (0.04–0.07)	0.040–0.055
QT interval, (s)	0.085 (0.08–0.1)	0.09 (0.08–0.11)	0.048–0.070
ST seg. amplitude (mV)	0.1 (0.05–0.15)	0.1 (0.05–0.15)	0.90–0.20

3. Cytology (blood smears for haemoparasites)
4. Blood culture and sensitivity
5. ECG
   a. Sinus rhythm normal
   b. Sinus dysrhythmias and second-degree heart block considered physiological in birds
   c. Partial fusion of P and T waves ('P on T' phenomenon) can be normal, especially in females
   d. Isoflurane anaesthesia may increase heart rate
   e. Normal ECG values after Casares et al (2000) and Musulin & Adin (2006) (Table 5.9)
6. Endoscopy
7. Biopsy (liver, kidney, pectoral muscles)
8. Ultrasonography
9. Echocardiography/Doppler.

Table 5.10 Normal values of some psittacine cardiac anatomy

Values for myocardium of left free wall	Sternal length (%)
Mean apical myocardium	2.3–2.85
Mean middle left myocardium	8.3–8.7
Mean basal myocardium thickness	7.9–9.0

From Krautwald-Junghanns et al (2004).

Management

1. Reduce stress as much as possible, e.g. remove affected birds from breeding programmes
2. Identify and treat underlying problems, e.g. chronic lung disease
3. Improve diet.

Treatment/specific therapy

• NSAIDs, e.g. meloxicam at 1 drop per 500 g s.i.d. may be useful for chronic pulmonary interstitial fibrosis
• Heart disease: once a diagnosis is achieved, drug regimes may be adapted from mammalian treatments. Examples would be:
  • Enalapril at 1.0–2.5 mg/kg p.o. s.i.d. or b.i.d. (Pees et al 2006)
  • Furosemide at 0.15 mg/kg i.m. s.i.d.
  • Digoxin at 0/05 mg/kg p.o. s.i.d.
• Haemoproteus: often considered asymptomatic and self-limiting, but can be a contributing factor to anaemia if present. Treat with chloroquinine at 250 mg per 120 mL drinking water for 14 days. Avoid ceratopogonid vectors
• Plasmodium
  • Primaquine at 0.75–1.0 mg/kg p.o. once only, combined with an initial loading dose of chloroquine at 25 mg/kg, reducing this to 15 mg/kg at 12, 24 and 48 h
• Leukocytozoon: may be asymptomatic, but can be fatal with acute hepatitis, renal tubular necrosis and myocardial haemorrhage. Chronic cases may present with wasting and vomiting. Treat as for plasmodium, above. Avoid exposure to vectors such as blackflies (*Simulium spp*) or Culicoides/hippoboscids
• Lymphoma/lymphosarcoma
  • Treatment is speculative and more modern regimes may be more appropriate. However, the following chemotherapeutic drugs have been used in cockatoos (France 1993):
    • Prednisolone at 25 mg/m^2 p.o. s.i.d.
    • Asparaginase at 400 IU/kg i.m. every 7 days. Premedicate with diphenhydramine at 2 mg/kg i.o. once only
    • Cyclophosphamide at 200 mg/m^2 i.o. every 7 days
    • Doxorubicin at 30 mg/m^2 i.o. every 2 days. Premedicate with diphenhydramine at 2 mg/kg i.o. once only
    • Vincristine sulfate at 0.75 mg/m^2 i.o. every 7 days for 3 weeks
• Atherosclerosis
  • Treat symptomatically
  • Linked to deficiency of n-3 polyunsaturated fatty acids, especially α-linolenic acid (Bavelaar et al 2005); supplement by feeding commercial diets, feeding small seeds, e.g. flax seeds.

Musculoskeletal disorders

Viral

• PBFD
• Retroviral infection (renal/gonadal tumours).

Bacterial

- Renal infections can spread to the adjacent lumbo-sacral plexus
- Septic arthritis
- Osteomyelitis.

Nutritional

- Metabolic bone disease (see *Nutritional Disorders*).

Neoplasia

- Renal tumour (possibly due to retroviral infection)
- Gonadal tumour (especially budgerigars; possibly due to retroviral infection)
- Osteosarcoma.

Other non-infectious problems

- Articular gout
- Limb bone fracture – tibio-tarsal fractures are particularly common
- Spinal trauma
- Identification ring too tight (especially closed rings)
- Developmental problems of chicks
- Juvenile osteodystrophy
- Metabolic or systemic problems, e.g. cardiovascular disease, hypoglycaemia, hypocalcaemia, anaemia.

Findings on clinical examination

- Weakness, ataxia
- Unwillingness or inability to move
- Leg paralysis – may be unilateral or bilateral
- Limb deformities including rotation around joints
- Flight disorders, see *Differential Diagnoses for Loss of Flight*.

Investigations

1. Radiography
   a. Radiograph not only the affected limb, but also the whole body, especially if there is obvious muscle wastage
   b. Contrast studies, e.g. with barium to assess for displacement of gut by intra-coelomic masses
      Note that reproductively active females stored excess calcium as deposits at the femur. These should not be mistaken for pathologic exostoses
2. Routine haematology and biochemistry
   a. Will need to differentiate from systemic or metabolic disorders
3. Culture and sensitivity
4. Endoscopy
5. Ultrasonography.

Management

1. Supportive treatment including covering antibiosis
2. Hospitalizing weakened birds on soft surfaces, e.g. towels to reduce the risk of trauma.

Treatment/specific therapy

- Renal infection – appropriate antibiosis
- Fractures – stabilization by external or internal fixation (Fig. 5.20). In small psittacines conservative management including analgesia may be more appropriate for femoral fractures
- Identification ring too tight – remove under general anaesthetic
- Neoplasia – treatment rarely viable
  - Osteosarcoma: treat has been attempted with doxorubicin at 60 mg/m^2 i.v. diluted with saline every 30 days (Doolan 1994)
- Juvenile osteodystrophy
  - In very young chicks, developmental problems such as valgus deformities (splay leg) can be corrected by hobbling the legs together before the skeleton becomes reasonably calcified. This should be done at no more than 5 days.

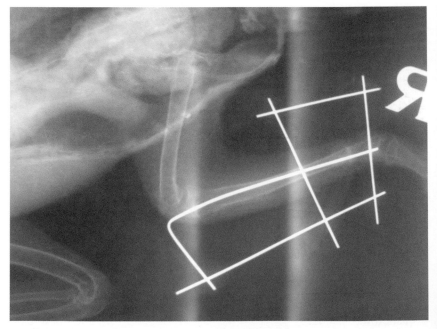

Fig. 5.20. Combined internal and external fixation repair of a fractured tibiotarsus.

Older chicks may require surgical correction once the bones have sufficiently calcified to withstand such surgery
• Reassess hand-rearing conditions, as these often reflect a poor rearing environment. Harcourt-Brown (2004) finds that dusky parrot chicks (*Pionus fuscus*) remain in the nest until day 53; the presence of several chicks in such a combined space may mutually support their growing skeletons and premature exercise may lead to pathologic deformity of the long bones.

Differential diagnoses for loss of flight

Viral

• Polyomavirus
• PBFD.

Bacterial

• Pathological fracture (from osteomyelitis).

Fungal

• Pathological fracture (from osteomyelitis).

Neoplasia

• Pathological fracture.

Other non-infectious problems

• Cardiovascular disease
• Respiratory disease
• Neurological disease
• Systemic disease (weakness)
• Fractured coracoid bone
• Other flight bone fractures, e.g. humerus
• Damage to the leading edge of the wing (propatagium)
• Prepatagial cutaneous ulcerative disease. Commonly seen in chronic self-mutilating African greys. Too painful to extend wings (see *Skin Disorders*).

Findings on clinical examination

• Unable to fly
  • Flight feathers absent or abnormal
    • Young budgerigars – polyomavirus
    • Older psittacines – PBFD
    • Self-mutilation
  • Flight feathers normal – consider traumatic injuries, etc.
• One wing may be held lower than the other
• Obvious traumatic injury, i.e. swelling, compound fracture. Check especially the wing tips
• Non-painful, immobile swelling, i.e. old, healed fracture.

Investigations

1. Radiography
2. Routine haematology and biochemistry
3. Culture and sensitivity
4. Endoscopy
5. Ultrasonography.

Treatment/specific therapy

- Propatagial damage: make sure that the tendon that supports the leading edge of the propatagium – the tendon of *m. tensor propatagialis longa* is repaired if severed
- Prepatagial CUD, see *Skin Disorders*
- Fracture repair where feasible.

Systemic disorders

Some conditions present with a variety of clinical signs that may be quite non-specific. In some cases, this results from immunosuppression, leading to secondary invasion of a variety of pathogens, or because of multi-organ involvement.

Viral

- PBFD (especially young African grey parrots)
- Retrovirus (leukosis/sarcoma viruses).

Bacterial

- *Staphylococcus aureus* (Hermans et al 2000)
- *Chlamydophilosis.*

Fungal

- *Aspergillosis* (see *Lower Respiratory Tract Disorders*).

Protozoal

- Sarcocystis.

Nutritional (see *Nutritional Disorders*)
Neoplasia

- Infiltrative neoplasia secondary to retrovirus infection. Any organ can be affected (Girling 2003).

Other non-infectious problems

- Amyloidosis
- Iatrogenic steroid prescription.

Findings on clinical examination

- Generalized ill-health
- Non-specific clinical signs
- Weight loss
- Anorexia
- Sudden death
- Obvious neoplasia.

Investigations

1. Radiography
2. Routine haematology and biochemistry
   a. Young birds with PDFD often profoundly leucopaenic
3. Serology (sarcocystis, chlamydophila)
4. Cytology
5. Culture and sensitivity
6. Chlamydophila PCR
7. Endoscopy
8. Ultrasonography
9. Biopsy.

Treatment/specific therapy

- PBFD. Experimentally, avian interferon has been used to aid elimination of PBFD in viraemic, young African grey parrots (Stanford 2003). The dose used was 1 000 000 units of avian γ-interferon i.m. s.i.d. for 90 days. Mammalian (feline) interferon was found to be unsatisfactory. *Note* PBFD infection is oral, with virus entering via the bursa of Fabricius, which in psittacines can take over 18–20 months for normal involution to occur (Schmidt 1997). Any bird testing positive should be immediately quarantined and retested 60–90 days later to assess degree of immunity (Girling 2003). Immune birds will not be viraemic and so will test negative.
- Steroids: gradually wean off steroids. Always use antibiotic and antifungal medications in conjunction with steroids to counter the marked immunosuppressive effects of exogenous steroids.
- Sarcocystis (see *Lower Respiratory Tract Disorders*).

Neurological disorders

Viral

- Paramyxovirus
- PDD
- Pacheco's disease
- Adenovirus (budgerigars)
- West Nile virus (flavivirus).

Bacterial

- Chlamydophilosis
- Bacterial meningitis.

Fungal

- Fungal meningitis.

Protozoal

- Sarcocystis.

Parasitic

- Cerebrospinal angiostrongyliasis due to nematode larvae of *Angiostrongylus cantonensis* (Monks et al 2005).

Dietary

- Hypocalcaemia/hypovitaminosis D_3 (African grey parrots especially)
- Hypoglycaemia.

Neoplasia
Other non-infectious problems

- Zinc toxicity
- Other heavy metal poisoning, e.g. lead
- Other toxicities
- Fractures
- Renal disease including neoplasia (see *Differential Diagnosis of Polydipsia/polyuria*)
- Other neoplasia
- Idiopathic epilepsy
- Hepatic encephalopathy (severe liver disease)
- Cerebrovascular accidents (atherosclerosis).

Findings on clinical examination

- Weight loss
- Depression
- Torticollis and head tilt
- Ataxia; unable to balance or support itself; may continually hang on to cage bars with beak for support
- Collapse
- Tremors and seizures
- Gastrointestinal signs (undigested seeds, loose droppings) suggestive of paramyxovirus.

Investigations

1. Radiography
   a. Standing radiographs in the conscious bird for detection of ingested heavy metals
2. Routine haematology and biochemistry

a. Serum calcium, zinc and lead. Alternatively, hepatic lead and zinc concentrations can be assessed from biopsy; these are thought to be much more reliable

b. Blood levels can be indicative of zinc toxicity, but as with lead, there is no absolute correlation between blood zinc levels and clinical signs. As a general rule, if zinc levels are >32.0–50.0 µmol/L and there are consistent clinical signs (see *Neurological Disorders* and *Gastrointestinal Tract Disorders*), then zinc toxicity should be suspected

c. Blood lead levels <9.6 µmol/L

d. Significant levels often accompanied by an absolute or relative monocytosis

e. Blood glucose levels; also check out other biochemical parameters as can be linked with liver disease, infection and endocrinological disorders

3. Serology for PMV (paired samples)
4. Serology for West Nile virus (paired samples)
5. PCR for Pacheco's disease
6. Culture and sensitivity
7. Endoscopy
8. Ultrasonography
9. Biopsy (see above).

Management

• Supportive treatment
• Fluids may be best given initially per cloaca rather than by crop tube in case of ataxic/seizuring birds due to high risk of regurgitation and aspiration pneumonia.

Treatment/specific therapy

• Zinc/lead poisoning
  • Flushing out of the proventriculus and gizzard
  • Performed under GA with the bird intubated and held head down so as to prevent aspiration of stomach contents
  • Surgical removal of ingested metals
  • Sodium calcium-edetate at 35 mg/kg b.i.d. for 5 days, stop for 3–4 days then repeat. Continue until zinc levels fall
  • Dimercaptosuccinic acid (DMSA) at 30 mg/kg p.o. b.i.d. for 10 days or 5 days/week for 3–5 weeks
  • Penicillamine at 55 mg/kg p.o. b.i.d. for 7–14 days
• PMV – not direct treatment; supportive therapy only. Paramyxovirus A (Newcastle disease) is notifiable in the UK
• West Nile virus – supportive treatment only
• Sarcocystis (see *Lower Respiratory Tract Disorders*)
• Cerebrospinal angiostrongyliasis due to nematode larvae of *Angiostrongylus cantonensis*. Supportive treatment plus consider ivermectin 0.2 mg/kg p.o., s.c., i.m. or fenbendazole at 50 mg/kg
  • Guarded prognosis.

Ophthalmic disorders

Sclerocorneal (ciliary) muscles along with the sphincter and dilator muscles of the iris are striated muscles that are under voluntary control. Movement of pupil can be extensive and rapid and is used in intraspecific displays. Such irides appear unresponsive to light so the lack of pupillary response should not be misinterpreted.

Conjunctivitis can appear as part a 'syndrome' of URT signs, e.g. periorbital swelling, conjunctivitis or intraocular disease because of interconnectedness of local structures; the infraorbital sinus connects with the caudal nasal concha, the nasal cavity and the cervicocephalic air sac that covers the head and neck caudally and dorsally. It also has diverticulae extending dorsal, ventral and caudal to the eye, as well as into the maxillary bill and mandible.

Viral

- Cutaneous papillomatosis
- Avian pox
- Ulceration and crusting of the eyelid margin especially Amazon parrots
- Conjunctivitis in lovebirds
- Adenovirus (lovebirds).

Bacterial

- Bacterial conjunctivitis
- Chlamydophilosis
- Mycoplasmosis
- Infraorbital sinusitis (see under 'Sinusitis', above).

Fungal

- Sinusitis.

Protozoal

- Encephalitozoon hellem (Phalen et al 2006).

Nutritional

- Hypovitaminosis A.

Neoplasia

- Space-occupying lesions, esp. pituitary adenomas
- Ocular neoplasia.

Other non-infectious problems

- Congenital atresia of the eyelids
- Cataracts
- Dermoids (Leber & Bürge 1999)
- Trauma
- Vascular accidents or ischaemic necrosis (esp. budgerigars)
- Heavy metal poisoning
- Hepatic encephalopathy.

Findings on clinical examination

- May be unilateral or bilateral
- Keratoconjunctivitis
- Crusty skin lesions on the eyelids
- Corneal ulceration
- Cataracts – can be normal in an aged macaw (35–45 years old)
- Periocular and cutaneous pox lesions suggest avian pox. May also see respiratory signs
- Intraocular haemorrhage (usually linked to head trauma)
- Loss of vision
- Ptosis–Horner's syndrome secondary to presumed trauma has been described (Gancz et al 2005).

Investigations

1. Standard ophthalmic examination
2. Topical fluorescein to assess for corneal damage
3. Routine haematology and biochemistry
4. Culture and sensitivity
5. Application of topical sympathomimetic agents, e.g. phenylephrine; if it ameliorates ptosis, this indicates Horner's syndrome
6. Biopsy
   a. Eyelid margin
   b. Conjunctiva
7. Ultrasonography.

Management

1. Covering topical and systemic antibiosis
2. Vitamin A supplementation at 10 000–25 000 IU/300 g daily.

Treatment/specific therapy

- Bacterial conjunctivitis – topical and systemic antibiosis
- Chlamydophilosis – systemic enrofloxacin or doxycycline
- Mycoplasmosis
  - Tylosin at 1 mg/mL drinking water for a minimum of 21 days
  - Enrofloxacin at 5–10 mg/kg i.m. s.i.d.
  - Topical ofloxacin eye drops
  - Tetracyclines
- Congenital atresia – attempt surgical repair but poorly responsive; long-term steroids may slow healing closure of the defect
- Corneal ulceration

- 3rd eyelid flap. The course of the nictitans is latero-dorsally, as opposed to latero-ventrally in small mammals. This is of limited use because the nictitans is constantly in motion and sutures tend to tear through eventually
  - Tarsorrhaphy for 2–4 weeks
  - Topical antibiosis and ophthalmic anaesthesia if analgesia required
- Cataract
  - Surgical removal, ideally phacoemulsification. Hypermature cataracts can degenerate, triggering a phacolytic uveitis
- Encephalitozoon hellem
  - Co-trimoxazole at 30 mg/kg b.i.d. p.o. for at least 3 weeks
  - Albendazole at 10 mg/kg p.o. for 6 weeks
  - Fenbendazole at 10 mg/kg p.o. for 1 month.

Endocrine disorders

Neoplasia

- Pituitary gland adenoma (especially budgerigars and cockatiels).

Other non-infectious problems

- Hypothyroidism
- Adrenal disease.

Findings on clinical examination

- Polydipsia/polyuria (pituitary gland adenoma).

Investigations

1. Radiography
2. Routine haematology and biochemistry
   a. Adrenal disease not reported in psittacines
   b. Corticosterone, not cortisol, is responsive to ACTH stimulation
   c. Experimental ACTH stimulation gave the results shown in Table 5.11 (Zenoble et al 1985):
   d. Serum thyroid hormone levels (non-moulting birds) (see Table 5.12):

Table 5.11 Parrots and related species: Experimental ACTH stimulation

	Corticosterone concentrations (mg/dL) before ACTH administration	Corticosterone concentrations (mg/dL) 90 min after ACTH administration
Red-lored Amazon	1.06	4.86
Blue-fronted Amazon	2.09	10.58
African grey parrot	2.33	4.69

Table 5.12 Parrots and related species: Serum thyroid hormone levels (non-moulting birds)

Species	T4 concentration			
	nmol/L		µg/dL	
	Range	Mean	Range	Mean
African grey parrot (*Psittacus e. erithacus*)	2.02–5.06	3.18	0.16–0.39	0.25
Moluccan cockatoos (*Cacatua moluccensis*)	2.04–6.29	4.66	0.16–0.49	0.36
Blue-and-gold macaws (*Ara ararauna*)	2.02–4.85	3.36	0.16–0.38	0.26
Umbrella cockatoos (*Cacatua alba*)	2.86–5.96	4.61	0.22–0.46	0.36
Yellow-headed Amazon (*Amazona ochrocephala*)	2.49–7.68	5.05	0.19–0.60	0.39
Blue-fronted Amazon (*Amazona aestiva*)	3.17–142	23.8	0.25–11.0	1.85
Lovebirds (*Agapornis spp*)	–	–	0.2–4.3	–

Adapted from Greenacre et al (2001).

3. Culture and sensitivity
4. Endoscopy
5. Biopsy/necropsy
6. Ultrasonography.

Treatment/specific therapy

- Hypothyroidism
  - L-thyroxine at 0.02 mg/kg p.o. s.i.d. or b.i.d.
- Goitre in budgerigars, see *Respiratory Tract Disorders*

Differential diagnosis of polydipsia/polyuria

Viral

- Paramyxovirus
- Avian influenza
- Adenovirus
- Herpesvirus.

Bacterial

- Pancreatitis
- Pyelonephritis.

Fungal

Protozoal

- *Encephalitozoon hellem.*

Nutritional

- Hypovitaminosis A
- Hypocalcaemia.

Neoplasia

- Renal tubules.

Other non-infectious problems

- Renal gout
- Diabetes mellitus
- Hepatitis
- Heavy metal poisoning especially zinc
- Amyloidosis (renal; hepatic)
- Trauma
- Physiological – egg laying.

Findings on clinical examination

(See also *Assessment of Droppings*)
- Weight loss
- Weakness
- Polydipsia and accompanying polyuria
- Marked wetting of the bottom of the cage
- Haematuria (especially with heavy metal poisoning)
- Urate fraction may have a strong 'fishy' smell common in the white cockatoos with renal disease (Stockdale 2004)
- Large, pale-coloured droppings suggestive of pancreatic damage
- Unilateral or bilateral lameness caused by pressure of renal tumours on adjacent lumbo-sacral plexus
- White uric acid tophi may be visible under the skin of the legs and feet. Joints may be swollen (articular gout)
- Neurological signs, e.g. ataxia, generalized tremors.

Investigations

1. Haematology and biochemistry
   a. Uric acid is secreted by the proximal tubule of the avian kidney and so is not dependent upon GFR, so blood uric acids levels may only rise in chronic renal disease. It may also crystallize out as gout tophi in the kidneys (renal gout) or other organs (visceral gout) which again may limit otherwise high blood uric acid levels. Most waste nitrogen is excreted as uric acid, not urea so urea levels tend to be low. There may be a rise in phosphorus and a change in the calcium/phosphorus ratio. Therefore, need to assess multiple values to assess renal disease, i.e. uric acid, urea, creatinine, calcium and phosphorus

b. Biochemistry for hepatic disease
c. Blood glucose: normal range cockatiel 12.76–24.4 mmol/L. Diabetic birds >55.5 mmol/L
d. Plasma glucagon to insulin ratio 5–10 times higher than in mammals
2. Urinalysis
   a. Glycosuria and/or ketonuria suggestive of diabetes mellitus, but may indicate mixing of faeces with urine
   b. Microscopy: white blood cells or renal casts suggest urinary tract disease
3. Radiography
   a. Plain and contrast (i.v. pyelogram with iohexol)
4. Endoscopy and biopsy
   a. On endoscopy (or postmortem) uric acid may be seen deposited on certain viscera such as the pericardium or the serosal surface of the liver
5. Cloacal swabs
   a. Bacteriology: culture and sensitivity
   b. Encephalitozoon hellem (special staining required).

Management

• Supportive treatment including fluid therapy (see *Differential Diagnosis of Gastrointestinal Disorders*).

Treatment/specific therapy

• Anabolic steroids, e.g. nandrolone 1 mg/kg s.c. may be of some benefit. *Note* some birds react badly to such oily injections
• Benazepril at <0.1 mg/kg p.o. s.i.d. *Note* that some birds may be susceptible to the hypotensive side-effects of benazepril
• Gout
  • Allopurinol at 10 mg/kg or given in drinking water: a stock solution is made from a 100 mg tablet crushed in 10 mL water; 1.0 mL (10 mg) of this solution is added to 30 mL of fresh drinking water daily. Long-term use may trigger xanthine deposition.
• Diabetes mellitus
  • Exogenous commercially available insulin rarely of use (disease due to excess glucagon? Failure to respond to mammalian insulin?). A small number of cases may respond to insulin therapy at 0.1–2 IU/kg b.i.d. (Rees Davies 2001)
  • Where possible change the diet to a low fat, low carbohydrate, high fat pelleted diet
• Encephalitozoon hellem
  • Treatment protocols include
  • Co-trimoxazole at 30 mg/kg b.i.d. p.o. for at least 3 weeks
  • Albendazole at 10 mg/kg p.o. for 6 weeks
  • Fenbendazole at 10 mg/kg p.o. for 1 month
  • Also consider anticoccidials, e.g. toltrazuril
  • Many birds are asymptomatic excreters. Often linked with immunosuppressive disorders such as PBFD (Barton et al 2003). Potentially zoonotic
• Hypocalcaemia – see 'Dietary'
• Hypovitaminosis A – see 'Dietary'.

Reproductive disorders

A female parrot will lay an egg every 48 h. The egg spends around 80% of this time in the shell gland, where it is palpable. Therefore, it useful to know both the normal clutch size for that species, and the interval since the last egg laid.

Bacterial

- Egg peritonitis (coelomitis).

Nutritional

- Hypocalcaemia (see *Nutritional Disorders*).

Neoplasia

- Oviductal adenocarcinoma.

Other non-infectious problems

- Dystocia (egg-binding)
- Intra-coelomic mass
- Skeletal abnormality
- Oviductal torsion
- Superovulation/excessive egg production (especially cockatiels)
- Egg peritonitis (sterile).

Findings on clinical examination

- Bird may be depressed, slightly dyspnoeic
- A coelomic mass may be palpable
- Partial leg paralysis
- History of multiple egg production
- Distended, fluid-filled coelom. Dyspnoea (egg serositis).

Investigations

1. Haematology and biochemistry
   a. Serum calcium (including ionized calcium)
2. Radiography
3. Ultrasonography
4. Examination under general anaesthetic
5. Coelomic tap and aspiration (midline)
   a. Cytology
   b. Culture and sensitivity
6. Endoscopy.

Management

1. Place bird somewhere darkened, warm and of high humidity
2. Give calcium and/or vitamin D_3 supplementation.

Treatment/specific therapy

● Dystocia (egg binding)
  ● Calcium supplementation: 100–500 mg of calcium given orally per bird in cases of hypocalcaemia
  ● Oxytocin 1–5 IU/kg i.m. Use judiciously as this can have a marked effect on blood pressure
  ● Dinoprost (Lutalyse) 20–100 μg/kg i.m. as a single dose
  ● Apply prostaglandin E_2 gel to the cloaca to stimulate contractions
  ● Under general anaesthetic the egg may be manipulated out
  ● If the egg is thin-shelled, then aspiration of the contents through the abdominal wall with a syringe and hypodermic needle will allow collapse of the egg and its subsequent delivery
● Superovulation
  ● Medroxyprogesterone acetate to inhibit ovulation at 10 mg/kg – titrate dose as precisely as possible as overdose likely to trigger a severe polydipsia/polyuria
  ● Leuprolide, as a single injection to give a dose of 52–156 μg/kg per day leuprolide acetate reversibly inhibits egg-laying in cockatiels by up to 31 days
  ● Surgical ovariectomy
● Egg serositis
  ● Abdominocentesis to alleviate dyspnoea
  ● Antibiotics and NSAIDS to reduce inflammation
  ● Surgery for abdominal lavage.

Growth and weaning

Psittacines (and many passerines) have altricial young, and display a characteristic growth curve. This curve rises rapidly to a peak body weight just before the time of weaning, then falls slightly to the weaning weight, before continuing up to the eventual adult weight.

Cockatiels younger than 1 week are unable to mobilize body tissues in the face of deficiencies and cockatiel chicks subjected to a low-protein diet fail to lose weight, maintaining their weight until death. Because of the expected growth curve, and this failure to lose weight in spite of nutritional problems, daily weighing is strongly recommended to monitor the chick's condition. Chicks should typically gain about 17% body weight daily in the first 7 days; all chicks should have doubled their body weight by day 7.

Psittacine chicks are ectothermic on hatching. Correct environmental temperatures are as follows:

Correct environmental temperatures for chicks

1. Newly hatched: 33.3–34.4°C.
2. Unfeathered: 32.2–33.3°C.
3. Partially feathered: 29.4–32.2°C.
4. Fully feathered: 23.9–26.7°C.
5. Weaned: 20.0–23.9°C.

- Retained yolk sac
  - Often accompanies umbilical infection
  - Debridement of infected material and antibiosis
  - Aspiration of yolk sac material
  - Surgical resection of yolk sac
- Failure to gain weight
  - Many possible problems but likely to be bacterial or fungal (Candida) infection
  - Start on Nystatin at 300 000 IU/kg p.o. b.i.d. for 10 days and a broad-spectrum antibiotic
  - May need crop tubing – switch from normal hand-rearing formula to a rehydrating/critical care formulation. This will need to be given more frequently to maintain the energy input that the chick requires. After 24 h, begin to introduce the hand-rearing formula back into the diet over a period or 2–3 days
  - Reassess environmental conditions
- Crop diseases of chicks – see *Differential Diagnosis for Vomiting/Regurgitation/Dysphagia*
- Hepatic lipidosis
  - Chicks fed on a too high-fat diet
  - Respiratory distress
  - Hepatomegaly
  - Reduce intake of food; reduce fat content of food; add lactulose to diet
  - Parenteral fluid administration
- Hepatic haematoma
  - Usually following trauma, e.g. dropping the chick
  - Often hepatic lipidosis concurrent (enlarged, friable liver)
  - Supportive treatment. Poor prognosis.

References

Barton C E, Phalen D N, Snowden K F 2003 Prevalence of microsporidian spores shed by asymptomatic lovebirds: evidence for a potential emerging zoonosis. J Avian Med Surg 17(4):197–202

Bavelaar F J, Beynen A C 2003 Plasma cholesterol concentrations in African grey parrots fed diets containing psyllium. J Appl Res Vet Med 1:97–104

Bavelaar F J, van der Kuilen J, Hovenier R et al 2005 Plasma lipids and fatty acid composition in parrots in relation to the intake of α-linolenic acid from two feed mixtures. J Anim Physiol Anim Nutr 89:359–366

Berrocal A 2004 Cryptococcal granulomatous dermatitis in an African parrot. ESVD and ACVD. Vet Dermatol 15(Suppl 1):68

Casares M, Enders F, Montoya J A 2000 Comparative electrocardiography in four species of Macaws (Genera Anodorhynchus and Ara). J Vet Med 47(5):277–281

De Voe, R S, Trogdon M, Flammer K 2004 Preliminary assessment of the effect of diet and L-carnitine supplementation on lipoma size and body weight in budgerigars (Melopsittacus undultatus). J Avian Med Surg 18(1):12–18

Diaz-Figueroa O, Garner M M, Tulley T N 2004 What is your diagnosis? J Avian Med Surg 18(1):51–53

Diaz-Figueroa O, Garner M M, Tulley T N 2005 What is your diagnosis? J Avian Med Surg 19(4):313–315 oneley R J T, Miller R I, Fanning T E 2007 Proventricular dilatation disease: an emerging exotic disease of parrots in Australia. Aust Vet J 85:119–123

Doolan M 1994 Adriamycin chemotherapy in a blue-front Amazon with osteosarcoma. Proc Annu Conf Assoc Avian Vet 88–91

Ferrer L, Ramis A, Fernández, J et al 1997 Granulomatous dermatitis caused by Mycobacterium genavense in two psittacine birds. Vet Dermatol 8:213–219

Flammer K, Trogdon M T, Papich M 2003 Assessment of plasma concentrations of doxycycline in budgerigars fed medicated seed or water. J Am Vet Med Assoc 223:993–998

France M 1993 Chemotherapy treatment of lymphosarcoma in a Moluccan cockatoo. Proc Annu Conf Assoc Avian Vet 15–19

Gancz A Y, Malka S, Sandmeyer L et al 2005 Horner's syndrome in a red-bellied parrot (Poicephalus rufiventris). J Avian Med Surg 19(1):3–34

Garner J P, Meehan C L, Famula T R et al 2005 Genetic, environmental, and neighbor effects on the severity of stereotypies and feather picking in orange-winged Amazon parrots (Amazona amazonica): An epidemiological study. Appl Anim Behav Sci 96(1–2):153–168

Girling S 2003 Diagnosis and management of viral diseases in psittacine birds. In Practice 25:396–407

Girling S 2004 Diseases of the digestive tract of psittacine birds. In Practice 26:146–153

Graham J E, Tell L A, Lamm M G et al 2004 Megacloaca in a Moluccan Cockatoo (Cacatua moluccensis). J Avian Med Surg 18(1):41–49

Greenacre C B, Young D W, Behrend E N et al 2001 Validation of a novel high-sensitivity radioimmunoassay procedure for measurement of total thyroxine concentration in psittacine birds and snakes. Am J Vet Res 62(11):1750–1754

Gregory C R, Latimer K S, Campagnoli R P et al 1996 Histologic evaluation of the crop for diagnosis of proventricular dilatation syndrome in psittacine bird. J Vet Diagn Invest 8:70–80

Grund C H, Werner O, Gelderblom H R et al 2002 Avian paramyxovirus serotype 1 isolates from the spinal cord of parrots display a very low virulence. J Vet Med B Infect Dis Vet Public Health 49(9):445–451

Hanley C S, Wilson G H, Latimer K S et al 2005 Interclavicular haemangiosarcoma in a double yellow-headed Amazon parrot (Amazona ochrocephala oratrix). J Avian Med Surg 19(2):130–137

Harcourt-Brown N H 1986 Diseases of birds in quarantine, with special reference to the treatment of Salmonella typhimurium by vaccination: a novel technique. Proc Vet Zoo Soc London

Harcourt-Brown N 2004 Development of the skeleton and feathers of dusky parrots (Pionus fuscus) in relation to their behaviour. Vet Rec 154:42–48

Hermans K, Devriese L A, De Herdt P et al 2000 Staphylococcus aureus infections in psittacine birds. Avian Pathol 29:411–415

Klaphake E, Beazley-Keane S L, Jones M et al 2006 Multisite integumentary squamous cell carcinoma in an African grey parrot (Psittacus erithacus erithacus). Vet Rec 158:593–596

Krautwald-Junghanns M, Braun S, Pees M et al 2004 Research on the anatomy and pathology of the psittacine heart. J Avian Med Surg 18(1):2–11

Leber A C, Bürge T 1999 A dermoid of the eye in a blue-fronted Amazon parrot (Amazona aestiva). Vet Ophthalmol 2:133–135

Lloyd C 2003 Control of nematode infections in captive birds 2003. In Practice 25:198–206

Malley D 1996 Handling and clinical examination of psittacine birds. In Practice 18:30, 311

Manucy T K, Bennet R A, Greenacre C B et al 1998. Squamous cell carcinoma of the beak in a Buffon's macaw (Ara ambigua). J Avian Med Surg 12:158–166

Meehan C L, Millam J R, Mench J A 2003a Foraging opportunity and increased physical complexity both prevent and reduce psychogenic feather picking by young Amazon parrots. Appl Anim Behav Sci 80:71–85

Meehan C L, Garner J P, Mench J A 2003b Isosexual pair housing improves the welfare of young Amazon parrots. Appl Anim Behav Sci 81:73–88

Meehan C L, Garner J P, Mench J A 2004 Environmental enrichment and development of cage stereotypy in orange-winged Amazon parrots (Amazona amazonica) Dev Psychobiol 44:209–218

Monks D J, Carlisle M S, Carrigan M et al 2005 Angiostrongylus cantonensis. As a cause of cerebrospinal disease in a yellow-tailed black cockatoo (Calyptorhynchus funereus) and two tawny Frogmouths (Podargus strigoides). J Avian Med Surg 29(4):289–293

Musulin S E, Adin D B 2006 Vet Med Today: ECG of the Month. J Am Vet Med Assoc 229 (4):505–507

Oglesbee B L, Lehmkuhl L 2001 Congestive heart failure associated with myxomatous degeneration of the left atrioventricular valve in a parakeet. J Am Vet Med Assoc 218 (3):360, 376–380

Pees M, Schmidt V, Coles B et al 2006 Diagnosis and long-term therapy of a right-sided heart failure in a yellow-crowned Amazon (Amazona ochrocephala). Vet Rec 158:445–447

Phalen D N, Logan, K S, Snowden K F 2006 Encephalitozoon hellem infection as the cause of a unilateral chronic keratoconjunctivitis in an umbrella cockatoo (Cacatua alba). Vet Ophthalmol 9:59–63

Philbey A W, Andrew P L, Gestier A W et al 2002 Spironucleosis in Australian king parrots (Alisterus scapularis) Aust Vet J 80(3):154–160

Pizarro M, Höfle U, Rodríguez-Bertos A et al 2005 Ulcerative enteritis (Quail disease) in Lories. Avian Dis 49:606–608

Polo F J, Peinado V I, Viscor G et al 1998 Hematologic and plasma chemistry values in captive psittacine birds. Avian Dis 42:523–535

Preziosi D E, Morris D O, Johnston M S et al 2006 Distribution of Malassezia organisms on the skin of unaffected psittacine birds and psittacine birds with feather-destructive behavior. J Am Vet Med Assoc 228:216–221

Rees Davies R 2001 Polyuria/polydipsia in parrots. UK VET 6(5):75–80

Rupiper D J, Carpenter J W, Mashima T Y 2000 Formulary. In: Olsen G H, Orosz S E (eds) Manual of avian medicine. Mosby, Philadelphia, p 560

Schmidt R E 1997 Immune system. In: Altman R B, Clubb S L. Dorrenstein G M et al. (eds) Avian medicine and surgery. Saunders, Philadelphia, p 645–652

Stanford M. 2003 Use of interferon to treat circovirus infection in grey parrots. Proceedings of the Autumn Meeting, British/Veterinary Zoological Society, p 35–36

Stockdale B 2004 Detecting avian malnutrition –part 2. Veterinary Times, 2nd August

Straub J, Pees M, Krautwald-Junghanns M 2002 Measurement of the cardiac silhouette in psittacines. J Am Vet Med Assoc 221(1):76–79

Torregrossa A, Puschner B, Tell L et al 2005 Circulating concentrations of vitamins A and E in captive psittacine birds. J Avian Med Surg 19(3):225–229

Van Hoek C S, King C E 1997 Causation and influence of environmental enrichment on feather picking of the crimson bellied conure (Pyrrhura perlata perlata). Zoo Biol 16:161–172

rstappen F A L M, Dorrestein G M 2005 Aspergillosis in amazon parrots after corticosteroid therapy for smoke-inhalation injury. J Avian Med Surg 19(2):138–141

Wade L 2004 Herbal therapy for liver disease: milk thistle (Silybum marianum). AAV
Newsletter and Clinical forum, March–May

Werquin G J D L, De Cock K J S, Ghysels P G C 2005 Comparison of the nutrient analysis
and calorific density of 30 commercial seed mixtures (in toto and dehulled) with 27
commercial diets for parrots. J Anim Physiol Anim Nutr 89:215–221

Wolf P, Rabehl N, Kamphues J 2003. Investigations on feathering, feather growth and
potential influences of nutrient supply on feather's regrowth in small pet birds (canaries,
budgerigars and lovebirds). J Anim Physiol Anim Nutr 87:134–141

Zandvliet M M J M, Dorrstein G M, van der Hage M 2001 Chronic pulmonary interstitial
fibrosis in Amazon parrots. Avian Pathol 30:517–524

Zenoble R D, Kemppainen R J, Young D W et al 1985 Endocrine responses of healthy parrots to ACTH and thyroid stimulating hormone. J Am Vet Med Assoc 187(11):1116–
1118

CHAPTER

6

Songbirds and softbills

The passerines (songbirds) and softbills are the other major groups of birds kept for ornamental purposes apart from psittacines, rather than utility species such as pigeons and birds of prey. There is inevitably an overlap between the disorders that occur in psittacines and those that occur in the passerines and softbills. This chapter deals with those diseases and disorders specific to various passerines and softbills, but diagnostic options should be considered in conjunction with the appropriate psittacine section, in *Parrots and Related Species*.

Commonly kept species include:

- Mynahs including the greater Indian hill mynah (*Gracula religiosa intermedia*), the lesser Indian hill mynah (*Gracula religiosa indica*) and the Bali or Rothschild mynah (*Leucopsar rothschildi*)
- Canaries (*Serinus spp*)
- Estrildidae finches including the waxbills (including the zebra finch *Poephila guttata*), parrot-finches (*Erythrura spp* and *Chloebia spp*) and mannikins (*Lonchura spp*)
- Toucans (e.g. the Toco toucan *Ramphastos toco*) and other Ramphastids.

Commonly encountered species are listed in Table 6.1.

Nursing care

(see *Parrots and Related Species*).

Analgesia and anaesthesia

(see *Parrots and Related Species*).

Skin disorders

Pruritus

- Ectoparasites (see below).

Alopecia

- Feather loss around head (toxoplasmosis)
- Feather picking – rarely self-mutilation; usually by other birds, especially zebra finches. May indicate iron storage disease in toucans
- Lice (canaries)
- Dermatomycosis (*Trichophyton spp* and *Microsporum spp*).

246

Table 6.1 Commonly encountered songbirds and softbills: Key facts

	Canary	Greater Indian hill mynah	Zebra finch	Toco toucan
Average life span (years)	5–15	12+	<17	6+
Weight (g)	18–30	210–270	10–16	450–500
Sexing	Young males will begin singing (sub-songs) at some point between weaning and first moult	Female wattles are smaller than those of the male	The beak is darker red in the male and large orange cheek spots	DNA; surgical sexing
Estimating age		<6–8 month-old-young have dull feathering plus poorly developed head wattles. The wattles take up to 12 months to develop	Young birds (<6 weeks) have black beaks and pronounced black 'tear line' running down from the eye (loses a first moult at 12 weeks old). The white variety lacks this pattern	
Normal clutch size	4–5	3–4	4–6	2–4
Incubation (days)	13–14	14	12.5–16	15–16

Scaling and crusting
- Dermatomycosis (*Trichophyton spp* and *Microsporum spp*).

Nodules and non-healing wounds
- Feather cysts (especially canaries)
- Intracutaneous keratinizing epithelioma has been described in the mynah bird (Rodríguez et al 2006)
- Papilloma virus – wart-like growths of the skin on the feet and legs of European finches
- Abscessation – typically due to *Staphylococci* and *Streptococci*
- Bumblefoot – typically chronic infection and abscessation of the feet, especially the plantar surfaces
- Head and beak lesions in toucans often the result of intraspecific aggression.

Changes in pigmentation
- Erysipelothrix (see 'Skin disorders in psittacines')
- Altered feather colouring
  - Nutritional
  - Hepatic disease.

Ectoparasites

- Flies. Hippoboscids (flat flies/louse flies) occasionally encountered especially with aviary birds. Can transmit haemoparasites such as *Haemoproteus* and *Leukocytozoon*, as well as transfer mites and lice between individuals
- Lice. Can reach significant numbers on debilitated birds. Particularly induce baldness in canaries secondary to irritation
- Ticks. Occasionally on new imports. Sudden death associated with tick attachment to head. Suggested aetiologies include hypersensitivity reactions, toxin injection or a tick-borne infection. Can also transmit other diseases such as haemoprotozoa, *Borrelia spp* and louping-ill.
- Red mite *Dermanyssus avium* and other species
- Northern fowl mite *Ornithonyssus sylviarum*
- Feather mites. Found between the barbs on the ventral surfaces of feathers. Often niche specific
- Quill mites such as *Syringophilus*, *Dermatoglyphus* and *Picobia spp.* Found inside quills. *Harpirhynchus* mites may induce hyperkeratotic epidermal cysts
- Skin mites
- Cnemidocoptid mites. Common one encountered is *Cnemidocoptes pilae* (scaley face/scaley leg).

Dermatitis

- Commensal bacterial numbers on the skin of birds are considered to be lower than those found on mammals
- Bacterial
  - *Staphylococci*
  - Streptococci
- Fungal
  - Candida.

Burns

Neoplasia

- Neoplastic-like lesions described in masked bullfinch (*Pyrrhula erythaca*) due to pox virus (Dorrestein et al 1993).

Non-cutaneous findings on clinical examination

- Respiratory distress, PCV <30% (red mites).

Investigations

1. Aseptic collection of samples for bacteriology/mycology
2. Cytology
3. Radiography. A standing view using horizontal beam is useful for detecting metallic foreign bodies in the conscious bird, otherwise lateral and VD views, under GA, are required for meaningful radiography
4. Endoscopy
5. Serology for *Aspergillus* antigen and *Chlamydophila* antigen
6. Fresh faecal samples for parasitic examination (*Giardia*, nematode eggs)

a. Smears can be dried and stained (Gram stain for bacterial assessment, Romanowsky stains for cytology)
7. Bulk faecal samples (collected over 3–5 days) can be submitted for *Chlamydophila* PCR
8. Diagnostic imaging including radiography and endoscopy
9. Biopsy.

Management

1. Optimize diet including the use of multivitamin supplements; reducing seed intake and increasing fruit and/or insect consumption where appropriate for the species
2. Where there is significant feather loss, consider supplementary heating to counter loss of insulation
3. Covering broad-spectrum antibiotics may be useful if there are obvious skin lesions
4. If pruritic consider analgesia – meloxicam (Metacam oral suspension) at 1 drop/500 g body weight twice daily. Do not use steroids
5. Avoid the use of collars except in extreme situations as these can be extremely stressful to the bird and can interfere with many normal behaviours including feeding, flight and climbing.

Treatment/specific therapy

● Ticks
  ● Ivermectin or fipronil. Remove ticks manually where possible
● Red mite and other species
  ● Ivermectin at 0.2 mg/kg p.o., s.c. or i.m. Light dusting with pyrethrin powder. Treat environment in case of red mite; painting woodwork may 'seal in' mites. *Note* some Estrilid finches appear hypersensitive to pyrethrin
● Quill mites
  ● Apply topical cis-permethrin powder (e.g. Harker's Louse Powder) or fipronil (Frontline) spray (applied to cotton wool and wiped on to bird). Beware hypothermia in small birds due to evaporation of carrier
● Cnemidocoptid mites, e.g. *Cnemidocoptes pilae*
  ● Ivermectin at 0.2 mg/kg p.o., s.c. or i.m. A small drop may be applied topically over the jugular vein or on to the back of the neck and seems to work well. Injection is not recommended in birds weighing <500 g due to problems with toxicity. Treat *Harpirhynchid*, *Epidermoptid* and *Cheyletiellid* mites as for *Cnemidocoptid* mites
● Feather cysts
  ● Manual expression with appropriate analgesia provides only temporary relief; ideally require surgical removal
● Abscesses
  ● Surgical removal
● Bumblefoot
  ● Usually requires surgical intervention; bird may need supportive dressing on affected foot to prevent reinfection of surgical site. If the condition is unilateral, be aware of pressure sores and other sequelae affecting the good leg due to bird shifting weight on to it

- Candidiasis
  - Amphotericin B at 1.5 mg/kg i.v. b.i.d. for 3–7 days, plus a topical antimycotic, e.g. clotrimazole
- Dermatomycosis (*Trichophyton spp* and *Microsporum spp*). Topical ketoconazole preparation and systemic antimycotic, e.g. itraconazole at 5 mg/kg s.i.d. p.o.
- Burns.
  - Treat as for other species, e.g. keep moist; may help to apply topical amorphous hydrogel dressings to encourage secondary healing, e.g. IntraSite Gel (Smith and Nephew Healthcare Ltd.); covering antibiosis; fluid therapy.

Systemic disorders

Bacterial

- Septicaemia.

Fungal

- *Aspergillosis.*

Neoplasia

Other non-infectious problems

- Carbon monoxide poisoning
- Polytetrafluoroethane (PTFE) toxicity from overheating of Teflon®
- Heavy metal poisoning.

Findings on clinical examination

- Non-specific signs (see *Consultation and Handling,* in *Parrots and Related Species*)
- Severe respiratory signs (carbon monoxide toxicity, PTFE toxicity)
- Vomiting, polyuria, possible CNS signs (heavy metal poisoning).

Investigations

1. Haematology and biochemistry
   a. Blood zinc or lead levels; liver heavy metal levels (biopsy or postmortem)
2. Postmortem
   a. Haemorrhagic, oedematous lungs (PTFE poisoning).

Treatment/specific therapy

- PTFE poisoning. If still alive (most birds die very quickly) remove from source of toxicity. NSAIDs, e.g. meloxicam, may be useful in the control of the pulmonary inflammation that is caused
- Zinc/lead poisoning
  - Sodium calcium edetate at 20–50 mg/kg b.i.d. given daily for 7 days, stopped for 7 days then repeated. This continues until blood levels fall to normal.

Respiratory tract disorders

Nasal tract

Rhinitis (see also 'Rhinitis', in *Parrots and Related Species*).

Viral

• Avian pox (see below).

Differential diagnoses for respiratory disorders

Viral

• Avian pox (septicaemic form, esp. canaries and other *Serinus* species)
• Coronavirus (tracheitis in canaries)
• Influenza virus A.

Bacterial

• *Pasteurella multocida*
• Staphylococci
• Streptococci
• Salmonellosis
• *Klebsiella pneumoniae*
• *Yersinia pseudotuberculosis* (esp. toucans and mynahs)
• *Aeromonas spp* and *Pseudomonas spp*
• Mycobacteriosis.

Fungal

• *Aspergillosis* (esp. mynahs)
• *Enterococcus faecalis*
• Candida
• Mucormycosis.

Protozoal

• Toxoplasmosis
• Trichomonas
• Sarcocystis.

Parasitic

• Blood-sucking mites (anaemia)
• *Sternostoma tracheacolum* (air sac mites) (esp. Australian finches)
• *Cytodites nudus* mites (also in respiratory tract). Rare
• Syngamus trachea (esp. mynahs and starlings).

Nutritional

• Hypovitaminosis A (see *Nutritional Disorders*).

Neoplasia

• Coelomic neoplasia, e.g. hepatic.

Other non-infectious problems

* Egg coelomitis
* Anaemia (see *Cardiovascular and Haematological Disorders*).

Findings on clinical examination

* Dyspnoea
* Tachypnoea
* Head swinging and neck stretching. Forward-leaning and extended neck strongly suggests tracheal obstruction
* Coughing occasionally encountered, but is uncommon
* Tail pumping
* Increased recovery time/exercise intolerance
* Increased inspiratory sounds often associated with upper respiratory tract disease
* Increased expiratory sounds often associated with lower respiratory tract disease
* Abdomen may be distended (fluid, neoplasia, haemorrhage)
* Subcutaneous air-filled swelling; may vary in size (ruptured air sac)
* Scabs and pox lesions on eyelids; commissure of mouth and skin. Diphtheritic lesions (Avipox)
* CNS signs, iridocyclitis and other ocular signs (toxoplasmosis)
* Loss of voice; abnormal squeaking or wheezing sounds (sternostomosis, aspergillosis)
* Other, non-respiratory signs
    * Regurgitation (trichomoniasis)
    * Debilitation and death. High mortality of 20–100%. Usually due to septicaemia (avian pox, *Yersinia pseudotuberculosis* (canaries and finches), pasteurellosis (mynahs).

Investigations

1. Transillumination of trachea (air sac mites)
2. Routine haematology and biochemistry
    a. Anaemia (blood sucking mites, anaemia of chronic illness)
3. Serology for *Chlamydophila*
4. Radiography
5. Endoscopy
    a. Culture of aseptically collected samples
6. Nasal discharge
    a. Tracheal wash
    b. Cytology of above samples
7. Faecal samples
    a. Modified Ziehl–Neelsen staining or PCR for mycobacteriosis
8. *Chlamydophila* PCR (collect bulk faecal samples over 5 days to identify intermittent excreters)
9. Biopsy
10. Postmortem
    a. Pneumonia
    b. Hepatomegaly with miliary abscessation; splenomegaly (*Yersinia pseudotuberculosis*, salmonellosis).

Management

1. Improve hygiene. Aeromonad and pseudomonad air sac infections have been associated with infected sprays or misters
2. General supportive care
3. Milk thistle (*Silybum marianum*) is hepatoprotectant. Dose at 4–15 mg/kg b.i.d. or t.i.d.

Treatment/specific therapy

- Avian pox – supportive care. Avoid access to blood-sucking insects (carriers). May also be spread by contact with infected blood; rarely in contaminated food and drinking water. Vaccination.
- Yersiniosis – appropriate antibiotics. Source of infection is often faecal contamination from wild birds and rodents
- Salmonellosis. Treatment as for *Yersinia*. Zoonotic potential
- Mycobacteriosis. Significant potential zoonosis so treatment rarely undertaken
- Sarcocystis
  - Treat with trimethoprim sulphadiazine (30 mg/kg s.i.d.) plus pyrimethamine 0.5–1.0 mg/kg p.o. b.i.d. for 30 days. May need to supplement with folic acid
  - The Virginia opossum is the primary host; cockroaches can act as paratenic hosts
- *Syngamus spp.* Indirect life cycle using earthworms, slugs and snails. Treat with fenbendazole at 50 mg/kg p.o. as a one off dose.
- *Sternostoma tracheacolum* (air sac mites)
  - Ivermectin at 0.1% ivermectin in propylene glycol applied as 1 drop to skin over pectoral musculature or lateral to thoracic inlet.

Cardiovascular and haematological disorders

Viral

- Polyoma-like virus (finches).

Bacterial

- Endocarditis.

Fungal

- Endocarditis.

Protozoal

- *Plasmodium spp*
- *Haemoproteus spp*
- *Leukocytozoon spp*
- *Trypanosoma spp.*

Parasitic

- *Schistosoma spp*
- Blood-sucking mites.

Neoplasia

Other non-infectious problems

- Congestive heart failure
- Atherosclerosis
- Endocardiosis.

Findings on clinical examination

- Pale mucous membranes (anaemia – if severe may present similar to respiratory disease)
- Exercise intolerance
- Weight loss
- Vague signs of ill-health.

Investigations

1. Auscultation
   a. Abnormal heart sounds
   b. Abnormal cardiac rhythms
2. Routine haematology and biochemistry
   a. Demonstration of parasites on stained smear
   b. Anaemia (*Plasmodium*, blood-sucking mites)
3. Radiography
   a. Hepatomegaly
4. Endoscopy
5. Ultrasonography and Doppler ultrasound
6. Electrocardiogram
7. Postmortem
   a. Myocarditis along with liver abnormalities (polyoma-like virus)
   b. Splenomegaly (*Plasmodium*)
   c. Lung congestion (*Plasmodium*).

Management

1. Reduce stress
2. Remove high perches
3. Supply oxygen.

Treatment/specific therapy

- *Plasmodium, Haemoproteus*
  - Chloroquine at 250 mg/120 mL fresh drinking water, daily for 14 days)
  - Pyrimethamine 0.5 mg/kg b.i.d. p.o. or in feed at 100 mg/kg of food. May need to supplement with folic acid
  - Control of vectors: mosquitos (*Plasmodium*); hippoboscid flies, biting midges or tabanids (*Haemoproteus*)

Leukocytozoon
- May be asymptomatic, but can be fatal with acute hepatitis, renal tubular necrosis and myocardial haemorrhage
- Chronic cases may present with wasting and vomiting
- Pyrimethamine 0.5 mg/kg b.i.d. p.o. or in feed at 100 mg/kg of food may be effective. May need to supplement with folic acid
- Avoid exposure to vectors such as blackflies (*Simulium spp*) or *Culicoides/hippoboscids*
- *Trypanosoma spp*
  - Treatment usually not required. Avoid exposure to vectors (hippoboscid flies, red mites, blackflies (*Simulium spp*) and mosquitos
- *Schistosoma spp* – praziquantel at 10 mg/kg
- Congestive heart failure. Attempt treatment as for other species
  - Furosemide at 0.5–2.0 mg/kg i.m. or s.c. b.i.d. or 5 mg/100 mL drinking water, fresh daily
  - Digoxin 0.02 mg/kg p.o. s.i.d.
  - Aminophylline 4.0 mg/kg p.o. or i.m. b.i.d.

Neurological disorders

Viral
- Paramyxovirus
- Adeno-like virus infection (canaries).

Bacterial
- Mycobacteriosis.

Fungal
- Mucormycosis.

Protozoal
- A toxoplasmosis (*Isospora serini*) (young canaries 2–9 months old).

Neoplasia

Other non-infectious problems
- Middle-ear disease
- Heavy metal poisoning especially zinc from galvanized caging, baths or drinking receptacles
- Haemochromatosis
- Convulsions similar to epileptic seizures (mynahs).

Findings on clinical examination

- Central nervous signs such as torticollis and opisthotonus
- Rhythmic nystagmus-like rotations of the head (middle-ear disease)
- Collapse
- Depression

- Anorexia
- Weight loss
- Green diarrhoea (paramyxovirus)
- Dark spot visible in 'abdominal' body wall (hepatomegaly due to a toxoplasmosis)
- Sudden death (paramyxovirus).

Investigations

1. Routine haematology and biochemistry
2. Radiography
3. Postmortem examination
4. Gram stain contents of any lesions
5. Modified Ziehl–Neelsen staining or PCR for mycobacteriosis
6. Histopathology.

Management

- Keep in quiet, darkened environment. Fluids may be given per cloaca if there is a risk of aspiration.

Treatment/specific therapy

- Zinc/lead poisoning
  - Sodium calcium edetate at 20–50 mg/kg b.i.d. given daily for 7 days, stopped for 7 days then repeated. This continues until blood levels fall to normal
- Viral infections: supportive treatment only. Give warmth, covering antibiotics and fluids if necessary
  - Mynahs infected with Newcastle disease excrete virus for 12–119 days post-infection (Panigrahy & Senne 1991)
- Mycobacteriosis
  - Potential zoonosis. Consider euthanasia
  - Two suggested treatment regimes (Rupiper et al 2000) are:
    - Ethambutol (200 mg), isoniazid (200 mg) and rifampin (300 mg) all crushed together and mixed with 10 mL of a simple syrup. This is administered s.i.d. according to Table 6.2
    - Combination therapy of:
      - Ethambutol (10 mg/kg p.o. b.i.d.)
      - Streptomycin (30 mg/kg i.m. b.i.d.)
      - Rifampin (15 mg/kg p.o. b.i.d.)

Table 6.2 Volumes required for suggested treatment regime for mycobacteriosis

Bird weight (g)	Volume of mixture (mL)
<100	0.1
100–250	0.2
250–500	0.3
500–1000	0.4

Mucormycosis. Usually diagnosed on postmortem. Linked to feeding damp, germinated seeds

- A toxoplasmosis
  - Toltrazuril at 5.0 mg in 100 mL drinking water for 2 days. Repeat after 12 days
  - Prevention of re-infection by removing access to their droppings. Clean flights regularly. Consider a false wire bottom to the flight
- Convulsions
  - Consider treatment initially with diazepam 0.5–1.0 mg/kg i.v. or i.m.
  - Phenobarbital 1.0–5.0 mg/kg p.o., i.m. i.v. b.i.d.

Ophthalmic disorders

Conjunctivitis can appear as part a 'syndrome' of URT signs, e.g. periorbital swelling, conjunctivitis or intraocular disease because of interconnectedness of local structures; the infraorbital sinus connects with the caudal nasal concha, the nasal cavity and the cervicocephalic air sac that covers the head and neck caudally and dorsally. It also has diverticulae extending dorsal, ventral and caudal to the eye, as well as into the maxillary bill and mandible.

Viral
- Pox virus (mynahs)
- Herpesvirus (esp. Australian and African finches).

Bacterial
- Mycoplasmosis
- Chlamydophilosis
- Nocardia.

Fungal
- Candida.

Protozoal
- Toxoplasmosis (Gibbens et al 1997).

Dietary
- Hypovitaminosis A (see *Nutritional Disorders*).

Neoplasia

Other non-infectious problems
- Trauma.

Findings on clinical examination

- Periocular and cutaneous pox lesions suggest avian pox. May also see respiratory signs
- Keratitis, conjunctivitis, distortion and depigmentation of eyelids (poxvirus in young mynahs)
- May be unilateral or bilateral
- Keratoconjunctivitis

- Crusty skin lesions on the eyelids
- Corneal ulceration (*Candida* keratitis in toucans, trauma)
- Cataracts
- Intra-ocular haemorrhage (usually linked to head trauma)
- Loss of vision
- Sunken eyes – can be unilateral or bilateral (toxoplasmosis). There may be feather loss around the head.

Investigations

1. Topical fluorescein to assess for corneal damage
2. Routine haematology and biochemistry
3. Serology (toxoplasma)
4. Culture and sensitivity
5. Cytology
6. PCR for chlamydophila
7. Biopsy
   a. Eyelid margin
   b. Conjunctiva
8. Ultrasonography
9. Necropsy and histopathology.

Treatment/specific therapy

- Toxoplasmosis
  - Potentiated sulphonamides
- Chlamydophilosis
  - Enrofloxacin (5.0 mg/kg p.o., i.m.)
  - Doxycycline (25–50 mg/kg p.o. s.i.d.) or 1.0 g/kg soft feed
- Mycoplasmosis
  - Tylosin at 1 mg/mL drinking water for a minimum of 21 days
  - Enrofloxacin 5.0 mg/kg p.o., i.m.
  - Topical ofloxacin ophthalmic drops
  - Tetracyclines
  - Doxycycline (as above)
- Nocardiosis. Blindness and lameness described in mynahs (Panigrahy & Senne 1991), along with postmortem signs of bacteraemic spread
- Candidiasis
  - Amphotericin B at 1.5 mg/kg i.v. b.i.d. for 3–7 days, plus a topical antimycotic, e.g. clotrimazole
- Trauma
  - As for other species.

Gastrointestinal tract disorders

Bacterial

- *E. coli* (normal cloacal inhabitant of toucans)
- *Citrobacter spp* (esp. weaver finches and waxbills)

- *Salmonella spp*
- *Campylobacter*
- *Erysipelothrix insidiosa* (Erysipelas)
- Chlamydophilosis
- Megabacteriosis (*Macrorhabdus ornithogaster*)
- Mycobacteriosis
- *Yersinia pseudotuberculosis.*

Fungal

- Candidiasis (esp. toucans and finches).

Protozoal

- Atoxoplasmosis (*Isospora serini*) in young canaries
- Coccidiosis (*Isospora spp, Eimeria spp, Dorisella spp* and *Wendyonela spp*)
- *Cryptosporidiosis*
- *Giardia*
- Trichomoniasis
- Cochleostoma (society finches).

Parasitic

- Nematodes
- Ascaridia (direct life cycle)
- Porrocaecum (indirect – needs invertebrate intermediate hosts, e.g. earthworms)
- Capillaria (direct or use earthworms as paratenic hosts)
- Spiruroids. Proventricular worm (*Geopetitia aspiculata*)
- *Acuaria skrjabini* (gizzard worm)
- Trematodes: *Prosthogonimus spp* (snails and dragonflies are intermediate hosts).

Dietary

Neoplasia

Other non-infectious problems

- Haemorrhagic diathesis (linked to starvation) (Dorrestein 2000)
- Liver disease.

<hr>

Findings on clinical examination

- Lethargy
- Weight loss
- Regurgitation, passing of whole or partially undigested seeds (megabacteriosis)
- Thickened crop wall with whitish lining, regurgitation, diarrhoea, moulting abnormalities
- Diarrhoea (see *Assessment of Droppings*, in *Parrots and Related Species*)
- Yellow droppings (esp. Estrilid finches with *Campylobacter*)
- Greenish droppings (liver disease, *Erysipelas* in mynahs)
- Dark patch in abdomen of canary chicks (black spot disease) due to hepatomegaly (atoxoplasmosis)
- Mortalities (usually resulting from septicaemia).

Investigations

1. Crop wash
2. Proventricular wash
3. Faecal examination
   a. Culture and sensitivity
   b. Parasitic examination
      i. Wet preparation
      ii. Floatation
         Note that *Isospora* carriers shed intermittently so negative results do not rule out infection (Table 6.3)
   c. Gram stain
   d. Modified Ziehl–Neelsen staining or PCR for mycobacteriosis.
4. Cytology
5. PCR for *Chlamydophila*
6. Radiography
7. Endoscopy
8. Ultrasonography
9. Postmortem
   a. Haemorrhagic enteritis (severe bacterial disease, protozoal). On postmortem differentiate from haemorrhagic diathesis
   b. Yellow gut contents, often with undigested seed (*Campylobacter*)
   c. Catarrhal enteritis (Mycobacteriosis).

Management

• See 'Management', in *Gastrointestinal Tract Disorders*, in *Parrots and Related Species*.

Treatment/specific therapy

• *Campylobacter* – antibiotics and improvements with hygiene
• Mycobacteriosis – potential zoonosis. Treatment rarely attempted
• Chlamydophilosis
   • Enrofloxacin at 5.0 mg/kg p.o., i.m.
   • Doxycycline
      • Doxycycline hyclate intravenous human preparation given at 60–100 mg/kg i.m. every 5–7 days for 45 days
      • Doxycycline hyclate as an in-water powdered medication. Use de-ionized water
      • Note birds may be intermittent excreters so at least three consecutive negative samples should achieved before ceasing treatment.

Table 6.3 Key to faecal coccidiosis

Isospora spp.	2 sporocysts and 4 sporozoites
Eimeria spp.	4 sporocysts and 2 sporozoites
Dorisella spp.	2 sporocysts and 8 sporozoites
Wendyonela spp.	4 sporocysts and 4 sporozoites

- Megabacteriosis (*Macrorhabdus ornithogaster*)
  - Amphotericin B at 5 mL/kg orally of 100 mg/mL suspension b.i.d. until organism is eliminated
  - Alternatively, ketoconazole at 10 mg/kg b.i.d.
  - Nystatin
    - 300 000 IU/kg p.o. b.i.d.
    - 100 000 IU/L drinking water
    - 200 000 IU/kg soft food.
- Atoxoplasmosis: 5 mg toltazuril in 100 mL drinking water for 2 days. Repeat after 12 days
  - Prevention of re-infection by removing access to their droppings
  - Clean flights regularly. Consider a false wire bottom to the flight
- Coccidiosis. Potentiated sulphonamides or as for a toxoplasmosis
- Cochlosomosis, trichomoniasis and *Giardia*
  - Ronidazole at 400 mg/kg in soft food and 400 mg/L in fresh drinking water daily for 5 days. Stop for 2 days then repeat
  - Metronidazole is reportedly toxic in some finches
- Parasites
  - Birds in outside aviaries should be wormed twice yearly (avoid breeding season) or have faecal screens every 6 months. All new birds should be wormed during quarantine
  - Suitable treatments for nematodes, proventricular worms and gizzard worms include fenbendazole at 50 mg/kg as a once only dose, or water soluble avermectins, e.g. moxidectin 0.1% added to drinking water at 20 mg/L for 48 h
  - *Capillaria*. Infection is direct, but intermediate stages can be carried by earthworms so remove faecal material regularly and prevent access to soil. Treat with fenbendazole at 50 mg/kg by crop tube; this may need repeating every 2 weeks until the bird is clear
  - *Ascaridia* and *Porrocaecum spp.* The life cycle is direct, although earthworms may act as transport hosts
  - Proventricular worms (*Geopetitia*). Indirect life cycle using insect intermediate hosts
    - Levamisole at 20–40 mg/kg p.o. once only or 1–2 g/4.5 L drinking water over 1–3 days. *Note* toxicities may be seen
  - *Acuaria skrjabini* (gizzard worm)
    - Levamisole at 20–40 mg/kg p.o. once only or 1–2 g/4.5 L drinking water over 1–3 days. *Note* toxicities may be seen
  - Cestodes and trematodes: single dose of praziquantel at 8–10 mg/kg p.o.

Hepatic disorders

Viral

- Polyoma-like virus (finches)
- Circovirus
- Avian leukosis.

Bacterial

- *Pasteurella multocida*
- *Salmonella spp.*

- *E. coli*
- *Erysipelothrix insidiosa* (Erysipelas)
- *Yersinia pseudotuberculosis*
- Chlamydophilosis.

Fungal

Protozoal

- Atoxoplasmosis
- Toxoplasmosis.

Dietary

- Hepatic lipidosis
- Haemochromatosis (iron storage disease).

Neoplasia

- Hepatocellular carcinoma
- Hepatoma
- Lymphosarcoma
- Pancreatic adenocarcinoma (possible metastatic spread).

Other non-infectious problems

- Lipogranulomata (canaries)
- Congestive heart failure.

Findings on clinical examination

- General malaise
- Poor appetite
- Loss of condition
- Ascites
- Yellow or green faeces
- 'Black spot' visible in nestling canary abdomen (a toxoplasmosis, circovirus)
- Nestling mortalities; beak deformities (polyoma-like virus)
- Respiratory distress (secondary to hepatomegaly).

Investigations

1. Haematology and biochemistry
   a. Raised liver enzymes
2. Radiography
   a. Hepatomegaly
   b. Ascites
3. Endoscopy
4. Biopsy
5. Ultrasonography
6. Postmortem
   a. Splenomegaly and hepatomegaly (chlamydophilosis, polyoma-like virus, avian leukosis)

b. Hepatomegaly with definite bronze to bluish appearance (haemachromatosis)
    c. Hepatomegaly with miliary abscessation; splenomegaly (*Yersinia pseudotuberculosis*)
    d. Hepatomegaly, mottled and multiple white foci (toxoplasmosis)
    e. Hepatomegaly, splenomegaly, yellowish discolouration of myocardium. In advanced cases there are pinpoint foci throughout these organs (a toxoplasmosis)
    f. Petechiae and ecchymotic haemorrhages of liver and other organs suggest septicemia/bacteraemia (*Pasteurella, Salmonella, E. coli,* erysipelas).

Management

1. Diuretics such as furosemide at 0.1–2.0 mg/kg i.m. s.c. b.i.d. may be useful in controlling ascites.
2. Milk thistle (*Silybum marianum*) is hepatoprotectant. Dose at 4–15 mg/kg b.i.d. or t.i.d. (Wade 2004).

Treatment/specific therapy

- Viral infections
  - Supportive treatment only
- Bacterial diseases
  - Appropriate antibiosis and supportive care
- Lipogranulomata are usually incidental findings on postmortem
- Yersiniosis – appropriate antibiotics. Source of infection is often faecal contamination from wild birds and rodents.

Renal disorders

See also *Differential Diagnosis of Polydipsia/Polyuria,* in *Parrots and Related Species.*

Bacterial
- Nephritis.

Fungal
- Nephritis.

Neoplasia

Other non-infectious problems
- Amyloidosis (esp. Gouldian finches).

Findings on clinical examination

- Weight loss
- Polydipsia and accompanying polyuria
- Marked wetting of the bottom of the cage
- Haematuria (especially with heavy metal poisoning)

- Unilateral or bilateral lameness (caused by pressure of renal tumours on adjacent lumbo-sacral plexus
- White uric acid tophi may be visible under the skin of the legs and feet. Joints may be swollen (articular gout)
- Neurological signs, e.g. ataxia, generalized tremors.

Investigations

1. Haematology and biochemistry
   a. Renal parameters can be difficult to interpret. Uric acid levels may only rise in chronic renal disease. Urea levels tend to be low. There may be a rise in phosphorus and a change in the calcium/phosphorus ratio. Therefore, need to assess multiple values to assess renal disease, i.e. uric acid, urea, creatinine, calcium and phosphorus
2. Urinalysis
   a. Microscopy: white blood cells or renal casts suggest urinary tract disease
3. Radiography
   a. Plain and contrast (i.v. pyelogram with iohexol)
4. Endoscopy and biopsy
   a. On endoscopy (or postmortem) uric acid may be seen deposited on certain viscera such as the pericardium or the serosal surface of the liver
5. Cloacal swabs
6. Bacteriology: culture and sensitivity.

Management

- Fluid therapy important.

Treatment/specific therapy

- Bacterial nephritis
  - Appropriate antibiotics
- Fungal nephritis
  - Appropriate antimycotics
- Amyloidosis
  - No specific treatment
  - Investigate possible underlying predisposition, e.g. chronic inflammatory disease such as bumblefoot.

Endocrine disorders

- Diabetes mellitus (toucans).

Findings on clinical examination

- Weight loss, polydipsia/polyuria (diabetes mellitus)
- Anorexia.

Investigations

1. Routine haematology and biochemistry
   a. Hyperglycaemia (>55.1 mmol/L; toucan normal: 11.0–19.3 mmol/L)
2. Urinalysis
   a. Glycosuria.

Treatment/specific therapy

● Diabetes mellitus
  ● Exogenous commercially available insulin rarely of use, possibly due to an excess of glucagon or a failure to respond to mammalian insulin
  ● A small number of cases may respond to insulin therapy at 0.1–0.5 IU/kg b.i.d. (Worell 1997).

Reproductive disorders

See *Reproductive Disorders*, in *Parrots and Related Species*.

Nutritional disorders

Malnutrition is a common underlying factor in disease occurrence in softbills. Those softbills that are granivorous (canaries, finches) do require supplementation with commercial 'softbill diets'.

● Hypovitaminosis A
  ● General ill-health
  ● Secondary bacterial and fungal infections
  ● Genetic disease in recessive white canaries (unable to absorb precursor carotenoids)
  ● Supplement with high dietary vitamin A levels (12 000 IU/kg food)
● Hypovitaminosis C
  ● Some passerines, e.g. shrikes and bulbuls require dietary vitamin C
  ● Lethargy, feather loss, intra-articular haemorrhage
● Metabolic bone disease
  ● Can be a marginal problem in aviary birds and only may during egg production
  ● Often a hypovitaminosis D_3 combined with a hypocalcaemia and hyperphosphataemia.

Clinical signs of metabolic bone disease in birds

● General weakness
● Pathological fractures and/or bending of bones
● Rickets
● Paralysis
● Tetany
● Dystocia

- Low clutch size, thin or soft shelled eggs and low hatchability. (Egg laying hens may have an episode of acute hypocalcemia that can result in partial paresis and perhaps egg binding.)
- Polydipsia/polyuria occasionally seen due too increased phosphorus turnover triggering a diuresis
- Birds, especially the young, with bone and joint deformities might be deficient in both calcium and vitamin D_3
- Young Ramphastids may present with folding fracture-like lesions of the beak
- Can occur in breeding females with concurrent tetracycline administration.

- Haemochromatosis (iron storage disease)
  - Common, especially in mynahs and toucans
  - Weight loss, dyspnoea, ascites, and weakness
- Hepatic lipidosis
  - Can occur in Estrildid finches, e.g. zebra finch.

Non-infectious problems

- Starvation. Often the result of mistaking seed husks in feed dishes as uneaten seed
- Avocado poisoning
- Green almond poisoning (cyanide)
- Ethanol toxicity (eating thawed frozen fruits – yeasts ferment sugars into ethanol).

Findings on clinical examination

- Check seed pots for husks mistaken for seed (and, therefore, not replenished)
- Dyspnoea, swollen abdomen (ascites) (haemochromatosis)
- Postmortem
  - Swollen liver, yellow or beige in colour; floats in formal saline (hepatic lipidosis)
  - Haemorrhagic diathesis (see *Gastrointestinal Tract Disorders*), apparent renal gout, lack of food in gut (starvation)
  - Lethargy, ataxia and incoordination (ethanol toxicity).

Investigations

1. Routine haematology and biochemistry
   a. Hypoproteinaemia, raised liver enzymes; serum iron levels (haemochromatosis)
   b. Serum iron levels (toucan normal values <6.27 μmol/L)
2. Analysis of crop contents
3. Radiography
   a. Hepatomegaly, ascites (haemochromatosis)
4. Biopsy
   a. Hepatic iron levels (haemochromatosis)
5. Postmortem
   a. Hydropericardium; subcutaneous oedema especially in region of pectoral muscle (avocado poisoning).

Management

- Provide supportive care.

Treatment/specific therapy

- Hypovitaminosis A
  - Supplement with vitamin A
  - For recessive white canaries, switch to canary foods high with dietary vitamin A levels (12 000 IU/kg food)
- Hypovitaminosis C
  - Supplement with 50–150 mg/kg vitamin C dry matter of food
- Metabolic bone disease
  - Supplement with calcium and vitamin D_3
  - Consider provision of UV light
  - Stop tetracycline administration
- Haemochromatosis
  - Low iron diet (<50 ppm)
  - Avoid citrus fruits and other sources of ascorbic acid – these may enhance iron uptake
  - Offer cold tea as water source – tannins bind strongly to iron and may reduce dietary uptake
  - Weekly phlebotomies equal to 1% body weight until iron levels normalized
  - Alternatively deferoxamine at 100 mg/k s.i.d. s.c. until liver levels normalized (Cornelissen et al 1995)
    Note that serum iron levels do not always reflect liver storage levels.

References

Cornelissen H, Ducatelle R, Roels S 1995 Successful treatment of a channel-billed toucan (Rhamphastos vitellinus) with iron storage disease by chelation therapy: sequential monitoring of the iron content of the liver during the treatment period by quantitative chemical and image analyses. J Avian Med Surg 9:131–137

Dorrestein G M 2000 Passerines and exotic softbills. In: Tully T N, Lawton M P C, Dorrestein G M (eds) Avian medicine, 7th edn. Butterworth-Heinemann, Oxford, 165

Dorrestein G M, Van der Hage M H, Grinwis G 1993 A tumour-like pox lesion in masked bullfinches (Pyrrhula erythaca). Proc 2nd Eur AAV, Utrecht, p 232–240

Gibbens J C, Abraham E J, MacKenzie G 1997 Toxoplasmosis in canaries in Great Britain. Vet Rec 140:370–371

Panigrahy B, Senne D A 1991 Diseases of mynahs. J Am Vet Med Assoc 199(3):378–381

Rodríguez F, Herráez H, Lorenzo H et al 2006 Intracutaneous keratinising epithelioma in a mynah bird (Gracula religiosa). Vet Rec 158:57–58

Rupiper D J, Carpenter J W, Mashima T Y 2000 Formulary. In: Olsen G H, Orosz S E (eds) Manual of avian medicine. Mosby, Philadelphia, p 560

Wade L 2004 Herbal therapy for liver disease: milk thistle (Silybum marianum). AAV Newsletter and Clinical forum, March–May

Worell A B 1997 Toucans and mynahs. In: Altman R B, Clubb S L, Dorrestein G M et al (eds) Avian medicine and surgery, Saunders, Philadelphia, p 910–917

7

Lizards

• •

A wide variety of lizards are available in the pet trade. The commonest species encountered are described in Table 7.1. The internal anatomy of a lizard is shown in Figure 7.1.

The long-term welfare of lizards is, more so than the majority of snakes, dependant upon correct environmental conditions.

Temperature

Many lizards are 'exercised' outside of their vivarium by well-meaning owners. This can lead to prolonged periods of the lizard being exposed to suboptimal temperatures, producing an immunosuppression and increased susceptibility to disease. Inside the vivarium, aggression between its inhabitants can mean some individuals are deprived of suitable basking opportunities, leading to immunosuppression. Some lizards require exceptionally high daytime temperatures. Bearded dragons, for example, need a basking spot set at around 38°C during the day; however, a nighttime temperature drop is no problem.

Ultraviolet exposure

Most diurnal lizards require exposure to ultraviolet B lighting (290–315 nm) for endogenous vitamin D_3 synthesis. Dietary supplementation alone is not sufficient for many species including iguanas, bearded dragons, monitor lizards (*Varanus spp*) and chameleons, so ultraviolet exposure is achieved by installing a full-spectrum light with a specified UVB output, e.g. 2%, 5% or 8%.

Common mistakes include:
1. Failure to provide full-spectrum lighting at all
2. Relying upon placing the reptile close to a sunny window (glass filters out UV light)
3. Use of an incorrect bulb (because glass filters UV light, the bulbs are made from quartz)
4. Failure to replace full-spectrum lights (UV output declines over time but we cannot see this, so replace every 6–8 months or according to manufacturer's instructions)
5. Allowing intra- and interspecific aggression preventing one or more lizards from gaining a suitable spot to bask beneath the full-spectrum light.

Table 7.1 Species of lizard most likely to be encountered: Key facts

Species	Notes	Common disorders
Bearded dragons (*Pogona vitticeps*)	Medium-sized, characterful lizards. They do like it warm, however, and the hot spot should be up to 38°C during the day	Metabolic bone disease, *Isospora* and foreign body ingestion. Secondary infections often are the result of inadequate temperatures
Leopard gecko (*Eublepharis macularius*)	An ideal beginner's lizard. Feeds well on supplemented insect prey including mealworms. Available in a wide variety of colour morphs, some of which carry very high prices	Cryptosporidiosis and foreign body ingestion
Crested gecko (*Rhacodactylus ciliatus*)	Popular because of its looks and wide natural colour variations, this gecko's wild diet is rich in fruits and so it can be kept using commercially available foods rather than live foods	Metabolic bone disease is occasionally seen, as is a muscular-dystrophy-like disease often mistaken for MBD
Green iguana (*Iguana iguana*)	A large stunning lizard as an adult, its vegetarian diet makes it prone to calcium deficiencies	Metabolic bone disease, abscessation (secondary to prolonged low environmental temperatures and aggression-related behavioral problems
Veiled chameleon (*Chamelo calyptatus*)	Chameleons are generally not good starter lizards, but the veiled chameleon, providing it is offered water via a spray and given supplemented foods will often do well	Metabolic bone disease and dystocia

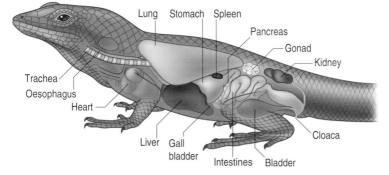

Fig. 7.1. Internal anatomy of a lizard (lateral).

Nutritional supplementation

Crickets, locusts, waxworms and mealworms are commonly fed to lizards not because they are nutritionally good, but because they are easy to farm commercially and they trigger normal feeding in insectivorous species. Insects are inherently low in calcium and so this must be balanced with commercial calcium supplements. These are applied to the insects either by dusting a calcium-rich powder on to the prey, or feeding it upon a calcium-rich food. Note that many commercial calcium supplements also contain vitamins, including vitamin D_3, as well as amino acids.

Consultation and handling

Small lizards such as leopard geckos can be examined relatively easily. Larger lizards may require a more managed technique involving assistance – iguanas and monitor lizards rarely bite, however (*note* this does not mean that they do not bite), and in preference, will attempt to fend you off by whipping with their tail.

Restraint involves grasping the animal from behind across the shoulders and across the pelvis, the handler holding the reptile away from the body. If a large lizard, such as an iguana, is especially aggressive, then placing a damp towel over its head is often sufficient to disorientate it and allow you to gain a hold (N. Highfield *pers. comm.*).

Many lizards, such as Chinese water dragons and young iguanas, can be temporarily immobilized by applying digital pressure to both eyes simultaneously. This technique, plus gentle handling, will allow many feisty lizards to be weighed and examined in a controlled fashion, before gentle stimulation (such as re-righting the reptile) returns it to a normal state of awareness. This may be a manifestation of the oculo-cardiac reflex.

In those lizards with hypocalcaemia/metabolic bone disease, the bones may be so fragile that fractures of the long bones, especially the femurs, can occur if excessive force is applied. A lizard that is presented as flaccid with little or no muscle tone is likely to be hypocalcaemic. Other causes can include septicaemia or poisoning but these are much less likely. In such cases, i.v. calcium is strongly recommended as soon as possible.

When beginning an examination, examine the head first. Most lizards can be induced to open their mouths even if it is in an attempt to bite you. With iguanas, firm traction on the dewlap will often induce them to open up.

Some lizards will shed their tails naturally if stressed or poorly handled (autotomy). These include iguanids, lacertids, geckos and some skinks. In these species, the tail will regrow but is usually a different shape and or markings. *Note* that the crested gecko (*Rhacodactylus ciliatus*) is an exception – unlike the other geckos in the *Rhacodactylus* genus, the tails do not regrow once shed.

Microchipping

- Left quadriceps muscle, or subcutaneously in this area (all species)
- In very small species, subcutaneously on the left side of the body
- Skin closure is achieved either by suture or with tissue glue.

Sexing

Many lizards are sexually dimorphic as adults and can be readily distinguished, typically by the presence of pronounced pores cranial to the cloaca (pre-analpores) or medial thigh (femoral pores), combined with the presence of hemipenile bulges

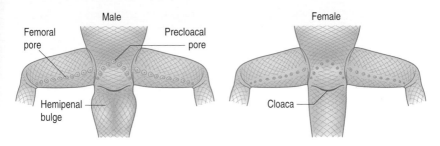

Fig. 7.2. Sexing lizards.

caudal to the cloaca (Fig. 7.2). Male veiled chameleons have a caudal spur on each hind foot, present from birth.

Nursing care

Provide appropriate environment including provision of:
1. Optimal temperature (basking lights, heat mats, etc., to allow thermoregulation). Use of max-min thermometers will assist in monitoring temperature ranges incumbent reptiles are exposed to
2. Full-spectrum lighting (provision of UV-A and UV-B)
3. Humidity
4. Ventilation
5. Easily cleaned accommodation; use paper substrate and disposable/sterilizable hides and other vivarium furniture (Fig. 7.3)
6. Keep individually to minimize intra-specific stress and competition for resources.

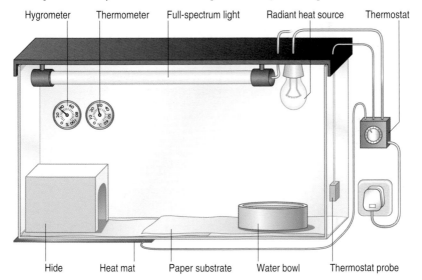

Fig. 7.3. A clinical vivarium setup for lizards and *Chelonia*.

Fluid therapy

Reptiles lack the Loop of Henlé and are, therefore, unable to produce hyperosmotic urine. Uric acid is excreted instead of ammonia; this is sparingly soluble and can be excreted at high concentration with minimal water loss as a sludge or paste.

The assessment of dehydration in reptiles can be difficult visually. Typically, signs of dehydration are sunken eyes, extensive skin folding and tenting.

Selection of fluids for reptiles

1. Isotonic fluids for blood loss, surgery and diarrhoea
2. Hypotonic in cases of prolonged anorexia
3. Hypertonic: there is little indication except in exceptionally large reptiles
4. Blood transfusions can be undertaken using blood from a lizard of the same species or closely related (same genus). Blood can be given i.o. or i.v.
5. Oxyglobin
6. Over hydration reptiles with compromised renal function can lead to vascular overload, heart failure and death.

Fluid replacement

1. Plasma volume in reptiles is around 6.0 mL/100 g.
2. Fluid replacement rates are suggested as:
   a. 0.5–1.0 mL/100 g/h, averaging around 1.5–3.0 mL/100 g/day
   b. Administer up to 0.5–2% body weight maximum of an isotonic replacement fluid, such as Hartman's solution, i.e. 5–20 mL/kg, reducing this once the hydration status becomes normal.
3. Daily bathing in shallow, warm water is often beneficial; it encourages many lizards to drink as well as defaecate and urinate.

Fluids administration

1. Stomach tubing is relatively straightforward in smaller lizards.
2. Oesophagostomy tubes can be used in some cases.
3. All parenteral fluids should be warmed to around 26°C.
4. Easiest vein to access is the ventral tail vein. If attempting to use this vein in male lizards, always allow a gap caudal to the cloaca for the hemipenes.
5. Alternatively a surgical cut-down onto the cephalic vein will allow catheterization.
6. For i.o. fluids the tibial cavity (via the tibial crest) is suggested.
7. Intra-coelomic should be used with caution:
   a. There is a large ventral midline abdominal vein that is likely to be pierced if one attempts to give fluids via the linea alba. There place the needle into a paramedian position – this should also avoid the dorsally positioned lungs
   b. There is no separation of the coelom into an abdomen and thorax, so excessive fluid build-up can compress the lungs.

Nutritional support

Liquidized normal diet or proprietary support diets can be used, given either by stomach tube or by oesophagostomy tube.

Analgesia

Table 7.2 Lizards: Analgesic doses

Analgesic	Dose
Buprenorphine	0.005–0.02 mg/kg i.m. every 24–48 h
Butorphanol	0.4–2.0 mg/kg s.c., i.m. b.i.d.
Carprofen	1.0–4.0 mg/kg s.c., p.o. every 24–72 h
Ketoprofen	2.0–4.0 mg/kg s.c., i.m. every 24–48 h
Meloxicam	0.1–0.5 mg/kg s.c. p.o. every 24–48 h
Morphine	0.05–5 mg/kg i.c. every 6–8 h
Pethidine	2–4 mg/kg i.c. every 6–8 h

Anaesthesia

All reptiles should be at their optimum temperature. Gaseous anaesthetics can be of limited use, as induction agents due to intracardiac shunting, tolerance of hypoxia and physiological diving reflexes (depending upon the species). Chameleons respond relatively quickly while semi-aquatic species may take some time.

Standard anaesthetic protocol

1. Pre-medication
    a. Atropine sulphate at 0.01–0.04 mg/kg i.m. or i.c. given 10–15 min prior to induction may help prevent intracardiac shunting.
Several anaesthetic protocols have been documented. The author has found the following the most useful:
2. Induction
    a. Propofol at 10 mg/kg i.v. delivered into ventral coccygeal (tail) vein (for alternative dose rates see *Chelonia* and *Snakes*).
3. Intubate and maintain with isoflurane.
4. Most reptiles cease to breathe during anaesthesia, therefore adopt intermittent positive pressure ventilation (IPPV) every 30 s, because high pO_2 inhibits ventilation.
5. In larger lizards such as iguanas and water dragons a jugular pulse can be seen sometimes; otherwise the use of pulse oximeters, ultrasound and/or ECG is required for monitoring.
6. For optimum anaesthesia it can be of benefit to infiltrate the surgical site with local anaesthetic.

Parenteral anaesthesia

1. Ketamine at 5.0 mg/kg i.m. plus medetomidine 100–150 µg/kg i.m.
2. Reverse with atipamezole at 5 times medetomidine dose (can take 25–90 min to take effect).

Recovery

1. Continue with IPPV until spontaneous respiration is resumed.
2. If using oxygen alone, switch to manual ventilation with air if possible.
3. Lizards are tolerant of anoxia, therefore continue with IPPV even if there is no obvious response.
4. Doxapram at 5–10 mg/kg i.v, i.o. or on to lingual mucosa may be beneficial.

Skin disorders

The epidermis of both lizards and snakes consists of two layers:
1. The *stratum corneum,* which consists of:
   a. Oberhautchen layer
   b. β-keratin layer
   c. α-keratin layer
   d. It is thickened plates of *stratum corneum* that form the scales. This layer also contains a complex mixture of neutral and polar lipids designed to reduce water loss across the skin
2. *Stratum germinativum.*

The dermis which is mainly connective tissue – may contain bony plates termed osteoderms.

Most lizards shed their skin piecemeal and uncoordinated – cellular proliferation and keratinization are continuous, however geckos normally shed their skin simultaneously over the whole of the body surface. Many lizards such as leopard geckos (*Eublepharis macularis*) will eat their shed skin.

Differential diagnoses of skin disorders

Shedding difficulties (dysecdysis)

- Humidity too low
- Other environmental problems – incorrect photoperiod, temperature, nutrition, etc.
- Lack of cage furniture to allow initiation of shedding
- Ectoparasites, e.g. *Hirstiella spp,* snake mites (*Ophionyssus natracis*)
- Scarring or other underlying dermal disease
- Hypovitaminosis A
- Hypothyroidism and possibly other endocrinopathies
- Secondary bacterial and fungal infections common.

Pruritus

* Ectoparasites.

Scaling and crusting

* Dysecdysis (see above)
* Bacterial dermatitis (*Aeromonas spp, Pseudomonas spp, Serratia spp*)
* Dermatophilosis
* Burns
* Hypovitaminosis A.

Erosions and ulceration

* Behavioural interactions with transparent barriers (ITB). Rostral nares and intermandibular joint often affected
* Lesions from hungry, uneaten crickets and other invertebrate prey
* Bites from conspecifics, especially during mating – these are typically over the shoulders and back of the neck.

Nodules and non-healing wounds

* Abscess
* Filarial nematodes (see also *Systemic Disorders*), esp. chameleons and day geckos.
* Granulomas (mycobacterial – see also *Systemic Disorders*, fungal, e.g. *Chrysosporium* anamorph of *Nannizziopsis vriesii* (CANV), *Trichophyton spp, Aspergillus spp, Geotrichium candidum, Cryptococcus neoformans, Aspergillus spp*)
* Poxvirus
* Viral papillomas (green lizard *Lacerta viridis* and occasionally other lacertids). Often very dark to black, and proliferative
* *Trichomonas spp* (subcutaneous abscesses in leopard gecko)
* Sebaceous cysts (green iguana)
* Pseudoaneurysm, especially on the head (bearded dragon)
* Calcinosis cutis and calcinosis circumscripta
* Endolymphatic glands in certain geckos, e.g. day geckos (*Phelsuma spp*).

Changes in pigmentation

* Scarring
* Yellowing of skin patches in bearded dragons (*Pogona spp*). Common following skin disease, e.g. burns, dysecdysis, infections but also linked to 'yellow fungus disease'
* Yellow fungus disease of bearded dragons. Dermatomycosis: Trichophyton, *Chrysosporium* anamorph of *Nannizziopsis vriesii* (CANV).

Ectoparasites

* Arthropods
* Ticks (*Aponomma exornatum, A. varanensis, A. fuscolineatum*, see Kenny et al 2004)
* Lizard mites (*Hirstiella trombidiiformis, Geckobiella spp, Pterygosoma spp*)
* Snake mite *(Ophionyssus natracis)* (Walter & Shaw 2002).

Burns

Neoplasia

* Fibrosarcoma
* Squamous cell carcinoma

- Liposarcoma
- Chromatophoroma (malignant).

Findings on clinical examination

- Distinct single or multiple swellings palpable in the skin
- Dysecdysis: patches of dull, thickened skin may indicate areas where several layers of skin have built up over successive dysecdysis episodes. Rings of unshed skin may form bands around the tips of extremities such as toes and tail tips. These may constrict as they dry, acting as tourniquets and compromising blood flow to the extremities. Lizards that have had previous problems may lack one or more digits
- Thickened skin, hyperkeratotic skin. History of high protein diet, e.g. rodents with no vegetable or vitamin supplementation fed long term to known omnivorous lizards, e.g. some monitors, tegus (hypovitaminosis A)
- Damage to rostral nares and intermandibular joint, linked to repetitive trauma against transparent barriers such as glass doors and sides. Particularly common in water dragons (*Physignathus spp*), which consistently attempt to leap through the barrier (ITB)
- Anaemia (heavy ectoparasitic infestations)
- Pseudoaneurysm – large fluctuant swelling on neck
- Burns
- Bilateral swellings on the neck of certain gecko species such as day geckos (*Phelsuma spp*). These are normal calcium storage sites and can be quite pronounced in healthy breeding females.

Investigations

1. Radiography
2. Routine haematology and biochemistry
3. Thyroid levels (Table 7.3)
4. Culture and sensitivity
5. Cytology
   a. Fine needle aspirate
   b. Aspiration – whole blood (pseudoaneurysm)

Table 7.3 Lizards: Thyroid levels

Species	Total T4 nM/L	Total T3 nM/L (Free T3 pM/L)
Sceloporus undulatus Adult	11.1–13.1	3.1–3.2
Ameiva undulata Adult	8.2	–
Dipsosaurus dorsalis Adult	3.2–14.5	–
Dipsosaurus dorsalis Hibernating adult	1.3	–
Dipsosaurus dorsalis Adult (spring)	13.0	0.5
Trachydosaurus rugosus Adult	3.0	0.3
Podarcis sicula Adult	–	0.15 (1.7)

After Hulbert (2000).

6. Endoscopy
7. Biopsy/necropsy
   a. Circulating microfilaria (Orós et al 2002)
8. Ultrasonography.

Treatment/specific therapy

- Dysecdysis
  - Moisten the affected areas in order to loosen the retained skin from the underlying epidermis
  - Retained spectacular scales in geckos are best removed using a damp cotton bud
  - Injection of vitamin A at 1000–5000 IU/kg i.m. will often trigger a further shed, allowing a closer management of the sloughing procedure such that both the old shed and the new are removed
  - Supplementation with thyroxine will often help with lizards showing dysecdysis. Serum thyroid levels may be useful, but normal ranges for comparison may not be available for your target species
- Abscess
  - Requires surgical removal if possible
- ITB
  - Treat lesions topically or systemically as required. May require removal of devitalized bone with associated teeth
  - Alter environment – attempt to remove to a larger, more naturalistic environment without transparent boundaries (Scott & Warwick 2002).
- Poxvirus. No treatment
- Viral papillomas
  - Usually self-limiting. May require surgical resection if present at a sensitive site, e.g. mouth where they may interfere with normal feeding
- Fungal dermatitis, granulomas, 'yellow fungus disease'
  - Ketoconazole at 10–30 mg/kg p.o. s.i.d.
  - Topical ketoconazole cream
  - Itraconazole 5 mg/kg p.o. e.o.d.
  - Topical chlorhexidine solution
  - Topical iodine solution
    Note that CANV can act as a primary reptile pathogen
- Filarial nematodes
  - Surgical resection where feasible
  - Ivermectin at 200 μg/kg s.c. (care with Solomon Island skinks, *Corucia zebrata*)
- Ticks
  - Individual removal of ticks
  - Ivermectin at 200 μg/kg s.c. (care with Solomon Island skinks, *Corucia zebrata*)
    Note that ticks are vectors for *Babesia/Hepatozoon* and *Ehrlichia*-like organisms
- Snake and lizard mites
  - Snake mites are parthenogenetic, so numbers can rapidly build up in vivaria; treatment must include the thorough cleansing of all affected vivaria. What cannot be sterilized with a mild bleach solution (5 mL/gallon) must be disposed
  - Replace usual substrate with paper (changed daily)

- Repeated washing with warm water will physically remove any mites
- Application of topical fipronil spray once weekly for at least 4 weeks. This is best first applied to a cloth and rubbed over the entire surface of the snake. Fipronil can also be used to treat the environment
- Injection of ivermectin at 200 μg/kg s.c. (*Note:* toxic to indigo snakes and chelonia) every 2 weeks will kill those that feed on the lizard
- Commercial imidacloprid (100 g/L) plus moxidectin (25 g/L) (Advocate Dog, Bayer) applied at double (32 mg/kg imidacloprid + 8.0 mg/kg moxidectin) to 10-fold dosages (160 mg/kg imidacloprid + 40 mg/kg moxidectin) according to thickness of skin (care with lacertids especially the six-lined grass lizard *Takydromus sexlineatus*) (Mehlhorn et al 2005a)
- Cultures of predatory mites (*Hypoaspis miles*) are commercially available for use in vivaria
- Pseudoaneurysm
  - Surgical repair
- Hypothyroidism
  - Supplement with levothyroxine at 0.02 mg/kg p.o. e.o.d.
- Calcinosis circumscripta and calcinosis cutis
  - Consider surgical resection if viable
  - May be linked with renal disease
- Neoplasia
  - Surgical resection
  - Chemotherapy in reptiles is in its infancy. Accessible cutaneous tumours can be treated by injecting cisplatin directly into the tissue mass on a weekly basis as a debulking exercise
  - Radiation has been used to treat an acute lymphoblastic leukaemia in a sungazer lizard (*Cordylus giganteus*), while surgical laser has been used in the treatment of a dermal melanoma in a green iguana
  - Chromatophoromas carry a poor prognosis with early metastasis.

Respiratory tract disorders

Viral

- Ophidian paramyxovirus (OPMV).

Bacterial

- Mycobacterial (see also *Systemic Disorders*)
- Bacterial pneumonia (especially water dragons).

Fungal

- Mycotic pneumonia
- Mycotic pleuritis.

Parasitic

- Lungworms (*Entomelas spp*) (verminous pneumonia)
- Pentastomids, e.g. *Raillietiella*, esp. monitors (*Varanus spp*).

Neoplasia
● Metastases.

Other non-infectious problems
● Sneezing in iguanas – normal removal of salts from nasal salt glands
● Firefly (*Photonis spp*) intoxication (see also *Systemic Disorders* and *Cardiovascular and Haematological Disorders*)
● Aspiration pneumonia (following oral administration of food or fluids; regurgitation after stomach tubing)
● Glottal foreign bodies
● Cardiovascular disease (see *Cardiovascular and Haematological Disorders*)
● Epistaxis (metastatic mineralization of nasal vasculature, trauma, infection, liver disease)
● Anaemia (various causes).

Findings on clinical examination
● Dyspnoea
● Tachypnoea
● Open-mouthed breathing and respiratory distress
● Oral and/or nasal discharge
● Unusual respiratory noises
● Altered colour of respiratory membranes (cyanosis, pallor)
● Neck extension
● Epistaxis
● Anorexia
● Depression
● Muscle wastage
● Sudden death.

Investigations
1. Microscopy
   a. Sputum examination (either from mouth, pulmonary lavage or endoscopic collection)
   b. Staining for cytology
   c. Gram stain
   d. Lungworm eggs and larvae
   e. Pentastomid eggs
2. Faecal examination
   a. Pentastomid eggs
   b. *Entomelas* eggs (swallowed from trachea)
3. Radiography
   a. Pneumonia – areas of increased opacity in the lung fields
4. Routine haematology and biochemistry
5. Serology for OPMV
6. Culture and sensitivity
7. Endoscopy
   a. Adult pentastomes present in lung

8. Biopsy/necropsy
9. Proliferative interstitial pneumonia (OPMV)
10. Ultrasonography.

Management

• If very cyanosed, provide oxygen. Otherwise normal supportive care (see *Nursing Care*).

Treatment/specific therapy

• OPMV
  • No direct treatment
  • Supportive treatment only
  • Often asymptomatic – frequently diagnosed and monitored serologically
• Lungworm
  • Fenbendazole at 50–100 mg/kg. Repeat every 2 weeks if necessary. *Note* that fenbendazole is metabolized to oxfendazole by the liver
  • Oxfendazole at 68 mg/kg. Repeat every 2 weeks if necessary
  • Ivermectin at 0.2 mg repeated every 2 weeks for 3 treatments (care with Solomon Island skinks, *Corucia zebrata*)
  • Lungworms have a direct life cycle; infective larvae can penetrate the skin or infect via the contaminated food and water
• Pentastomids
  • Ivermectin at 0.2 mg repeated every 2 weeks for 3 treatments (care with Solomon Island skinks, *Corucia zebrata*)
• Foreign body
  • Attempt surgical removal. Likely to need tracheotomy
• Epistaxis
  • Investigate possible causes
• Anaemia
  • Investigate causes, e.g. haemorrhage, high ectoparasite load, gastrointestinal disease, renal disease, etc.

Gastrointestinal tract disorders

Disorders of the oral cavity

In crested geckos, calcium is stored in bilaterally symmetrical endolymphatic glands dorsally at the back of the pharynx. In breeding females on a good calcium intake these can appear as quite pronounced whitish to greyish swellings and should not be mistaken for pathological lesions.
• Periodontal disease
  • Especially affects acrodont lizards (agamids – including bearded dragons, water dragons and chameleons)
  • May be related to feeding soft insects, e.g. crickets, waxworms
  • Discolouration, loss of tissue and teeth, osteomyelitis
  • Radiography to assess underlying osteomyelitis
  • Culture of lesions

- Appropriate antibiosis
- Ultrasonic and instrument scaling
- Regular cleaning with oral cleansing product as control measure
- Metabolic bone disease
  - Softening or pathological fractures of the mandibles
  - The weakened bone is unable to support orthopaedic techniques; in some cases supporting the jaw closed with strong adhesive plaster (taking care to leave the nares open) accompanied by placement of an oesophagostomy tube may allow healing to occur
- Ossifying fibroma
  - Usually unilateral; typically affects mandibles
  - Occasionally seen in iguanas
  - Surgical debulking and/or cryosurgery
  - Usually self-limiting
- Other neoplasia (Fig. 7.4)

Fig. 7.4. Oral mass in a pink-tongued skink.

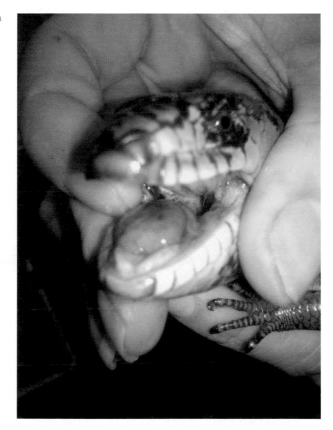

- Fungal mandibular periodontal osteomyelitis
  - Attempt systemic antimycotics such as:
    - Ketoconazole at 10–30 mg/kg p.o. s.i.d.
    - Topical ketoconazole cream
    - Itraconazole 5 mg/kg p.o. e.o.d.
- Stomatitis
  - Uncommon. Often linked with respiratory or gastrointestinal diseases (see *Gastrointestinal Disorders*). See *Snakes* for further advice on treatment of stomatitis
    - Mycotic (*Emmonsia spp*)
    - Herpesvirus (Wellehan et al 2003c)
    - Infection of the temporal glands on chameleons
- Swellings dorso-lateral to the angle of the jaw. Requires debridement under general anaesthetic and appropriate antibiosis
- Pharyngeal oedema
  - Renal disease
  - Cardiovascular disease
- Icterus (see *Hepatic Disorders; Cardiovascular* and *Haematological Disorders*). Adult bearded dragons naturally have very yellow mucous membranes
- Cyanosis (see *Respiratory Tract Disorders*)
- Disorders of the tongue
  - In many lizards including the green iguana the rostral tip of the tongue bears a symmetrical darker patch that may be mistaken for an ulcer or inflammatory condition
  - Chameleons and monitor lizards have long tongues that are vital for food location and prehension
  - Lingual sheath may become infected and adhesions may result. Debride under general anaesthetic and instigate appropriate antibiosis
  - Hypocalcaemia/metabolic bone disease in chameleons may present as partial or complete paralysis of the tongue
  - In some old chameleons there is a failure of the tongue protruding mechanism. These must be hand-fed.

Differential diagnoses for gastrointestinal disorders

Viral

- Reovirus (Drury et al 2002)
- Adenovirus (fat-tailed gecko *Hemitheconyx caudicinctus*) (Wellehan et al 2003b)

Bacterial

- *Salmonella spp*
- *E. coli*
- Other bacteria.

Fungal

- Mycotic enteritis (esp. chameleons)
- Yeast infections (in some cases may be linked with long-term antibiosis).

Protozoal

- *Cryptosporidium spp*
- Flagellates, e.g. *Trichomonas, Trichomonas*

- *Giardia*
- *Isospora* (esp. *I. amphiboluri* in bearded dragons)
- *Eimeria spp*
- Cilates, e.g. *Nyctotherus* (green iguana), *Clevelandellida spp*

Parasitic

- Hookworms: *Oswalsocruzia spp*
- Spirurids (stomach worms), e.g. *Abbreviata spp, Physaloptera spp* (in ant-eating lizards, e.g. horned lizard (*Phrynosoma*)
- Pinworms
- Oxyurids, e.g. *Pharyngodon spp.*
- Capillaria
- Strongyloides
- Trematodes – esp. molluscivores, e.g. pink-tongued skinks.

Nutritional

- Metabolic bone disease
- Intestinal tympany secondary to excessive fermentable carbohydrate intake in folivorous lizards.

Neoplasia

- Colonic adenocarcinoma (Patterson-Kane & Redrobe 2005).

Other non-infectious problems

- Foreign body/impaction (especially large/inappropriate pieces of substrate)
- Cloacal prolapse.

Findings on clinical examination

- Progressive weight loss (tail shrinkage in leopard geckos and related fat-tailed geckos)
- Inappetence
- Very wet or fluidy faeces (flagellates, strongyloides)
- Lack of faeces
- Haemorrhagic and/or mucousy faeces (Hookworms)
- Chronic wasting, mortalities, high parasitism levels (possible reovirus – see Drury et al 2002)
- Gastrointestinal stasis and bloating may occur as part of metabolic bone disease, often accompanied by more typical signs (see *Nutritional Disorders*)
- Vomition (uncommon)
- Cloacal prolapse
  - Cloacitis
  - Cloacoliths
  - Intestinal foreign body
  - Intussusception
  - Extra-intestinal mass, e.g. renal neoplasm
  - Dystocia
  - Hypocalcaemia/metabolic bone disease
  - Parasitism.

Investigations

1. Faecal examination
   a. Wet prep:
      i. Worm eggs (Fig. 7.5)
         (1) Ascarid eggs
         (2) Capillaria (vase shaped eggs with two poles)
         (3) Hookworm eggs (thin walled, oval eggs)
         (4) Oxyurid eggs; note that rodent pinworm eggs may be seen in lizards fed on infested prey rodents
         (5) Spiruroid eggs (medium walled; contain larvae)
         (6) Strongyloides (larvae in *fresh* faecal samples; eggs are thin-walled and similar to *Entomelas*)
         (7) Flagellates (seen as motile protozoa)
         (8) Pentastomid eggs (see *Respiratory Tract Disorders*)
         (9) Trematode eggs
         (10) Protozoal cysts (Table 7.4).
   b. Gram stain
2. Radiography
   a. Contrast studies with 25 mL/kg of 25% barium sulphate in the green iguana (*Iguana iguana*) (Table 7.5)

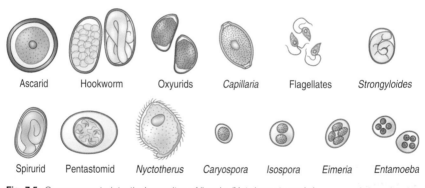

Ascarid   Hookworm   Oxyurids   *Capillaria*   Flagellates   *Strongyloides*

Spirurid   Pentastomid   *Nyctotherus*   *Caryospora*   *Isospora*   *Eimeria*   *Entamoeba*

Fig. 7.5. Common gastrointestinal parasites of lizards. (Not drawn to scale.)

Table 7.4 Lizards: Protozoal cysts

Protozoa	Description
Eimeria	4 sporocysts each containing 2 sporozoites
Isospora	2 sporocysts containing 4 sporozoites
Caryospora	1 sporocyst
Cryptosporidium	Very small (2.5–6.0 μm). Identify using special stain, e.g. MZN
Giardia	Double anterior nuclei (resemble eyes)
Entamoeba invadens	Circular cyst containing 1–4 nuclei

Table 7.5 Radiography contrast studies with 25 mL/kg of 25% barium sulphate in the green iguana (Iguana iguana).

Position of barium sulphate	Iguanas at 29.4°C	Iguanas at 24°C
Complete gastric emptying (h)	6–12	24
Small intestinal transit time (h)	4–6	7
Complete small intestine emptying (h)	16	23–29
Colon transit time (h)	3–27	18–40
Complete colon emptying (h)	33–68	112–147

Adapted from Smith et al (2001).

    b. Recommended timing for serial radiographs in iguanas is zero, 1, 2, 3, 4, 5 and 6 h post-gavage, then every 12 h until barium is present within the distal descending small colon
       Note that the total gut transit time for carnivorous lizards will be significantly shorter than for a herbivorous lizard such as the green iguana
    c. Herbivorous lizards, e.g. green iguana, have a large sacculated colon adapted as a fermentative vat which may normally appear as a large, gas-filled viscus on radiography
    d. Enteritis – gas-filled intestine especially obvious in carnivorous (= simple gut) lizards
    e. Radiodense foreign bodies, e.g. stones, gravel and sand impactions (Fig. 7.6)
    f. Radiolucent foreign bodies, e.g. bark chippings may require contrast studies to identify
3. Routine haematology and biochemistry
4. Culture and sensitivity
5. Endoscopy
6. Biopsy/necropsy
    a. Cryptosporidium – especially the large intestine/colon
7. Ultrasonography.

Management

• Good nursing care including fluid therapy (see *Nursing Care*).

Treatment/specific therapy

• Adenovirus
    • No treatment. Supportive therapy only
• Reovirus
    • No treatment. Supportive therapy only
• Salmonellosis
    • Probably best considered as a normal constituent of lizard cloacal/gut microflora.
    • Rarely pathogenic to lizards
    • Excretion likely to increase during times of stress, e.g. movement, illness

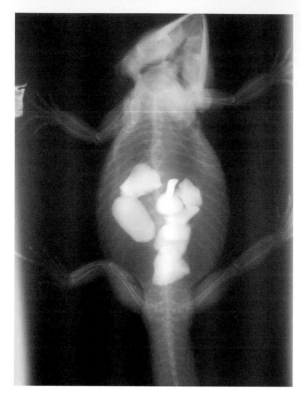

Fig. 7.6. Radiograph of a bearded dragon following ingestion of large pieces of gravel.

- Treatment usually not appropriate as unlikely to be effective long-term and may encourage resistance
- Recommendations for prevention of salmonellosis from captive reptiles issued by the Center for Disease Control in the USA. These are:
  - Pregnant women, children <5 years of age and persons with impaired immune system function (e.g. AIDS) should not have contact with reptiles
  - Because of the risk of becoming infected with Salmonella from a reptile, even without direct contact, households with pregnant women, children <5 years of age or persons with impaired immune system function should not keep reptiles. Reptiles are not appropriate pets for childcare centres
  - All persons should wash hands with soap immediately after any contact with a reptile or reptile cage
  - Reptiles should be kept out of food preparation areas such as kitchens
  - Kitchen sinks should not be used to wash food or water bowls, cages or vivaria used for reptiles, or to bath reptiles. Any sink used for these purposes should be disinfected after use.

- *Cryptosporidium*
  - Direct life cycle; infection by exposure to water or faeces containing infective oocysts
  - There is no recognized effective treatment
  - Try metronidazole at 100–275 mg/kg p.o. once only
  - Nitazoxanide at 5 mg/kg s.i.d.
  - Paromomycin at 300–800 mg/kg p.o. s.i.d. for 10 days
  - Oocysts (*C. parvum*) in water can be viable after 7 months at 15°C
  - Disinfect by exposing to water above 64°C for >2 min
  - Cryptosporidium oocysts are very resistant to chlorine or iodine
- *Isospora* and *Eimeria spp*
  - Direct life cycle
  - Sulfadimethoxine at 90 mg/kg (loading dose) then 45 mg/kg s.i.d. for 7 days plus thorough cage cleaning (Stahl 2000)
  - Trimethoprim-sulfa at 30 mg/kg daily for 5 days then every other day until elimination
  - Prey insects not eaten within 24 h should be discarded and not recycled
  - Treatment may be needed for several (2–6) weeks
  - Quarantine all new introductions and undertake repeat faecal examinations
- Flagellates and ciliates
  - Metronidazole
    - 100–257 mg/kg body weight. Repeat after 2 weeks if necessary
    - 50 mg/kg every 5–7 days as necessary
  - Fenbendazole at 50 mg/kg daily for 5 days
    Note: may occur simultaneously with cryptosporidium (Taylor et al 1999)
- *Giardia*
  - Metronidazole at 125–250 mg/kg p.o. every 48–72 h for 7–14 days
  - Potential zoonosis
- Ascarids, hookworms, stomach worms, and oxyurids
  - Fenbendazole at 50 mg/kg weekly for 3 weeks. *Note* that fenbendazole is metabolized to oxfendazole by the liver
  - Oxfendazole at 68 mg/kg. Repeat every 2 weeks if necessary
  - Ivermectin at 200 µg/kg s.c. (*care with Solomon Island skinks, Corucia zebrata*)
  - Topical emodepside plus praziquantel preparations (Profender, Bayer) at 56 µL/100 g body weight (Mehlhorn et al 2005b)
  - *Note* that *Oxyuris* worms usually have a direct life cycle
  - Hookworms have a direct life cycle; infective larvae can penetrate the skin or infect via the contaminated food and water
- Trematodes
  - Praziquantel at 10 mg/kg; repeat after 2 weeks
- Intestinal tympany
  - Pass stomach tube to release gas from stomach if present
  - Stomach tube activated charcoal or simethicone
  - Typically linked to an excess intake of fermentable carbohydrate; may be linked with abnormal gut motility or obstruction
- Cloacal prolapse
  - Purse-string suture around cloaca for several weeks
  - Limit feeding to reduce straining during defaecation
  - If repeated prolapses consider cloacopexy
- Foreign body
  - Surgical removal.

Nutritional disorders

- Obesity (see also 'Hepatic lipidosis', in *Hepatic Disorders*) esp. bearded dragons, monitor lizards
- Metabolic bone disease (MBD) (see *Musculoskeletal Disorders*)
- White muscle disease (esp. in herbivorous reptiles) vitamin E and selenium deficiency
- Hypovitaminosis A (see *Skin Disorders*)
- Biotin deficiency (see *Neurological Disorders*).

Findings on clinical examination

- Gross enlargement of the coelom
- Anorexia
- Constipation (due to compression of gut by fat pads)
- Weakness
- Swollen long bones; mandibles, weakness, knuckling, inability to lift body, fractures (MBD).

Investigations

1. Radiography
   a. Enlarged abdominal fat pads
   b. Assess skeletal integrity and bone density
2. Routine haematology and biochemistry
   a. Obesity: AST and bile acids may be elevated
   b. Serum ionized and non-ionized calcium, blood vitamin D_3 (25-hydroxycholecalciferol) levels
3. Culture and sensitivity
4. Endoscopy
5. Biopsy/necropsy
6. Ultrasonography
   a. Hepatic enlargement
   b. Ascites.

Treatment/specific therapy

- Obesity
  - Fluid therapy and nutritional support
  - Attempt to reduce calorific intake if still feeding
  - Vitamin E supplementation to reduce risk of steatitis.

Hepatic disorders

Viral

- Adenovirus (esp. bearded dragons *Pogona spp,* water dragons *Physignathus spp*) (see *Systemic Disorders*)
- Herpesvirus (Chuckwalla *Sauromalus varius*) (Wellehan et al 2003a)

Bacterial
- Mycobacteriosis (granulomas – may be multifocal).

Fungal
- Protozoal
- Microsporidae (see *Systemic Disorders*).

Nutritional
- Hepatic lipidosis.

Neoplasia
- Cholangiocarcinoma
- Spindle-cell sarcoma (Martorell et al 2002)
- Hepatoma.

Other non-infectious problems
- Biliary hyperplasia (Wilson et al 2004)
- Melanomacrophage hyperplasia
- Amyloidosis.

Findings on clinical examination

- Lethargy
- Anorexia
- Vomiting
- Coelomic distension (there may be an associated dyspnoea) (see also *Swollen/ distended Body Cavity*)
- Oedematous swelling at back of pharynx
- Jaundice (icterus) Note that bearded dragons (*Pogona spp*) naturally have yellow-pigmented oral mucous membranes
- Yellow urates
- Neurological signs
- Petechial to ecchymotic haemorrhages (adenovirus)
- Severe postoperative haemorrhage (loss of clotting factors).

Investigations

1. Radiography
   a. Hepatomegaly (will often displace lungs and intestines dorsally)
2. Transillumination
   a. Useful in small, lightly pigmented lizards such as leopard geckos
   b. Direct a small bright light, e.g. from otoscope, through the body so as to view the underside of the lizard. The liver is usually readily identified and its relative size assessed
3. Routine haematology and biochemistry
   a. Bile acids (fasting) <60 μmol/L

Bile acid stimulation test in the green iguana (*Iguana iguana*)

- 48 h fast
- Initial blood sample taken
- Gavage with 4 mL of enteric herbivore diet (257 mg fat)
- Blood sample taken at 3 h (emergence of food from pylorus)
- Blood sample taken at 8 h (complete emptying of stomach)
- Results: Average bile acids (µmol/L) ($n = 11$). 0 h, 7.5 µmol/L; 3 h, 33.3 µmol/L; 8 h, 32.5 µmol/L.

From McBride et al (2004), undertaken on iguanas weighing between 356 g and 496 g.

4. Coelomic tap and cytology
   a. Avoid midline as likely to puncture ventral vena cava
5. Culture and sensitivity
6. Endoscopy
7. Biopsy/necropsy
   a. Pale-coloured liver (hepatic lipidosis)
   b. Hepatomegaly (Fig. 7.7)
8. Ultrasonography
   a. Hepatomegaly
   b. Ascites.

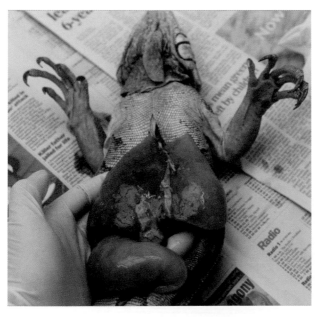

Fig. 7.7. Hepatomegaly in a green iguana (postmortem).

Management

- Milk thistle (*Silybum marianum*) is a hepatoprotectant. Dose at 4–15 mg/kg b.i.d. or t.i.d.
- For ascites try furosemide at 2–5 mg/kg s.i.d. if ascitic
- Lactulose 0.05 mL/100 g p.o. s.i.d.

Treatment/specific therapy

- Adenovirus
  - Supportive therapy only
- Herpesvirus
  - Attempt treatment with acyclovir at 80 mg/kg s.i.d. Very guarded prognosis
- Mycobacteriosis
  - Potential zoonosis. Consider euthanasia
  - No successful treatment for mycobacteriosis in reptiles reported
- Hepatic lipidosis
  - Fluid therapy and nutritional support
  - Covering antibiotics
  - Lactulose 0.05 mL/100 g p.o. s.i.d.
  - Oesophagosty tube may be appropriate in some cases
- Neoplasia. Treatment unlikely
- Amyloidosis
  - No treatment. Address possible initiating factors, e.g. chronic inflammatory conditions.

Pancreatic disorders

Diabetes mellitus (see *Endocrine Disorders*)

Cardiovascular and haematological disorders

Viral

- Iguana herpesvirus
- Chameleon erythrocyte virus (iridovirus).

Bacterial

- Vegetative endocarditis, e.g. *Salmonella*, *Streptococcus*.

Fungal

- Protozoal
- *Haemogregarina spp*
- *Haemoproteus spp*
- *Plasmodium spp*
- *Shellackia spp*

Parasitic

- Filarial nematodes (esp. chameleons).

Nutritional

- Calcification of major vessels including the aorta.

Neoplasia

- Lymphoproliferative disorders, e.g. lymphoid and monocyte leukaemia (see *Systemic Disorders*).

Other non-infectious problems

- Endocardiosis
- Myocardiosis
- Cardiomyopathy
- Myocardial infarction
- Metastatic calcification esp. of aorta
- Visceral gout (uric acid in pericardial sac) see *Renal Disorders*.
- Firefly (*Photonis spp*) intoxication esp. in bearded dragons (see also *Systemic Disorders* and *Respiratory Tract Disorders*)
- Autoimmune haemolytic anaemia (Boyer 2002).

Findings on clinical examination

- Lethargy
- Anorexia
- Oedema, esp. in back of pharynx
- Pale mucous membranes
- Exophthalmia (see also *Ophthalmic Disorders*)
- History of exposure to fireflies, linked with clinical signs of gaping, head shaking, blackened colouration, breathing difficulties and death
- Swollen pharynx; hepatomegaly, depression, anorexia
- Murmurs may be heard in cases with marked heart disease, e.g. endocarditis. In most reptiles nothing will be heard
- Necrosis of the extremities secondary to septicaemic thrombi (often resulting from vegetative endocarditis – see *Systemic Disorders*) (Fig. 7.8).

Investigations

1. Auscultation
   a. For many lizard species no heart beat is audible with standard stethoscopes, except in cases of severe cardiac disease such as endocarditis. However, larger lizards such as bearded dragons can often be auscultated
   b. Frequency (HBF) per minute in reptiles can be estimated at:
      i. HBF = 33.4 (Weight$_{kg}$$^{-0.25}$) assuming the reptile is at its correct body temperature
2. Radiography
   a. In many lizards the heart lies in the thoracic girdle and is, therefore, obscured somewhat radiographically
   b. Mineralization of the aorta and intrapulmonary airways (metastatic calcification)

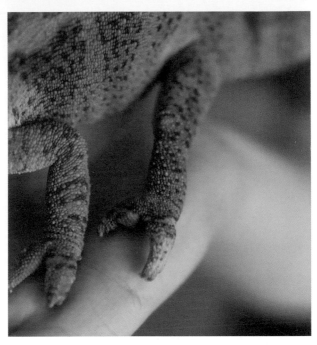

Fig. 7.8. Necrosis of the digits in a Parson's chameleon secondary to septicaemic thrombi.

3. Ultrasonography and Doppler blood-flow detectors
4. Electrocardiogram
   a. ECG values recorded from lacertid lizard (*Gallotia bravoana*) (Table 7.6)
   b. In this study higher temperatures increased the P segment and decreased the ST duration, RR duration and cardiac axis
5. Routine haematology and biochemistry
6. Cytology: may find filarial worms on blood smear
   a. Iguana blood:clear spherical intracytoplasmic lesions (iguana herpesvirus)
   b. Chameleon blood: intracytoplasmic inclusions (iridovirus)
7. Autoagglutination, Rouleaux formation, anisocytosis (auto-immune haemolytic anaemia)
8. Culture and sensitivity
   a. Blood culture
9. Endoscopy
10. Biopsy/necropsy.

Treatment/specific therapy

- Iguana herpesvirus
  - Acyclovir 80 mg/kg s.i.d. for 6 weeks
  - Often associated with severe hepatic fibrosis and interstitial nephritis

Table 7.6   ECG values recorded from lacertid lizard (Gallotia bravoana)

	Mean	Range	SD
Weight (g)	166	105–244	53
Ambient temperature (°C)	20	20–21	0
Internal temperature (°C)	21	18–24	3
Heart rate (beats/min)	44	35–60	9
R–R interval (s)	1.43	1.05–1.78	0.3
P duration (s)	0.09	0.08–0.1	0.01
P amplitude (mV)	0.08	0.05–0.1	0.3
P–R interval (s)	0.15	0.1–0.18	0.03
R amplitude (mV)	0.15	0.1–0.18	0.03
QRS duration (s)	0.08	0.05–0.1	0.02
Q–T interval (s)	0.21	0.1–0.32	0.09
S–T interval (s)	0.14	0.02–0.2	0.07
S amplitude (mV)	0.03	0.02–0.05	0.01
T duration (s)	0.12	0.1–0.15	0.03
T amplitude (mV)	0.07	0.03–0.14	0.04
SV amplitude (mV)	0.12	0.04–0.2	0.05
SV duration (s)	0.13	0.08–0.2	0.05
Mean electrical axis (°)	80	45–135	44
QT:RR ratio	0.15	0.06–0.26	0.07
PR:RR ratio	0.1	0.09–0.13	0.02

From Martinez-Silvestre et al (2003).

- Chameleon erythrocyte virus. No treatment
- Filarial nematodes – see *Skin Disorders*
- Firefly (*Photonis spp*) intoxication
  - Fireflies contain cardiac glycoside-like cardenolides that suppress heart rate
  - Supportive treatment including gavage with activated charcoal
- Haemoparasites
  - Loading dose of chloroquine phosphate (5 mg/kg p.o.) and primaquine phosphate (0.5 mg/kg p.o.)
  - Continue with chloroquine at 2.5 mg/kg p.o. once weekly and primaquine at 0.5 mg/kg once weekly for 12–16 weeks
- *Shelackia spp* rarely pathogenic – may indicate immunosuppression consistent with concurrent disease or poor environmental conditions
- Leukaemia
  - Treatment potentially difficult and untried
  - Radiation therapy was used by Martin et al (2003). Single low dose whole body radiation treatment of 1 Gray. A reduction in WBC was noted after 1 month and was normal, with normal differential by 3 months

- Autoimmune haemolytic anaemia
  - Prednisolone at 0.5 mg/kg s.i.d. for 2 weeks then e.o.d. until PCV stable
  - Cimetidine 4 mg/kg p.o. s.i.d. if evidence of gastric haemorrhage
  - Covering antibiosis
  - Blood transfusion
- Cardiomyopathies and other cardiac disorders
  - Furosemide at 2–5 mg i.m., i.v. p.o. s.i.d. or b.i.d.
  - Pimobendan at 0.2 mg/kg s.i.d.
- Metastatic calcification
  - See *Musculoskeletal Disorders.*

Systemic disorders

Viral

- Adenovirus (inland bearded dragon *Pogona vitticeps* and Rankin's dragon *P. henrylawsonii*)
- Iguana herpesvirus (see *Cardiovascular and Haematological Disorders*)
- Iridovirus.

Bacterial

- Septicaemia/bacteraemia
- *Chlamydophila* and *Chlamydophila*-like organisms
- Mycobacteriosis (see also *Respiratory Disorders* and *Skin Disorders*)
- Streptococci (bacteraemia)
- *Salmonella arizona*
- *Listeria monocytogenes* (Girling & Fraser 2004).

Fungal

Protozoal

- Intranuclear coccidiosis
- Microsporidae (see also *Hepatic Disorders*) esp. bearded dragons.

Parasitic

- Filarial nematodes (see also *Skin Disorders* and *Cardiovascular and Haematological Disorders*).

Neoplasia

- Lymphoma and leukaemia
- Mesothelioma
- Haemangiosarcoma.

Other non-infectious problems

- Cardiac disease (see *Cardiovascular and Haematological Disorders*)
- Intracoelomic haemorrhage
- Firefly (*Photonis spp*) intoxication (see also *Cardiovascular and Haematological Disorders* and *Respiratory Tract Disorders*)
- Gout (visceral, articular and renal). See *Renal Disorders*
- Amyloidosis.

Findings on clinical examination

- Lethargy
- Anorexia (see *Anorexia* notes in *Snakes* for a differential list)
- Oedema
- Sudden mortalities
- Neurological signs
- Anorexia, lethargy and death especially in bearded dragons (Adenovirus). Petechial to ecchymotic haemorrhages may occur
- Necrosis of the extremities secondary to septicaemic thrombi (often resulting from vegetative endocarditis – see *Cardiovascular and Haematological Disorders*).

Investigations

1. Radiography
2. Routine haematology and biochemistry
3. Cytology: may find filarial worms on blood smear
4. Culture and sensitivity
   a. Blood culture
5. ZN staining and PCR for mycobacteria
6. Immunohistochemistry and PCR for *Chlamydophila* and *Chlamydia*-like organisms (Soldati et al 2004)
7. Endoscopy
8. Biopsy/necropsy
   a. Single or multiple granulomas (Mycobacteria, fungi, *Chlamydophila pneumoniae*, *Chlamydia*-like organisms)
   b. Microsporidea (G +ve, acid fast) found in liver, kidneys, lung gonads and CNS
   c. Adenovirus
   d. Neoplasia.
9. Ultrasonography.

Treatment/specific therapy

- Adenovirus
  - Symptomatic treatment only
  - Exclude parents and siblings from breeding groups to eliminate potential carriers
- Iridovirus
  - Symptomatic treatment only
  - Some may actually be invertebrate iridoviruses, originating from infected crickets
- Bacterial infections
  - Appropriate antibiosis
  - Supportive therapy
  - Symptomatic management of necrotic extremities. May require surgical amputation

- Listeriosis
  - Not normally a part of reptile gut flora
  - Case described in Girling & Fraser 2004 linked to feeding contaminated mouse pups that had been frozen and defrosted
- Mycobacteriosis
  - Potential zoonosis. Consider euthanasia
  - No successful treatment for mycobacteriosis in reptiles reported
- Microsporidae
  - No effective treatment
  - Albendazole at 10 mg/kg s.i.d. p.o. may prevent replication
- Intranuclear coccidiosis
  - Potentiated sulphonamides at 30 mg/kg s.i.d.
- Filarial nematodes
  - Ivermectin at 200 μg/kg s.c. (care with Solomon Island skinks, *Corucia zebrata*)
  - Surgical resection of associated skin granulomas
- Neoplasia
  - Surgical resection if feasible
- Lymphoma and leukaemia (see *Cardiovascular and Haematological Disorders*).

Swollen/distended body cavity

Infections may cause organopathies that in turn result in a swollen or distended coelom.

Neoplasia

- Hepatic neoplasia
- Renal neoplasia.

Other non-infectious problems

- Obesity (enlarged coelomic fat pads)
- Distension of the gastro-intestinal tract, e.g. secondary to foreign body obstruction, intussusception, hypocalcaemia (intestinal atony)
- Distension of the bladder (bladder calculi, bladder atony, CNS lesions)
- Hepatomegaly
- Ascites
- Liver disease
- Hypoproteinaemia
- Cardiovascular disease
- Septicaemia
- Renomegaly.

Reproductive causes

- Gravid
- Dystocia (see *Reproductive Disorders*).

Findings on clinical examination

- Swollen coelom
- Constipation (secondary to external compression of the gut by enlarged fat pads)
- Dyspnoea
- Other clinical signs may be present depending upon underlying cause.

Investigations

1. Radiography
   a. Distended viscus
   b. Bladder calculi
   c. Foreign bodies, e.g. sand or stone impactions
2. Routine haematology and biochemistry
3. Coelomic tap
4. Culture and sensitivity
5. Endoscopy
6. Biopsy/necropsy
7. Ultrasonography
   a. Coelomic fluid
   b. Distended viscus.

Management

- Fluid can be drawn from the coelom to relive the distension, but this may interfere with the fluid balance of the lizard
- Furosemide at 2–5 mg i.m., i.v. p.o. s.i.d. or b.i.d.

Treatment/specific therapy

- See individual headings.

Musculoskeletal disorders

Bacterial
- Septic arthritis
- Osteomyelitis
- Cellulitis
- Myositis.

Fungal

Parasitic
- Heavy parasite burden especially haemoparasites (anaemia) or gastrointestinal parasites (protozoa, helminths).

Nutritional

- Metabolic bone disease (MBD)
- Nutritional secondary hyperparathyroidism (dietary calcium deficiency, dietary calcium/phosphorus imbalance, hypovitaminosis D_3 [lack of exposure to ultraviolet light, lack of dietary vitamin D_3 protein deficiency] see also 'Other noninfectious problems', below).
- Metastatic calcification of smooth muscle of various organs including cardiovascular system, pulmonary system, gut and urogenital system. Typically linked to excess dietary vitamin D_3 intake, e.g. over supplementation, feeding with dog and cat food. Especially problematical in herbivorous reptiles, e.g. iguanas (but see *Treatment*)
- Hypovitaminosis E (often combined with selenium deficiency).

Neoplasia

- Fibromas (esp. mandibles in green iguana)
- Liposarcoma
- Myeloma
- Osteosarcoma.

Other non-infectious problems

- Metabolic bone disease
- Renal secondary hyperparathyroidism
- Also liver and intestinal disease – see also 'Nutritional' above)
- Autotomy (geckos, iguanids, lacertids and some skinks)
- Fractures (traumatic) especially long-toed lizards such as green iguanas and water dragons
- Spondylosis/spondylitis
- Hypertrophic osteopathy (HO) (also known as hypertrophic pulmonary osteoarthropathy, HPOA)
- Osteopetrosis
- Kyphosis/scoliosis (genetic; disease of the associated musculature (myopathies); nutritional disorders)
- 'Floppy-tail' – a particular form of kyphosis associated with small arboreal lizards, esp. day geckos and crested geckos
- Dysecdysis with resultant sloughing of distal extremities, e.g. toes and tail-tip (see *Skin Disorders*)
- Avascular necrosis of the distal tail
- Swelling at tail base in males (seminal plugs – see *Reproductive Disorders*)
- Congenital defects – typically abnormal incubation environment.

Findings on clinical examination

- Any limb or spinal swelling, fracture or paralysis should be considered as a possible sign of a pathologic fracture (Fig. 7.9)
- Soft mandibles, foreshortening of the maxillae, swollen mid-shaft of long bones, kyphosis/scoliosis, weakness, inability to support own body weight (MBD)
- Muscle weakness, inability to support body or hunt/locate food (Fig. 7.10)

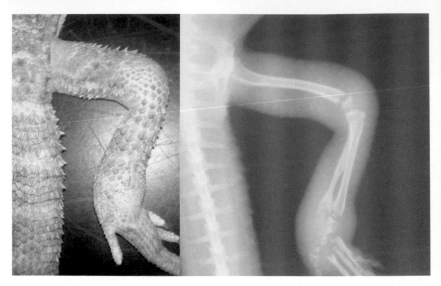

Fig. 7.9. Swollen tarsus with osteolysis arising from a septic arthritis in the bearded dragon above. *Note* the pathologic fracture in the distal femur.

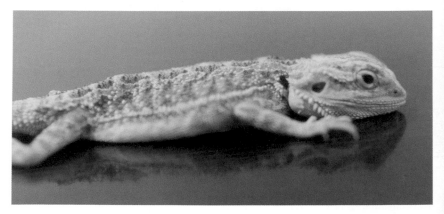

Fig. 7.10. A young bearded dragon with extreme muscle weakness secondary to metabolic bone disease.

- Muscle fasciculations and other neurological signs
- Withering and fracture of distal tail
- Loss of digits
- Scoliosis in crested geckos, often accompanied by kinking of the tail
- In arboreal geckos the tail hangs either to the side or over the back when resting in a head-down position ('floppy-tail').

Investigations

1. Husbandry
   a. Discuss re: access to full-spectrum lighting, frequency of light bulb changing, provision of calcium/provision in suitable form, intra- or interspecific interactions that may influence access to basking sites and/or food/calcium sources
2. Radiography
   a. Pathologic (MBD, neoplasia) or traumatic fractures (Fig. 7.11)
   b. Osteolysis (osteomyelitis, myeloma, osteosarcoma)
   c. Fibrous osteodystrophy (MBD)
3. Other signs of MBD. Loss of bone density and cortical bone thinning
   a. Fibromas and other neoplasia
   b. HO
   c. Osteopetrosis – excessive thickening of the bones

Fig. 7.11. Traumatic fracture of the radius in a green iguana.

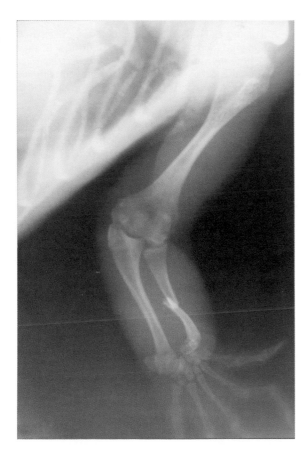

    d. Septic arthritis
    e. Gout – radiolucent uric acid accumulation
4. Routine haematology and biochemistry
    a. Blood vitamin D_3 (25-hydroxycholecalciferol) levels: normal plasma levels for Pogonids = 105 nmol/L; for green iguana (*Iguana iguana*) = 265 nmols/L
    b. Total calcium, ionized calcium, phosphate)
    c. Hyperphosphataemia (renal secondary hyperparathyroidism)
5. Culture and sensitivity
6. Spondylitis, osteomyelitis
7. Cytology (FNA)
8. Endoscopy
9. Biopsy
10. Ultrasonography.

Treatment/specific therapy

- Autotomy
  - For those species that naturally autotomize, then no treatment beyond minimizing blood loss is necessary; suturing will prevent normal tail regeneration – note that the crested gecko (*Rhacodactylus ciliatus*) is an exception – unlike the other geckos in the *Rhacodactylus* genus the tails do not regrow once shed. For other species with traumatic or surgical tail amputation then skin closure is necessary
- Metabolic bone disease
  - Usually due to secondary nutritional hyperparathyroidism linked with either failure to provide sufficient calcium supplementation or exposure to UV-B
  - Parenteral calcium gluconate or lactate at 1.0–2.5 mg/kg daily
  - Oral vitamin D_3 at 1–4 IU/kg daily
  - Dietary calcium supplementation
  - Exposure to full spectrum lighting as a UV-B source
  - Calcitonin at 1.5 IU/kg s.c. s.i.d. if is normocalcaemic
- Metastatic calcification
  - No effective treatment
  - Reduce hypercalcaemia by:
    - Calcitonin at 1.5 IU/kg s.c. s.i.d.
    - Fluid therapy at 15 mL/kg Hartman's solution intracoelomic until normocalcaemic
  - Although often linked to excessive vitamin D3 supplementation, many cases may be due to low levels of calcitrol, commonly secondary to renal disease. This leads to toxic levels of PTH production with associated abnormal tissue mineralization and further renal damage
- Osteopetrosis
  - Hereditary disorder. Symptomatic treatment
- Hypertrophic osteopathy
  - Symptomatic treatment
  - Usually terminal
- Heavy parasite burden
  - Treat as described under relevant sections

- Septic arthritis
  - Surgical investigation and treatment. May require partial or complete amputation. Consider underlying possibility of vegetative endocarditis (see *Cardiovascular and Haematological Disorders*)
- Abscessation and osteomyelitis, myositis
  - Appropriate antibiosis
  - Consider amputation if damage is extensive
- Spondylosis – no treatment
- Spondylitis
  - Appropriate antibiosis
  - Consider NSAIDs, e.g. meloxicam at 0.2 mg/kg once daily or every other day (in the green iguana, see Hernandez-Divers 2006b)
- Kyphosis/scoliosis/ 'floppy-tail'
  - No specific treatment
  - Assess for underlying MBD (see above)
  - Can occur in crested geckos without obvious MBD. May be a muscular-dystrophy-like disorder
  - 'Floppy-tail' is an acquired disorder seen in certain arboreal lizards and is related to excessive time resting head-down on completely vertical surfaces, e.g. vivarium sides. It is not always associated with MBD, but is associated with pelvic and sacral abnormalities which are presumed to be linked to the mechanical stress of the weight of the tail on the tail base musculature and underlying skeleton
- Hypertrophic pulmonary osteopathy
  - Likely linked to multiple organ disorders. Very guarded prognosis
- Neoplasia
  - Surgical resection if possible, e.g. amputation of distal extremities.

Neurological disorders

Viral

- Paramyxovirus (PMV)
- Adenovirus (rare).

Bacterial

- Septicaemia
- CNS granuloma.

Fungal

- CNS granuloma.

Protozoal

- Microsporidae (see *Systemic Disorders*), esp. bearded dragons
- *Acanthamoeba*
- *Toxoplasma.*

Parasitic

- Larval migrans.

Nutritional

- Biotin deficiency
- Hypovitaminosis E (often combined with selenium deficiency – see *Musculoskeletal Disorders*)
- Hypocalcaemia (see 'Metabolic bone disease' in *Musculoskeletal Disorders*)
- Hypoglycaemia.

Neoplasia

- Schwannoma.

Other non-infectious problems

- Hepatic disease (see *Hepatic Disorders*)
- Toxins
- Iatrogenic, e.g. aminoglycosides, ivermectin, metronidazole
- Nicotine
- Cedar wood shavings
- Ingestion of toxic plants, e.g. *Diffenbachia*, azaleas.

Findings on clinical examination

- Twitching of toes, occasionally tail tip, muscle fasciculations (hypocalcaemic tetany). May be pronounced or complete muscle flaccidity. Often accompanied by other signs of MBD (see *Musculoskeletal Disorders*)
- Varied neurological may be seen with PMV infections in lizards, but infections are often asymptomatic
- Weakness
- Head tilt (vestibular disease)
- Convulsions
- Death
- History of prolonged intake of raw eggs (biotin deficiency).

Investigations

1. Radiography
2. Routine haematology and biochemistry
   a. Blood vitamin D_3 (25-hydroxycholecalciferol) levels; also total calcium, ionized calcium, phosphate)
   b. Serology for PMV
3. Culture and sensitivity
4. Endoscopy
5. Biopsy/necropsy
6. Ultrasonography.

Treatment/specific therapy

1. *Acanthamoeba* and *Toxoplasma*
   a. Treatment difficult
   b. Metronidazole at 100–275 mg/kg p.o. once only

   c. Trimethoprim/sulphadiazine at 15 mg/kg p.o. daily
   d. Potential zoonoses
2. Biotin deficiency
   a. Described in monitor lizards (*Varanus spp*) fed on raw eggs
   b. Supplement diet
   c. Treat symptomatically
3. Hypoglycaemia
   a. Uncommon
   b. Parenteral and oral glucose therapy
4. Larval migrans
   a. Treat as for endoparasites. Poor prognosis
5. Toxins
   a. Remove from source of toxin
   b. For ingested toxins flush out stomach under GA or perform gastrotomy
   c. Supportive care.

Ophthalmic disorders

Ophthalmic examination

Diurnal lizards have all cone retinae while nocturnal lizards have both rods and cones. Lizards have one or two fovea and have a conus papillaris (analogous to the avian pecten). The lacrimal and Harderian glands are well developed.

Most lizards have eyelids but many geckos instead possess a snake-like spectacle (an exception to this is the commonly kept leopard gecko, *Eublepharis macularis*). The eyelids may be fused as in chameleons. These lizards also lack a nictitating membrane.

For examination, the posterior segment of the eye is difficult as the iris muscle fibres are striated and partly under voluntary control. Therefore, parasympatholytics, e.g. atropine, and sympathomimetics, e.g. phenylephrine, will not work. Consider examination by:
1. Using low light levels
2. General anaesthesia
3. Non-parasympatholytic mydriatics such as vecuronium. These are inappropriate in lizards which possess a spectacle.

Differential diagnoses

Bacterial
● *Pseudomonas*
● *Aeromonas*.

Fungal
● Keratitis
● Panophthalmitis.

Protozoal
● *Trichomonas spp* (subspectacular abscess).

Nutritional

• Hypovitaminosis A (chameleons).

Neoplasia

Other non-infectious problems

• Trauma
• Foreign body
• Retained spectacle
• Occlusion of nasolacrimal duct
• Congenital absence of nasolacrimal duct
• Stenosis due to or following inflammation
• Cardiovascular disease (bilateral exophthalmus)
• Congenital defects
• Microphthalmia – often associated with head abnormalities
• Some Caribbean iguanas have red sclerae; this should not be mistaken for pathology.

Findings on clinical examination

• Conjunctivitis
• Blepharitis
• Blepharospasm (foreign body, ulceration)
• Ocular discharge
• Corneal ulceration
• Deep ulceration followed by perforation and iris collapse
• Hypopyon
• Uveitis
• Keratitis
• Whitish material in eye (hypovitaminosis A, secondary infection)
• Cataracts
• Retinal degeneration
• Exophthalmia
• Distension of the subspectacular space (in species with a spectacle).

Investigations

1. Ophthalmic examination
   a. For those species with a spectacle:
      i. Space beneath spectacle distended with *clear* fluid (occlusion of naso-lacrimal duct)
      ii. Subspectacular abscess: The eye appears *opaque* and the spectacle may be bulge due to increased pressure in the corneo-spectacular space. This condition may be unilateral or bilateral
2. Radiography
3. Routine haematology and biochemistry
4. Culture and sensitivity
5. Endoscopy
6. Biopsy/necropsy
7. Ultrasonography.

Treatment/specific therapy

- Bacterial keratitis
  - Topical ophthalmic antibiotics; may also benefit from systemic antibiotics
- Fungal keratitis
  - Topical ophthalmic antimycotics
- Corneal ulceration
  - Topical antibiosis and lubrication
  - Suturing of eyelids together may be of benefit
  - Excoriation followed by topical tissue glue may be of use
  - Deep ulceration followed by perforation and iris collapse
  - Enucleation if ocular penetration and uveitis
- Subspectacular abscess
  - Treatment involves surgical incision into the spectacle to allow an assessment for any corneal lesions
  - All debris should be flushed from the corneal surface, and if possible the nasolacrimal duct cannulated and flushed
  - Topical ophthalmic antibiotic or antimycotic preparations should be used
  - A new spectacle should form at the next skin shed. To prevent dessication, consider attempting to suture contact lens in place
- Nasolacrimal duct occlusion
  - Treatment is similar to subspectacular abscess
- Congenital defects
  - No treatment
  - Consider incubation parameters (temperature, humidity, etc.) as well as genetic factors when considering cause.

Endocrine disorders

Endocrine disorders are poorly investigated in reptiles
- Hypothyroidism (see *Skin Disorders*)
- Diabetes mellitus.

Findings on clinical examination

- Anorexia
- Polydipsia/polyuria
- Weight loss
- Dysecdysis (see *Skin Disorders*).

Investigations

1. Radiography
2. Routine haematology and biochemistry
   a. Hyperglycaemia (differentiate from stress hyperglycaemia)
   b. Serum insulin
   c. Serum glucagon (may be more important in glucose regulation than insulin)
3. Coelomic tap

4. Culture and sensitivity
5. Endoscopy
6. Biopsy/necropsy
7. Ultrasonography.

Treatment/specific therapy

- Diabetes mellitus
  - Symptomatic therapy
  - Start on high-fibre, low-protein diet
  - Consider use of insulin.

Renal disorders

Impairment of fluid balance, or renal disease, causes pathological crystallization of uric acid crystals which presents as visceral or articular gout.

Viral

- Iguana herpesvirus (see *Cardiovascular and Haematological Disorders*).

Bacterial

- Bacterial nephritis.

Fungal

- Fungal nephritis.

Neoplasia

Other non-infectious problems

- Gout (renal, visceral and articular)
- Bladder calculi
- Renal failure of middle-aged iguanas
- Iatrogenic (nephrotoxic drugs, e.g. aminoglycosides).

Findings on clinical examination

- Anorexia
- Lethargy
- Weight loss
- Polydipsia/polyuria (see also 'Diabetes mellitus', in *Pancreatic Disorders*)
- Anuria
- Oedema and swellings (Fig. 7.12)
- Hind-limb weakness (see also *Neurological Disorders*)
- Constipation (swollen kidneys may occlude pelvic canal)
- Pale mucous membranes
- Pharyngeal oedema
- Mortalities
- Vague ill-health, anorexia in iguanas of 3–8 year old (renal failure of middle-aged iguanas).

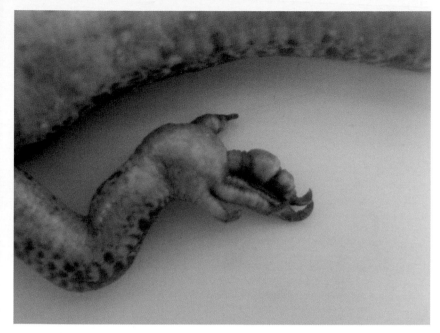

Fig. 7.12. Severe gout in the foot of a pink-tongued skink.

Investigations

1. Radiography
   a. Renomegaly. The kidneys of many lizards, especially iguanids, are located in the pelvic cavity. Difficult to see normally; they can extend into the coelomic cavity if enlarged
2. Routine haematology and biochemistry
   a. No good single test
   b. Lizards with renal disease may show hyperuricaemia, hyperuraemia, hyperphosphataemia, hyperkalaemia, hyponatrimia and hyper- or hypoproteinaemia, although none of these are consistent findings.

Renal failure of middle-aged Iguanas

1. High serum phosphorus (normal range 1.0–3.0 mmol/L; can be up to 5.7 in gravid female iguanas) and Ca:PO_4 <1.
2. Serum urea and creatinine levels usually normal. Uric acid levels only elevated in terminal disease.
3. CPK and SGOT often high.
4. May be hypo- or hypercalcaemic.

Estimation of renal clearance in the green Iguana

1. Fast the reptile for 24 h (allow normal access to water).
2. Maintain at PBT.
3. Inject intravenous iohexol at 75 mg/kg.
4. Collect blood samples (minimum 0.5 mL) at 4 h, 8 h and 24 h.
5. Centrifuge and submit plasma on ice for analysis.
6. Mean GFR for healthy iguanas is 14.8–18.3 mL/kg per h.

(Hernandez-Divers 2006a).

3. Urinalysis
   a. Renal casts
   b. Inflammatory cells
4. Culture and sensitivity
5. Endoscopy
   a. Abnormalities in shape, colour or size of kidneys
6. Biopsy/necropsy
7. Ultrasonography
   a. Hyper- or hypoechoic, focal or multifocal changes; alteration of size
   b. Renomegaly (renal failure of middle-aged iguanas, chronic interstitial fibrosis (may be associated with iguana herpesvirus; renal gout).

Management

- For fluid therapy, see *Nursing Care*.

Treatment/specific therapy

- Renal failure of middle-aged iguanas
  - Aetiology probably dietary (excessive animal protein) and may include chronic mild dehydration
  - Fluid therapy
  - Other renal therapeutic drugs could, with caution, be tried
- Gout
  - Fluid therapy
  - Allopurinol at 10 mg/kg s.i.d. *Note* this will only prevent subsequent uric acid deposition
  - Very guarded prognosis
  - May be linked to excess dietary protein, renal disease, chronic dehydration, use of nephrotoxic drugs).

Reproductive disorders

Nutritional
- Hypocalcaemia (with subsequent oviductal inertia).

Neoplasia

Other non-infectious problems

- Haemorrhage from ovarian artery
- Dystocia
- Preovulatory ovarian stasis (POOS)
- Egg stasis (post-ovulatory)
- Egg yolk peritonitis
- Ovarian necrosis
- Seminal plugs (caseous debris accumulating in the inverted hemipenes).

Findings on clinical examination

- Inappetence, anorexia
- History of reproductive activity, e.g. mating, burrowing in nesting chamber or other areas of vivarium. Some eggs may have been laid. *Note* that some healthy females (esp. iguanas, water dragons, bearded dragons, veiled chameleons) will spontaneously ovulate without the presence of a male or others of the same species
- Restlessness
- Obvious swelling of the coelomic cavity (not always obvious)
- Hind-limb weakness
- Signs of metabolic bone disease (see *Systemic Disorders*)
- Dehydration in neglected cases (especially veiled chameleons)
- Swelling caudal to cloaca in males (seminal plugs)
- Sudden death (haemorrhage from ovarian artery).

Investigations

1. Radiography
   a. The hemipenes are calcified and therefore visible in some lizard species especially monitor lizards (*Varanidae*)
   b. Eggs may be reasonably well calcified (many geckos) or poorly calcified (iguanas, water dragons); these latter are visible as circular to oval opacities. Typically these are in the caudal coelom but because there is no diaphragm, in extreme cases they can occupy much of the coelomic cavity, displacing other organs dorsally. Eggs that are heavily mineralized, excessively large or irregular in shape are usually abnormal (Fig. 7.13)
   c. Ensures there are no obvious obstructions, e.g. pelvic deformities from metabolic bone disease
   d. Foetal skeletons may be visible in advanced gestation in live-bearing lizards, e.g. Solomon Island skinks (*Corucia zebrata*)
2. Transillumination
   a. Useful in small, lightly pigmented lizards such as leopard geckos
   b. Direct a small bright light, e.g. from an otoscope, through the body so as to view the underside of the lizard. The liver is usually readily identified and its relative size assessed. Eggs, bladder size and fat pads can all be identified and assessed
3. Routine haematology and biochemistry
   a. Blood calcium levels

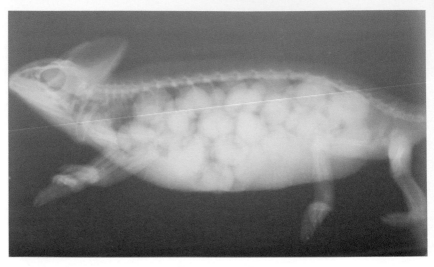

Fig. 7.13. Dystocia complicated by superovulation in a veiled chameleon.

4. Culture and sensitivity
5. Endoscopy
6. Biopsy/necropsy
   a. Haemorrhage in periovarian tissue
7. Ultrasonography
   a. Useful for preovulatory ovarian stasis.

Treatment/specific therapy

- Seminal plugs
  - Gentle removal
  - May be linked with hypovitaminosis A
- Dystocia
  - Provision of correct environment including appropriate temperature, humidity and nesting chamber may induce normal egg-laying. Supplement with calcium, e.g. calcium gluconate at 1 mL/kg p.o. b.i.d.
  - Medical induction
    - Calcium at 100 mg/kg every 6–12 h
    - 5–20 IU/kg oxytocin given 1 h after last calcium
    - Repeat over 2–3 cycles if lizard is otherwise healthy
    - If some eggs still retained after 48 h, consider surgery
    - Argipressin at 0.01–1.0 μg/kg (more potent than oxytocin in reptiles)
  - Percutaneous ovocentesis (Hall & Lewbart 2006). Only useful in small lizards with small numbers of eggs. Performed under anaesthesia with sterile 23 gauge butterfly catheter. Beware of yolk leaking into coelomic cavity, aspiration of the viscera or their contents, both of which will trigger a serositis. Allow lizard to pass collapsed eggs

- Salpingotomy
- Ovariosalpingectomy. Make a paramedian incision: avoid incising into the ventral midline due to ventral vena cava (visible with transillumination).

Neonatal disorders

See *Neonatal Disorders* in *Snakes*.

Behavioural disorders

- Behavioural interactions with transparent barriers (ITB) (see *Skin Disorders*)
- Aggression in adult male iguanas.

Signs

- Heightened aggression; iguanas may attack owner or passersby through the vivarium glass
- Some male iguanas show heightened aggression at particular times of their female owner's menstrual cycle. Thought to be pheromonal in origin.

Treatment/specific therapy

- Behavioral management is difficult due to restricted space available to give each iguana its personal space
- With sexually motivated behaviour, temporary improvement may be achieved with regular injections of delmadinone acetate at 1 mg/kg i.m. Repeat as necessary
- If delmadinone is effective, consider castration.

References

Boyer T H 2002 Autoimmune haemolytic anemia in a Parson's chameleon, Calumma parsonii parsonii. Proc Assoc Reptil Amphib Vet 81–85

Drury S E N, Gough R E, Welschman D. de B 2002 Isolation and identification of a reovirus from a lizard, Uromastyx hardwickii, in the United Kingdom. Vet Rec 151:637–638

Girling S J, Fraser M A 2004 Listeria monocytogenes septicaemia in an Inland Bearded dragon Pogona vitticeps. J Herpet Med Surg 14(3):6–9

Hall A J, Lewbart G A 2006 Treatment of dystocia in a leopard gecko (Eublepharus macularius) by percutaneous ovocentesis. Vet Rec 158:737–739

Hernandez-Divers S J 2006a Advances in reptile renal diagnostics: identifying changes in renal function, not renal failure. Br Vet Zoo Soc Proc May:70–71

Hernandez-Divers S J 2006b Single-dose oral and intravenous pharmacokinetics of meloxicam in the green iguana (Iguana iguana). Br Vet Zoo Soc Proc May:54–55

Hulbert A J 2000 Thyroid hormones and their effects: a new perspective. Biol Rev 75:519–631

Kenny M J, Shaw S E, Hillyard P D et al 2004 Ectoparasite and haemoparasite risks associated with imported exotic reptiles. Vet Rec 154:434–435.

Martin J C, Moore A S, Ruslander D et al 2003 Successful radiation treatment of leukaemia in a sungazer lizard (Cordylus giganteus). Proc Assoc Reptil Amphib Vet 8

Martinez-Silvestre A, Mateo J A, Pether J 2003 Electrocardiographic parameters in a Gomeran Giant Lizard (Gallotia bravoana). J Herpet Med Surg 13(3):22–25

Martorell J, Ramis A, Espada Y 2002 Use of ultrasonography in the diagnosis of hepatic spindle-cell sarcoma in a savannah monitor (Varanus exanthematicus) Vet Rec 150:282–284

McBride M, Koch T F, Hernandez-Divers S et al 2004 Preliminary evaluation of resting and post-prandial bile acid levels and a novel biliverdin assay in the green iguana (Iguana iguana). Proc Assoc Reptil Amphib Vet 105

Mehlhorn H, Schmahl G, Mevissen I 2005a Efficacy of a combination of imidacloprid and moxidectin against parasites of reptiles and rodents: case reports. Parasitol Res 97:S97–S101

Mehlhorn H, Schmahl G, Frese M et al 2005b Effects of a combination of emodepside and praziquantel on parasites of reptiles and rodents. Parasitol Res 97:S64–S69

Orós J, Ruiz A, Castro P et al 2002 Immunohistochemical detection of microfilariae of Foleyella species in an Oustalet's chameleon (Furcifer oustaleti). Vet Rec 150:20–22

Patterson-Kane J C, Redrobe S P 2005 Colonic adenocarcinoma in a leopard gecko (Eublepharis macularis). Vet Rec 157:294–295

Scott S, Warwick C 2002 Behavioural problems in a monitor lizard. UK Vet 7(3):73–75

Smith D, Dobson H, Spence E 2001 Gastrointestinal studies in the green iguana: technique and reference values. Vet Radiol Ultrasound 42(6):515–520

Soldati G, Lu Z H, Vaughan L et al 2004 Detection of mycobacteria and chlamydiae in granulomatous inflammation of reptiles: A retrospective study. Vet Pathol 41:388–397

Stahl S 2000 Diseases of Bearded Dragons (Pogona vitticeps). Exotic Animal Medicine and Surgery BSAVA Continuing Education Course, 3 November–5th November

Taylor M A, Geach M R, Cooley W A 1999 Clinical and pathological observations on natural infections of cryptosporidiosis and flagellate protozoa in leopard geckos (Eublepharis macularis). Vet Rec 145:695–699

Walter D E, Shaw M 2002 First record of the mite Hirstiella diolii Baker (Prostigmata Pterygosomatidae) from Australia, with a revue of mites found on Australian lizards. Aust J Entomol 41(1):30–34

Wellehan J F X, Jarchow J L, Regiardo C et al 2003a A novel herpesvirus associated with hepatic necrosis in a San Esteban chuckwalla, Sauromalus varius. J Herpet Med Surg 13(3):15–19

Wellehan J F X, Johnson A J, Jacobson E R et al 2003b Nested PCR amplification and sequencing of reptile adenoviruses including a novel gecko adenovirus associated with enteritis. Proc Assoc Reptil Amphib Vet 14

Wellehan J F X, Johnson A J, Jacobson E R et al 2003c Novel herpesviruses associated with stomatitis in lizards. Proc Assoc of Reptil Amphib Vet 57

Wilson G H, Fontenot D K, Brown C A et al 2004 Pseudocarcinomatous biliary hyperplasia in two green iguanas, Iguana iguana. J Herpet Med Surg 14(4):12–18

Snakes

· ·

Snakes are popular reptile pets, and there has been a resurgence in their popularity with the breeding of a variety of colour morphs. A huge number of species are available in the pet-trade, but the commonly kept species are listed in Table 8.1.

The internal anatomy of a snake is shown in Figure 8.1 (see also 'Radiography', in *Musculoskeletal Disorders*).

Consultation and handling

A healthy snake should be reasonably alert and responsive to touch. If it is flaccid or exhibiting CNS signs, such as 'star-gazing' it is likely to be suffering a septicaemia, poisoning or possibly a protozoal infection such as acanthamoeba.

Start the examination at the head and work backwards. Larger snakes such as the pythons and boas may require one or more people to hold them while you perform your examination. A gag is usually required to open the mouth – wooden spatulas work reasonably well and are less traumatic than metal equivalents. Do not encourage staff or clients to drape large constricting snakes across the shoulders and around the neck because if the snake feels insecure, it may well tighten its grip unexpectedly.

Venomous snakes require specialist handling equipment and should only be handled by a competent herpetologist or while under an anaesthetic.

Microchipping

● Left nape of the neck, subcutaneously placed at twice the length of the head from the tip of the nose
● Skin closure is achieved either by suture or with tissue glue.

Sexing

Many snakes are not obviously sexually dimorphic or dichromatic. The safest and most popular way of sexing monomorphic snakes is by 'probe-sexing', where a small, well-lubricated and blunt-ended rod is gently inserted into the cloaca and then directed caudally to one side of the midline so as to slot into the inverted hemipenes of the male, if present. If female, the probe will only travel a few subcaudal scales, while in a male it will pass a significant distance (Fig. 8.2).

Table 8.1 Commonly kept species of snake: Key facts

Species	Notes	Common disorders
The royal python (*Python regius*)	This is a small python, growing to 90–120 cm. It has a not undeserved reputation for prolonged fasting, probably as a result of poor husbandry and endogenous cycles, although this is less pronounced with the modern captive-bred individuals and colour morphs	Dermatitis, dysecdysis and pneumonia. Anorexia, especially in wild caught or captive farmed individuals
The Burmese python (*Python morulus bivittatus*)	This python is a potentially very large snake; adults can reach up to 5–7 m long with a large muscular cross-section. Adults are usually reasonably behaved but hatchlings and youngsters can be aggressive	Dysecdysis, burns, pneumonia, inclusion body disease (IBD)
Boa constrictor (*Constrictor constrictor*)	A large snake up to 1.8–3.0 m long. Usually handleable but some individuals can be aggressive. Several colour morphs available and there is some selective breeding to reduce size using naturally occurring dwarf island subspecies	Snake mites, dysecdysis, inclusion body disease (IBD)
Corn snake (*Elaphe guttata guttata*)	Moderate-sized rodent-eating snakes that make excellent introductions to snake-keeping. This is probably the nearest there is to a domestic snake; it is available in a very wide range of colour morphs, grows to a manageable size (around 1.0 m) and readily takes frozen-defrosted prey	Dysecdysis, cryptosporidium
King snakes (*Lampropeltis spp*)	King snakes are natural predators of snakes and other reptiles and so are usually kept individually	Dysecdysis, obesity
Garter snakes (*Thamnophis spp*)	Small to medium-sized snakes. Can be nervous on handling. Many of these are earthworm, fish and amphibian predators, although they can be readily converted on to mammalian prey	Septicaemia, thiamine deficiency

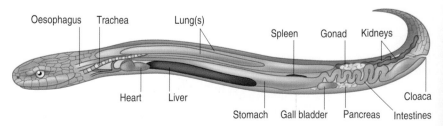

Fig. 8.1. Internal anatomy of a snake (lateral).

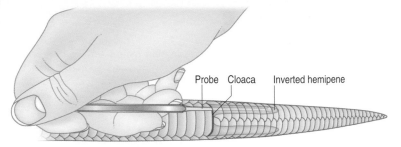

Fig. 8.2. Sexing snakes.

Nursing care

Provide an appropriate environment, including provision of:
1. Optimal temperature (basking lights, heat mats, etc., to allow thermoregulation). Use of max–min thermometers will assist in monitoring temperature ranges incumbent reptiles are exposed to
2. Full-spectrum lighting appears to be relatively unimportant for snakes with some exceptions, e.g. rough green snake (*Opheodrys aestivus*)
3. Humidity
4. Ventilation
5. Easily cleaned accommodation; use paper substrate and disposable/sterilizable hides and other vivarium furniture (Fig. 8.3)
6. Keep individually to minimize intra-specific stress and competition for resources.

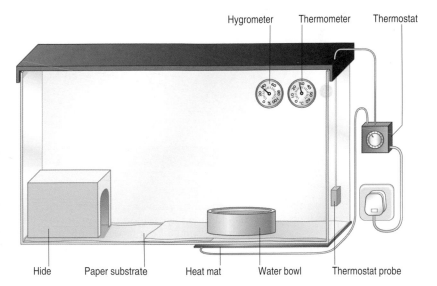

Fig. 8.3. Clinical vivarium setup for snakes (lighting is optional – see text).

Fluid therapy

See 'Fluid Therapy', in *Lizards*.

Dehydrated snakes typically show an increase in skin tenting and folding, especially longitudinal folding. Daily bathing in shallow, warm water is often beneficial; it encourages many snakes to drink as well as defaecate and urinate.

Fluids administration in snakes

1. Stomach tubing is relatively straightforward in snakes as the cardia is relatively weak.
2. Oesophagostomy tubes can be used in some cases.
3. Intracoelomic fluids can be given, but try for the ventral tail vein or even the palatine vein.
4. A jugular cut down can be performed if the snake is anesthetized and a catheter inserted, and small volumes may be administered as a bolus into the ventricle.
5. Small volumes may be given per cloaca.

Nutritional support

Liquidized normal diet or proprietary support diets can be used, given either by stomach tube or by oesophagostomy tube. Force-feeding of prey species may prove traumatic in inexperienced hands.

Analgesia

See 'Analgesia', in *Lizards*.

Anaesthesia

1. For general notes, see 'Anaesthesia', in *Lizards*.
2. Induction: Propofol at 10 mg/kg i.v. into the ventral tail vein, or 1.0–2.0 mg/kg intraventricular.
3. Otherwise as for *Lizards*.

Skin disorders

Normal ecdysis in snakes

Shedding in snakes is a cyclical event with synchronous replacement of the whole epidermis at the same time. Snakes should shed their skin in one continuous sheet, starting rostrally, and any deviation from this should be considered abnormal. Ecdysis is under both environmental and endocrinologic control. Ecdysis in snakes follows the following sequence:

1. Resting phase. There is only one *stratum corneum* and *stratum germinativum*.
2. The *stratum germinativum* undergoes intense proliferation to form a new *stratum corneum*, but there is no outward visible change in the snake.

3. The new *stratum corneum* begins to differentiate and keratinize. At this point there is a slight dulling of the skin of the snake, and the spectacle may appear slightly cloudy.
4. A new layer – *the stratum intermedium* – is now apparent. This lies between the inner and outer layers of strata cornea. The epidermis is thickest now and so the snake's colours are at their dullest; the spectacle is cloudy.
5. The stratum intermedium is dissolved away by lymph carrying enzymes – this leaves a cleavage plane between the two *strata cornea*. The snake's colours will be seen to brighten and the spectacle will clear.
6. Approximately 4–7 days after the spectacles clear, the outer *stratum corneum* is shed.

Differential diagnoses of skin disorders

See also *Skin Disorders*, in *Lizards*

Shedding difficulties (Dysecdysis)

- Humidity too low
- Other environmental problems – incorrect photoperiod, temperature, nutrition, etc.
- Lack of cage furniture to allow initiation of shedding
- Snake mites *(Ophionyssus natracis)*
- Scarring or other underlying dermal disease
- Hyperthyroidism (excessive, repeated skin shedding)
- Secondary bacterial and fungal infections common.

Pruritus

- Snake mites
- Irritation; large numbers can be associated with anaemia, dysecdysis, depression and anorexia.

Erosions and ulceration

- Rodent bites
- Adhesive tape (Fig. 8.4)
- Blisters and sores, especially on the ventral scales (ventral dermal necrosis, vesicular dermatitis, blister disease). Typically bacterial – *Pseudomonas spp, Aeromonas spp, Proteus spp*
- Mycotic dermatitis, e.g. *Chrysosporium* anamorph of *Nannizziopsis vriesii* (CANV)
- *Kalicephalus* larvae.

Nodules and non-healing wounds

- Granulomas (bacterial, mycobacterial, fungal)
- Dermatophilosis (*Dermatophilus chelonae*)
- Dermatophytosis, include *Penicillium spp, Trichophyton mentagrophytes, Candida albicans, Aspergillus spp, Fusarium spp.*
- Filarial worms (*Oswaldofilaria, Foleyella, Macdonaldius spp*)
- Pentastomids (esp. *Armillifer armillifer, Porocephalus spp, Kiricephalus spp*) (see also *Respiratory Tract Disorders*)
- Cestodes: *Diphyllobothrium* and *Spirometra* (sparganosis).

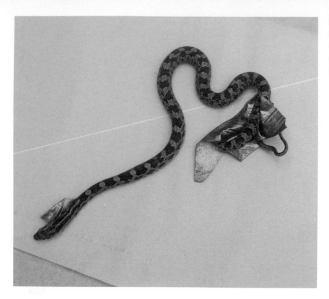

Fig. 8.4. A young anerythristic cornsnake caught up in duct tape used on the electrics in a home-made vivarium.

Changes in pigmentation

- Petechial haemorrhages: septicaemia (see *Systemic Disorders*) *Kalicephalus spp* (see *Gastrointestinal Tract Disorders*).

Ectoparasites

- Helminths
  - *Kalicephalus* (hookworm) larvae (see *Gastrointestinal Tract Disorders*)
  - Filarial worms (*Oswaldofilaria, Foleyella, Macdonaldius spp*)
- Cestodes: *Diphyllobothrium* and *Spirometra* (sparganosis)
- Arthropods
  - Ticks (*Aponomma latum* and *Amblyomma spp*, see Kenny et al 2004)
  - Snake mite *(Ophionyssus natracis)*
  - Pentastomids, e.g. *Raillietiella.*

Burns

- Many snakes are thigmotherms; powerful unprotected heating equipment can cause severe localized burning of the dermis.

Spontaneous rupture of skin (hypovitaminosis C)

Neoplasia

- Squamous cell carcinoma
- Fibrosarcoma
- Chromatophoroma (malignant)
- Liposarcoma
- Lipoma (esp. cornsnakes, *Elaphe guttata*).

Findings on clinical examination

- Dysecdysis: One or more patches of retained skin. In some areas the skin will appear dull and thickened where several layers of skin have built up over successive dysecdysis episodes. In some cases rings of unshed skin may form bands around the tip the tail. As these dry they constrict, acting as tourniquets and compromising blood flow to the extremity. The spectacles may be retained (see *Ophthalmic Disorders*)
- Small mites found on snakes; tend to accumulate under the scales, the postorbital area, labial pits and any skinfolds around the mouth or cloaca. Snake may spend much of time submerged in water bowl (snake mites)
- Large arthropod parasites (ticks)
- Red patches resembling bruising (haemorrhages – septicaemia, trauma)
- Anaemia (heavy ectoparasitic infestations)
- Swellings (neoplasia, subcutaneous parasites, e.g. filarial nematodes, but also consider coelomic disorders).

Investigations

1. Cytology (fine needle aspirate)
   a. Faecal or sputum examination
   b. Pentastomid eggs
2. Routine haematology and biochemistry
   a. Thyroid levels (see *Endocrine Disorders*)
3. Aseptic collection of samples
   a. Culture and sensitivity
4. Endoscopy
   a. Adult pentastomids (look like strange caterpillars)
5. Radiography
6. Biopsy
7. Ultrasonography.

Treatment/specific therapy

- Dysecdysis
  - Moisten the affected areas in order to loosen the retained skin from the underlying epidermis. If the skin feels firmly attached, leave it and try again after further moistening
  - Placing the snake in a warm, damp towel, pillow case or duvet cover (for large snakes) provides rehydration, lubrication and soft, slightly abrasive surfaces against which to rub. Enforced bathing in warm water may also help but beware the possibility of drowning
  - Retained spectacular scales are best removed using a damp cotton bud (see *Ophthalmic Disorders*)
  - Vitamin A at 1000–5000 IU/kg i.m. will often trigger a further shed, allowing a closer management of the sloughing procedure such that both the old shed and the new are removed

- Hyperthyroidism
  - Antithyroid drugs, e.g. methimazole at 2 mg/kg s.i.d.
  - Possible try other antithyroid drugs such as carbimazole
  - Partial or complete thyroidectomy may also be appropriate dependant upon the case
- Ventral dermal necrosis
  - Usually associated with too damp an environment – in semi-aquatic species, it can be initiated by the dermal penetration of hookworm larvae. If left untreated it may progress to a septicaemia
  - Treatment is with topical povidone-iodine plus appropriate systemic antibiosis – successful antibiotics include enrofloxacin, amikacin or even gentamicin
  - Parenteral vitamin A at 1000–5000 IU will induce ecdysis helping to remove much of the infected skin and necrotic material
- Abscess/granuloma
  - Any abnormal swelling should be investigated as a potential abscess or granuloma and may require surgery plus systemic antibiosis
- Dermatophytosis and fungal mycoses
  - Topical chlorhexidine (0.26 mL/L)
  - Topical antifungals, e.g. miconazole, terbinafine
  - Ketoconazole at 15 mg/kg every 72 h p.o.
  - Griseofulvin at 15 mg/kg every 72 h p.o.
- *Kalicephalus*
  - Fenbendazole at 25 mg/kg weekly for at least 2–3 weeks)
- Filarial nematodes and pentastomids
  - Ivermectin at 200 µg/kg s.c. (toxic to indigo snakes)
  - Surgical resection of associated skin granulomas
  - Adult pentastomids usually present in lung following extensive tissue migration
- Cestodes
  - Surgical removal where feasible
  - Praziquantel at 5 mg/kg p.o., s.c. or i.m. Repeat after 2 weeks
- Adhesive tape entanglement
  - The outer epithelial layers may be removed and owners may tear the skin in their efforts to remove the tape
  - Use a solvent (such as halothane or isoflurane) to gradually remove the adhesive; an anaesthetic may be required especially if tape is adhered to the spectacle (see *Ophthalmic Disorders*)
  - Repair any skin lesions; small lesions can be sealed with tissue glue, larger may require suturing
  - Covering antibiosis if necessary
- Burns
  - Debride necrotic material (may require anaesthetic)and treat with a topical amorphous hydrogel dressings, e.g. IntraSite Gel (Smith and Nephew Healthcare Ltd., and/or Povidine-iodine
  - Covering antibiotic or antifungal medication
  - If the burns are extensive then fluid therapy should be instigated (see *Gastrointestinal Tract Disorders*)
  - Scaring will eventually result which may lead to localized areas of dysecdysis; if scarring is extensive then can lead to problems
  - Restrictive scarring may mean that constricting snakes have difficulty completing the behavioural repertoire necessary for normal feeding

- Spontaneous rupture of skin
  - Clean, debride and suture edges of lesion
  - Supplement with ascorbic acid. May be linked to feeding starved and, therefore, vitamin C deficient rodent prey
- Ticks
  - Individual removal of ticks
  - Ivermectin at 200 µg/kg s.c. (toxic to indigo snakes)
    Note that ticks are vectors for *Babesia/Hepatozoon* and *Ehrlichia*-like organisms
- Snake mites
  - Parthenogenetic so numbers can rapidly build up in vivaria; treatment must include the thorough cleansing of all affected vivaria. What cannot be sterilized with a mild bleach solution (5 mL per gallon) must be disposed
  - Replace usual substrate with paper (changed daily)
  - Repeated washing with warm water will physically remove any mites
  - Application of topical fipronil spray once weekly for at least 4 weeks. This is best first applied to a cloth and rubbed over the entire surface of the snake. Fipronil can also be used to treat the environment
  - Injection of ivermectin at 200 µg/kg s.c. (*Note:* toxic to indigo snakes and chelonia) every 2 weeks will kill those that feed on the snake.
  - Commercial imidacloprid (100 g/L) plus moxidectin (25 g/L) (Advocate Dog, Bayer) applied at double (32 mg/kg imidacloprid + 8.0 mg/kg moxidectin) to 10-fold dosages (160 mg/kg imidacloprid + 40 mg/kg moxidectin) according to thickness of skin (care with garter snakes *Thamnophis spp.*) (Mehlhorn et al 2005b)
  - Cultures of predatory mites (*Hypoaspis miles*) are commercially available for use in vivaria
  - Linked to septicaemia and IBD outbreaks (see *Systemic Disorders*) as possible vector
- Neoplasia
  - Surgical resection
  - Chromatophoromas carry a poor prognosis with early metastasis
  - Chemotherapy in reptiles is in its infancy and most tumours are managed surgically. Accessible cutaneous tumours can be treated by injecting cisplatin directly into the tissue mass on a weekly basis as a debulking exercise.

Respiratory tract disorders

Viral

- Reovirus
- Paramyxovirus.

Bacterial

- Abscesses
- Granulomas
- Pneumonia/air sacculitis (Fig. 8.5).

Fungal

- Abscesses
- Granulomas

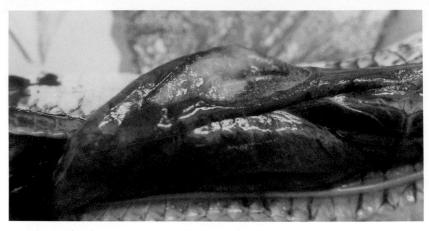

Fig. 8.5. Accumulation of purulent material in the lungs of a Royal python with pneumonia.

- Pneumonia/air sacculitis
- *Cryptococcus neoformans* (see also *Systemic Disorders* and *Neurological Disorders*)
- *Coccidiomycosis*
- *Aspergillus spp, A. niger.*

Parasitic

- Lungworm; *Rhabdias spp.*

Neoplasia

- Metastases, e.g. from renal carcinomas
- Chondroma (tracheal).

Other non-infectious problems

- Occluded nostrils.

Findings on clinical examination

- Nasal discharge/rhinitis
- Open mouthed breathing
- 'Wet' or unusual respiratory noises
- Discharge around the glottis or inside the proximal trachea. Must differentiate from oesophageal discharge (gastritis/enteritis) or secondary to stomatitis. Some conditions may occur concurrently
- Snake mucus is often thick and tenacious. Mucus may be found as gobbets in the vivarium
- Snakes have limited ability to cough and the trachea is long so obstructions due to mucus can be serious and may require flushing
- Occluded nostrils
- Sudden death.

Investigations

1. Microscopy
   a. Sputum examination (either from mouth, pulmonary lavage or endoscopic collection)
   b. Staining for cytology
   c. Gram stain
   d. Lungworm eggs and larvae
2. Radiography
3. Routine haematology and biochemistry
4. Serology for *Cryptococcus* (also consider isolation from lung lavage)
5. PCR and HI serology for paramyxovirus
6. Culture and sensitivity
7. Endoscopy
8. Biopsy
9. Ultrasonography
10. CT scan
    a. Pees et al (2007) offer the measurements in Table 8.2 for CT examinations of the lungs of healthy Indian pythons (*Python morulus*) and pythons with respiratory tract disease
    b. Also the mean (±SD) measurements of attenuation in defined lung areas for CT examinations of healthy pythons and pythons with respiratory tract disease (Table 8.3).

Management

- If respiratory disease is severe provide a high oxygen atmosphere
- Aminophylline at 2.0–4.0 mg/kg i.m.

Treatment/specific therapy

- Viral infections
  - No treatment. Supportive therapy only. Those diagnosed with paramyxovirus should be removed from the collection
- Bacterial infections
  - Appropriate antibiosis. Consider nebulizing
- Fungal infections
  - Ketoconazole at 15 mg/kg every 72 h p.o.
  - Griseofulvin at 15 mg/kg every 72 h p.o.
- Lungworm
  - Fenbendazole at 50–100 mg/kg. Repeat every 2 weeks if necessary. *Note* that fenbendazole is metabolized to oxfendazole by the liver
  - Oxfendazole at 68 mg/kg. Repeat every 2 weeks if necessary
  - Ivermectin at 0.2 mg s.c. or p.o. repeated every 2 weeks for 3 treatments (*toxic to indigo snakes*)
  - Lungworms have a direct life cycle; infective larvae can penetrate the skin or infect via the contaminated food and water
- Chondroma
  - Surgical debulking/resection

Table 8.2 Measurements for CT examinations of the lungs of healthy Indian pythons (Python molurus) and pythons with respiratory tract disease

Pythons	Length (mm) (mean ± SD)		Mean area in cross section (mm²) (mean ± SD)	Mean thickness value at each location for the dorsal, left, right, and ventral part of the lung (mm) (mean ± SD)		
	Right lung	Left lung		At point 25% of the length of the respiratory tissue	At point 50% of the length of the respiratory tissue	At point 75% of the length of the respiratory tissue
Healthy	222 ± 86 (89–348)	188 ± 69 (89–295)	279 ± 188 (79–594)	5.1 ± 2.1 (2.2–9.4)	4.2 ± 1.2 (2.2–6.0)	2.7 ± 0.8 (2.2–5.6)
Respiratory disease	307 ± 23 (283–336)	244 ± 29 (205–286)	483 ± 133 (347–675)	6.8 ± 1.8 (2.2–6.0)	5.0 ± 1.0 (4.0–6.0)	2.8 ± 0.8 (3.5–6.0)

Pees et al (2007).

Table 8.3 Mean ± SD measurements of attenuation in defined lung areas for CT examinations of healthy pythons and pythons with respiratory tract disease

Pythons		Entire lung tissues		Dorsal part of lungs		Left part of lung		Right part of lung		Ventral part of lungs	
		Attenuation	Variability of attenuation	Attenuation	Variability of attenuation	Attenuation	Variability of attenuation	Attenuation	Variability of attenuation	Attenuation	Variability of attenuation
Healthy	Mean ± SD	−744.4 ± 47.1	94.8 ± 9.7	−761.0 ± 43.1	48.4 ± 8.0	−756.3 ± 53.0	50.6 ± 18.0	−755.4 ± 51.3	54.3 ± 17.0	−761.8 ± 50.0	61.4 ± 6.9
	Range	−805.3–672.0	82.2–111.9	−819.1–693.7	34.8–63.8	−819.9–670.0	28.8–84.1	−831.2–664.0	28.1–85.7	−847.6–706.0	49.9–72.3
Respiratory disease	Mean ± SD	−613.7 ± 176.4	160.9 ± 56.4	−655.5 ± 155.0	99.6 ± 61.6	−624.4 ± 173.9	102.0 ± 65.1	−604.3 ± 193.1	121.4 ± 77.2	−555.9 ± 214.5	165.3 ± 56.9
	Range	−789.0–359.0	98.9–226.2	−808.1–424.9	44.2–192.1	−770.2–350.1	39.9–198.1	−829.7–372.6	44.9–213.2	−771.8–266.7	73.3–211.9

Pees et al (2007).

- Occluded nostrils
  - Flush and remove as much debris as possible. May require anaesthesia to undertake.

Gastrointestinal tract disorders

Disorders of the oral cavity

Note that mucus may be seen in the mouth as part of respiratory disease and should be differentiated.

Bacterial

- Stomatitis (a variety of G −ve bacteria, esp. *Aeromonas, Pseudomonas, Proteus, Morganella*)
- Intermandibular cellulitis (*Pseudomonas* and *Aeromonas*)
- Venom gland infection (venomous snakes).

Fungal

- Stomatitis.

Parasitic

- Ocheostomid trematodes.

Neoplasia

- Undifferentiated sarcoma (Abou-Madi et al 1994) (see also *Systemic Disorders*).

Other non-infectious problems

- Fractures (traumatic, pathological).

Findings on clinical examination

- Discharge from the mouth and nares
- Fluid respiratory noises
- Inflammation of the oral and pharyngeal membranes; may progress to ulcerative lesions of the palatine area, the trachea and the tongue sheath. A diphtheritic membrane may be present (stomatitis)
- Occasionally infection may track up the lachrymal duct resulting in a subspectacular abscess over one or both corneas (stomatitis) (see *Ophthalmic Disorders*)
- Obvious flat helminth-like parasites in oral cavity (trematodes)
- Gross swelling of the lower jaw and intermandibular area (intermandibular cellulitis)
- Permanent apparent dislocation of the mandible/swelling of one or both mandibles (fracture)
- Abnormal colouring of mucous membranes (icterus, cyanosis)
- Unilateral (or occasionally bilateral) swelling on the face, below eye and/or along maxilla (venom gland infection/abscess).

Investigations

1. Radiography
   a. Stomatitis with possible underlying osteomyelitis
2. Routine haematology and biochemistry

3. Cytology (may need FNA) including Gram staining
4. Culture and sensitivity
5. Endoscopy
6. Biopsy
7. Ultrasonography.

Treatment/specific therapy

- Stomatitis
  - Snakes may not feed while suffering from stomatitis, so may require fluid support such as Hartman's at 15–25 mL/kg; nutritional support should be given by stomach tube during this time
  - The stomach tube should be lubricated and coated with appropriate antibiotic to try to prevent iatrogenic spread of infection to the oesophagus and further
  - Topical antibiotics plus topical povidone-iodine daily may be sufficient
  - Surgical debridement of necrotic tissue followed by systemic and topical treatments may be required
- Intermandibular cellulitis
  - A synergistic infection of both *Pseudomonas fluorescens* and *Aeromonas hydrophila*
  - Supportive treatment
  - Appropriate antibiotics
- Fractured jaw
  - Pathologically weakened bone, or mandibles of small snakes, may be unable to support orthopaedic techniques; in some cases taping the jaw closed with strong adhesive plaster (taking care to leave the nares open) accompanied by placement of an oesophagostomy tube may allow healing to occur (Fig. 8.6)
- Trematodes
  - Often asymptomatic; may cause snake to gape
  - Praziquantel at 5 mg/kg p.o., s.c. or i.m. Repeat after 2 weeks
  - Freeze food items, e.g. frogs, fish for 3 days prior to feeding to eliminate intermediate stages
- Icterus (see *Hepatic Disorders; Cardiovascular and Haematological Disorders*)
- Cyanosis (see *Respiratory Tract Disorders*)
- Neoplasia (see 'Treatment', under *Skin Disorders*)
- Venom gland infection
  - Surgical removal of infected venom gland
  - Covering antibiosis
  Note that removal of both venom glands renders the snake incapable of taking live prey, may alter the shape of the head and may affect digestion.

Differential diagnosis for gastrointestinal disorders

Viral
- Reovirus (Reavil et al 2003).

Bacterial
- *Salmonella spp.*
- *E. coli*
- *Chlamydophila spp* (see also *Systemic Disorders*).

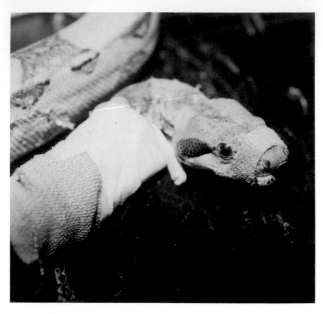

Fig. 8.6. Taping the jaw of a young boa constrictor with a fractured mandible. *Note* the oesophagostomy tube in place.

Fungal

- Candidiasis.

Protozoal

- *Cryptosporidium serpentis*
- *Entamoeba invadens*
- *Eimeria*
- *Caryospora*
- *Isospora*
- Flagellates, e.g. *Trichomonas, Trichomonas.*

Parasitic

- Ascarids
- *Ophiascaris*
- *Polydelphis*
- *Hexametra*
- *Ophiostrongylus*
- Hookworms
- *Kalicephalus*
- Capillaria
- Strongyloides
- Oxyurids
- Tapeworms
- Flukes
- Pentastomids (esp. *Armillifer armillifer, Porocephalus spp, Kiricephalus spp*) (see also *Skin Disorders*).

Neoplasia
- Adenocarcinomas.

Other non-infectious problems
- Foreign body ingestion or impaction
- Constipation
- Dystocia (as a cause of constipation)
- Cloacal prolapse
- Cloacitis
- Cloacoliths
- Intestinal foreign body
- Intussusception
- Extra-intestinal mass, e.g. renal neoplasm
- Dystocia
- Hypocalcaemia/metabolic bone disease (see *Nutritional Disorders*)
- Parasitism.

Findings on clinical examination

- Vomiting/regurgitation
- Weight loss
- Lethargy
- Chronic regurgitation, extreme weight loss, depression, mucus-laden stools and an obvious abdominal bulge caused by hypertrophy of the gastric mucosa (*Cryptosporidiosis*)
- Dysentery (mucus-laden, bile stained and/or showing frank blood), anorexia, dehydration, wasting and death (*Entamaeba invadens*)
- A coelomic mass may be palpable
- Petechial skin haemorrhages (*Kalicephalus*) (see *Skin Disorders*)
- Cloacal prolapse (differentiate from prolapse of the colon or hemipenes).

Investigations

1. Microscopy
   a. Fresh faecal sample – 'wet prep' (Fig. 8.7 and Table 8.4)
2. Radiography
   a. Plain radiographs
   b. Contrast studies, e.g. for hypertrophic gastritis (*Cryptosporidiosis*)

Contrast studies in snakes

1. Barium sulphate suspension given by gavage at 5 mL/kg
2. Double contrast: immediately follow barium with 45 mL/kg air
3. Take first radiograph after 15 min.

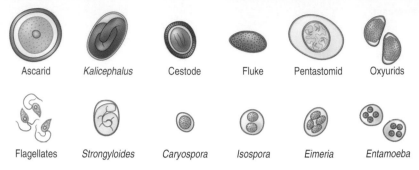

| Ascarid | *Kalicephalus* | Cestode | Fluke | Pentastomid | Oxyurids |

| Flagellates | *Strongyloides* | *Caryospora* | *Isospora* | *Eimeria* | *Entamoeba* |

Fig. 8.7. Common gastrointestinal parasites of snakes. (Not drawn to scale.)

Table 8.4 Parasites found in fresh faecal samples

Faecal parasite	Comments
Ascarid eggs (*Ophiascaris, Polydelphis*)	Typical ascarid eggs
Oxyurid eggs	Rodent pinworm eggs may also be seen in snakes fed on infested prey rodents
Hookworm eggs	Thin walled, oval eggs
Strongyloides	Larvae in *fresh* faecal samples; eggs are thin-walled and similar to *Rhabdias*
Capillaria	Typical urn-shape with operculae at either end (see *Hepatic Disorders*)
Tapeworm eggs	Thick walled with several dark hooklets in the centre
Fluke eggs	Thin-shelled, often with single operculum. Orange or deep yellow colour. Miracidium may be visible
Flagellates	Numerous motile pear-to-circular-shaped protozoa approximately 8 × 5 µm
Cryptosporidium	Oocysts may be visible using phase contrast microscopy after floatation. Otherwise consider MZN staining
Isospora oocysts	Circular
Eimeria oocysts	Elongate
Entamoeba	Cysts and amoeboid protozoa

3. Routine haematology and biochemistry
4. Culture and sensitivity
5. Endoscopy
6. Biopsy/necropsy
7. Electromicroscopy
    a. Reovirus
8. Ultrasonography.

Management

- For fluid therapy and general management, see *Nursing Care*.

Treatment/specific therapy

- Reovirus
  - Supportive treatment only
- Salmonellosis
  - Probably best considered as a normal constituent of the snake cloacal/gut microflora
  - Occasionally pathogenic to snakes. May cause erosive gut lesions with subsequent bacteraemia/septicaemia
  - Excretion likely to increase during times of stress, e.g. movement, illness
  - Treatment usually not appropriate as unlikely to be effective long term and may encourage resistance
  - Recommendations for prevention of salmonellosis from captive reptiles issued by the Center for Disease Control in the USA. These are:
    - Pregnant women, children <5 years of age and persons with impaired immune system function (e.g. AIDS) should not have contact with reptiles
    - Because of the risk if becoming infected with Salmonella from a reptile, even without direct contact, households with pregnant women, children <5 years of age or persons with impaired immune system function should not keep reptiles. Reptiles are not appropriate pets for childcare centres
    - All persons should wash hands with soap immediately after any contact with a reptile or reptile cage
    - Reptiles should be kept out of food preparation areas such as kitchens
  - Kitchen sinks should not be used to wash food or water bowls, cages or vivaria used for reptiles, or to bath reptiles. Any sink used for these purposes should be disinfected after use
- *Cryptosporidium serpentis*
  - Direct life cycle; infection by exposure to water containing infective oocysts
  - There is no recognized effective treatment
  - Metronidazole
    - In general, 100–257 mg/kg body weight. Repeat after 2 weeks if necessary
    - For colubrids, 40 mg/kg repeated after 2 weeks
    - *Boidae, Elaphidae* and *Viperidae* 125–250 mg/kg repeated after 2 weeks
    - Alternatively 20 mg/kg e.o.d. until eradication
  - Nitazoxanide at 5 mg/kg s.i.d.
  - Paromomycin at 300–800 mg/kg p.o. s.i.d. for 10 days
  - Oocysts (*C. parvum*) in water can be viable after 7 months at 15°C
  - Disinfect by exposing to water above 64°C for >2 min. *Cryptosporidium* oocysts are very resistant to chlorine or iodine
- *Isospora, Caryospora* and *Eimeria*
  - Sulphadimethoxine at 50 mg/kg daily for 3 days; stop for 3 days then repeat 3 day course.
  - Toltrazuril at 7.5 mg/kg p.o. s.i.d. for 2 days. Repeat after 12 days
  - Young/stressed snakes more susceptible
  - Rodent prey may be source of contamination.

- *Entamoeba invadens*
  - Ingestion of faeces-contaminated water or food with the infective cysts
  - Often commensally present in gut of herbivorous reptiles, e.g. terrestrial *Chelonia* so do not keep snakes with such reptiles
  - Metronidazole (as for *Cryptosporidium* above)
  - Chloroquine
    - 125 mg/kg p.o. every 48 h for three treatments
    - 50 mg/kg i.m. every 7 days for 3 weeks
  - Iodoquinol/diiodohydroxyquin 50 mg/kg p.o. s.i.d. for 21 days. *Note* possibly toxic to black rat snakes
  - Paromomycin
    - 300–360 mg/kg e.o.d. for 14 days
    - 25–100 mg/kg daily for 4 weeks
  - Potential zoonosis
- Ascarids, hookworms and oxyurids
  - Fenbendazole at 50–100 mg/kg. Repeat every 2 weeks if necessary. *Note* that fenbendazole is metabolized to oxfendazole by the liver
  - Oxfendazole at 68 mg/kg. Repeat every 2 weeks if necessary
  - Ivermectin at 0.2 mg s.c. or p.o. repeated every 2 weeks for 3 treatments (*toxic to indigo snakes*)
  - Topical emodepside plus praziquantel preparations (Profender, Bayer) at 56 µL/100 g body weight (Mehlhorn et al 2005a)
  - *Note* that *Oxyuris* worms usually have a direct life cycle
  - Hookworms have a direct life cycle; infective larvae can penetrate the skin or infect via the contaminated food and water.
- Tapeworms
  - Praziquantel at 5 mg/kg p.o., s.c. or i.m. Repeat after 2 weeks
- Foreign body/intussusception
  - Surgical enterotomy/enterectomy
- Faecal impaction (constipation)
  - Investigate for underlying cause, e.g. foreign body, dystocia, neoplasia
  - Fluid therapy (see *Nursing*)
  - Gut motility enhancers, e.g. metoclopramide at 60 µg/kg; cisapride at 1.0 mg/kg s.i.d.
  - Enema under GA
  - Surgical enterotomy
- Cloacal prolapse
  - Purse-string suture around cloaca for a minimum of 14 days weeks
  - Limit feeding to reduce straining during defaecation
  - If repeated prolapses consider cloacopexy.

Anorexia

Environmental factors

- Inappropriate environment
  - Temperature too high/low
  - Humidity too high/low
  - Failure to provide adequate (size and/or number) of hiding places (insecurity)
  - Excessive handling especially in the days to weeks following purchase

- Excessive lighting and/or light duration. At least 10 h dark required
- Excessive disturbance outside the vivarium.

Physiological

- Preparatory to brumation (hibernation) in temperate snakes
- Preparatory to ecdysis.

Reproductive

- Prior to egg laying
- Reproductive seasonality in both sexes; note that male snakes exhibiting anorexia linked with reproductive activity may have large numbers of spermatozoa present in their urine
- For wild Royal pythons (*Python regius*) a reproduction-associated anorexia occurs naturally in the spring, which corresponds to autumn in northern latitudes, so loss of appetite in captive Royal pythons at this time may be normal. Males become sexually mature at weights above 650 g, while females are usually over 1000 g.

Stress

- Overcrowding
- Inappropriate species combinations
- Interference from uneaten prey animals.

Inappropriate feeding

- Not weaned on to dead food
- Wrong food offered
- Food offered not identified as food, e.g. white mice ignored whereas agouti-coloured mice taken. This may depend upon previous experience
- Poorly prepared food, e.g. partly defrosted/refrozen prey offered
- Offering food at inappropriate time of day, e.g. during day for nocturnal species.

Disease (see relevant sections)

Findings on clinical examination

- Snakes with a physiological anorexia tend to lose body condition slowly. This applies especially to the large constricting boas and pythons
- Snakes with disease processes often lose condition comparatively quickly and obviously
- Loss of muscle mass especially along the epaxial musculature
- Other obvious clinical signs, e.g. masses, stomatitis, ectoparasites, etc.

Treatment/specific therapy

- Weigh regularly and record – once weekly is usually sufficient
- Re-evaluate the snake's environment and husbandry based upon research of that particular species' need
- In physiological cases no remedial action is necessary and provided the snake maintains reasonable condition it should resume feeding, although this may persist until either endogenous or exogenous stimuli alter. This may take up to 3–4 months in some species

- If the snake is losing condition or if a physiological cause has been eliminated, then investigate as for other disease problems
- Force feeding
  - Liquidized diet
  - Lubricated whole prey.

Nutritional disorders

- Obesity
- Hepatic lipidosis (see *Hepatic Disorders*)
- Steatitis
- Vitamin B12 deficiency
- Metabolic bone disease (uncommon in snakes – see under *Lizards* if suspected)
- Hypoglycaemia (see *Neurological Disorders*).

Findings on clinical examination

- Gross, swollen appearance to body (obesity); head may appear unnaturally small. In extreme cases fat may appear partially sectioned giving a 'string of doughnuts' appearance
- Coelomic and subcutaneous fat becomes hard (steatitis)
- CNS signs (B12 deficiency, see *Neurological Disorders*).

Investigations

1. Faecal examination
   a. Capillaria eggs: typical urn-shape with operculae at either end (see 'Investigations', in *Gastrointestinal Tract Disorders*)
2. Radiography
   a. Hepatomegaly
   b. Evidence of extreme soft tissue covering
3. Routine haematology and biochemistry
   a. Cholesterol and triglyceride levels
4. Endoscopy
5. Biopsy/necropsy
6. Ultrasonography.

Treatment/specific therapy

- Obesity
  - Gradual weight loss
  - Long-term starvation likely to generate a ketoacidosis
  - Supplement with vitamin E to reduce the risk of steatitis
- Steatitis
  - Secondary to a diet high in saturated fats, e.g. obese rodents
  - Treat with vitamin E at 50 mg/kg p.o. or i.m.
  - Offer a diet low in saturated fats.

Hepatic disorders

Viral

- Adenovirus (boids)
- Reovirus (King snakes) (Reavil et al 2003).

Bacterial

- Mycobacteriosis (granulomas – may be multifocal).

Fungal

Parasitic

- *Capillaria spp* (esp. earthworm-fed garter and water snakes).

Nutritional

- Hepatic lipidosis.

Neoplasia

- Hepatocellular adenoma (garter snake, *Thamnophis radix*)
- Secondaries from other tumours.

Other non-infectious problems

- Biliary cysts.

Findings on clinical examination

- Loose faeces (see also *Gastrointestinal Tract Disorders*)
- Large swelling mid-body (hepatomegaly, biliary cysts)
- Neurological signs (hepatic encephalopathy – see *Neurological Disorders*)
- Jaundice (icterus).

Investigations

1. Faecal examination
    a. Capillaria eggs: typical urn-shape with operculae at either end (see 'Investigations', in *Gastrointestinal Tract Disorders*)
2. Radiography
    a. Hepatomegaly
    b. Hepatic masses
3. Routine haematology and biochemistry
4. Culture and sensitivity
5. Endoscopy
6. Biopsy/necropsy
    a. Adenoviral inclusions
    b. ZN staining and PCR for mycobacteria
7. Electromicroscopy
8. Ultrasonography.

Management

- Milk thistle (*Silybum marianum*) is hepatoprotectant. Dose at 4–15 mg/kg b.i.d. or t.i.d.
- For ascites try furosemide at 2–5 mg/kg s.i.d. if ascitic.

Treatment/specific therapy

- Mycobacteriosis – see *Systemic Disorders*
- Capillaria
  - Fenbendazole at 25 mg/kg p.o. every 2 weeks for 3 treatments
- Biliary cysts
  - Removal of fluid percutaneously
  - Surgical resection
- Hepatic lipidosis
  - Fluid therapy and nutritional support
  - Covering antibiotics
  - Lactulose 0.05 mL/100 g p.o. s.i.d.

Pancreatic disorders

Viral

- Paramyxovirus.

Investigations

1. Radiography
2. Routine haematology and biochemistry
3. Culture and sensitivity.
4. PCR and HI testing for paramyxovirus
5. Endoscopy
6. Biopsy/necropsy
   a. Pancreatic ductular lesions (paramyxovirus)
7. Ultrasonography.

Treatment/specific therapy

- Paramyxovirus – No specific treatment.

Cardiovascular and haematological disorders

Bacterial

- Vegetative endocarditis
- Granulomatous pericarditis.

Protozoal

* *Haemogregarina spp*
* *Hepatozoon spp.*

Parasitic

* Filarial worms (*Oswaldofilaria, Foleyella, Macdonaldius spp*) (see also *Skin Disorders*).

Nutritional

* Visceral gout (uric acid in pericardial sac) see *Renal Disorders*
* Neoplasia
  * Leukaemia.

Other non-infectious problems

* Anaemia
* Cardiomyopathy
* Myocardial mineralization
* Thromboembolism.
* Myocardial ischaemia
* Congestive heart failure
* Developmental abnormalities.

Findings on clinical examination

* Lethargy
* Apparent respiratory disease (see also *Respiratory Tract Disorders*)
* Pale mucous membranes
* Oedema
* Cardiomegaly – may be visible externally as a mass around 22–35% of the snout-vent length. It may be seen to be beating (differentiating the heart from pericardiac masses, e.g. granulomas). *Note* that very thin, anorexic snakes may appear to have a large heart secondary to loss of surrounding tissue
* Avascular necrosis of the tail tip (thromboembolism).

Investigations

1. Radiography
   a. Cardiomegaly
   b. Calcification of blood vessels
2. Ultrasonography and Doppler blood-flow detectors
   a. Cardiomyopathy
   b. Pericardial effusions
   c. Vegetative endocarditis
3. Electrocardiogram
   a. Valentinuzzi et al (1969b) suggest that an ECG can be taken with two leads:
      i. A longitudinal lead that consists of a rostral electrode located at 10% of the body length and a caudal electrode at 50% of the body length; both electrodes are on the ventral surface of the animal

      ii. Two transverse electrodes are located bilaterally at the level of the heart (approximately 24% of the body length)

      iii. Changes in the position of the heart, either during handling or by artificial respiration, may cause significant changes in the magnitude and orientation of the vectors. During recording of the transverse leads, rotation around the YY-axis usually produces large variations in the amplitudes of the ECG waves. Spontaneous changes in T-amplitude are relatively common

   b. ECG of the boa constrictor at rest and at room temperature (Table 8.5).

      i. The ventricular T wave is generally in the same direction as the major deflection R; Q and S are poorly developed. The T wave also varies greatly in amplitude and may become completely inverted without apparent change in the position of the leads relative to the heart

      ii. There is an SV complex preceding the P wave

      iii. Valentinuzzi et al (1969a) found experimentally that as the heart deteriorates and dies the relative and absolute amplitude of the SV complex markedly increases.

4. Routine haematology and biochemistry
   a. Anaemia
   b. May be artefactual due to lymph contamination and dilution
5. Cytology: may find filarial worms on blood smear
6. Culture and sensitivity
7. Endoscopy
8. Biopsy/necropsy.

Management

- Provide high oxygen environment.

Table 8.5   ECG of the boa constrictor, at rest and at room temperature

Variable	Value
Heart rate (beats/min)	24
SV–P (s)	0.50
P–R (s)	0.55
SV–P/SV–SV	0.18
P–R/P–P	0.20
SV (ms)	100
P (ms)	80
QRS (ms)	140
Q–T (s)	1.4

After Valentinuzzi et al (1969c).

Treatment/specific therapy

- Haemoparasites
  - Loading dose of chloroquine phosphate (5 mg/kg p.o.) and primaquine phosphate (0.5 mg/kg p.o.)
  - Continue with chloroquine at 2.5 mg/kg p.o. once weekly and primaquine at 0.5 mg/kg once weekly for 12–16 weeks
- Filarial nematodes (see *Skin Disorders*)
- Thromboembolism
  - No established treatment. Possibly try NSAIDs
  - Necrotic extremities may require surgical amputation
  - Investigate underlying factors, e.g. septicaemia, low temperatures
- Cardiomyopathies
  - Furosemide at 2–5 mg i.m., i.v. p.o. s.i.d. or b.i.d.
- Leukaemia
  - Treatment potentially difficult and untried
  - Radiation therapy has been used with lizards (see *Lizards*) with a single low dose whole body radiation treatment of 1 Gray
- Anaemia
  - The underlying cause should be investigated
  - Blood transfusion from a conspecific, or possibly a close relative (same genus) could be attempted
  - Oxyglobin.

Systemic disorders

Viral

Bacterial

- Septicaemia/bacteraemia
- *Salmonella arizona*
- *Chlamydophila pneumoniae*
- *Chlamydophila spp* (Jacobson et al 2002)
- Mycobacteriosis.

Fungal

- *Cryptococcus neoformans*
- *Zygomycete* fungi.

Neoplasia

- Sarcoma (Abou-Madi et al 1994)
- Mesothelioma
- Lymphocytic leukaemia (Raiti et al 2002)
- Multicentric T-cell lymphoma (Raiti et al 2002).

Other non-infectious problems

- Cardiac disease (see *Cardiovascular and and Haematological Disorders*)
- Gout (see *Renal Disorders*)
- Amyloidosis.

Findings on clinical examination

- Anorexia
- Weight loss
- Lethargy
- Altered behaviour, e.g. shunning normal basking areas, constantly hiding
- Inappetence, petechial haemorrhages visible in the skin, especially the ventral scales, may show central nervous signs such as incoordination, frantic movements or loss of the righting reflex (septicaemia)
- Swellings (neoplasia)
- Clinical signs may vary with organ system affected.

Investigations

1. Radiography
2. Routine haematology and biochemistry
   a. High actual or relative heterophila (inflammatory)
   b. Multiple abnormal leukocytes (leukaemia)
3. Culture and sensitivity
   a. Blood culture (septicaemia/bacteraemia)
4. Serology for *Cryptococcus*
5. Cytology
   a. ZN staining and PCR for mycobacteria
   b. Immunohistochemistry and PCR for *Chlamydophila* and *Chlamydia*-like organisms (Soldati et al 2004)
   c. Tracheal washings or cerebrospinal tap to isolate *Cryptococcus*
6. Endoscopy
7. Biopsy/necropsy
   a. Single or multiple granulomas (mycobacteria, fungi, *Chlamydophila pneumoniae*, *Chlamydia*-like organisms)
8. Ultrasonography.

Management

- Fluid therapy, see *Nursing Care*.

Treatment/specific therapy

- Septicaemia
  - Supportive treatment
  - Antibiotics
- Mycobacteriosis
  - Potential zoonosis. Consider euthanasia
  - No successful treatment for mycobacteriosis in reptiles reported
- Cryptococcosis
  - Difficult to treat. Consider using:
    - Ketoconazole at 10–30 mg/kg p.o. s.i.d.
    - Topical ketoconazole cream
    - Itraconazole 5 mg/kg p.o. e.o.d.

- Lymphoma and leukaemia
  - Treatment potentially difficult and untried, but see *Lizards*
- Sarcoma (see *Musculoskeletal Disorders*).

Musculoskeletal disorders

Bacterial
- Osteomyelitis
- Abscessation.

Fungal
- Granulomata.

Protozoal

Parasitic
- Cestodes: *Diphyllobothrium* and *Spirometra* (sparganosis).

Nutritional
- Prolonged anorexia.

Neoplasia
- Sarcoma
- Spinal neoplasia
- Fibrosarcoma
- Osteosarcoma.

Other non-infectious problems
- Traumatic fractures
- Spondylitis/spondylosis
- Myopathies
- Congenital abnormalities
- Steatitis
- Faecal impaction – see *Gastrointestinal Tract Disorders*
- Congenital deformities due to incorrect incubation temperatures; drug-administration while gravid; in-breeding
- Osseous dysplasia (inheritable)
- Muscle wastage secondary to chronic anorexia (see *Anorexia*).

Findings on clinical examination

- Severe kinking of the spine (myopathies, spondylitis/spondylosis, fractures)
- Obvious abnormalities especially of the skull
- Swellings and/or erosions (neoplasia, osteomyelitis, abscessation, osseous dysplasia)
- Extreme muscle wastage.

Investigations

1. Radiography
   a. Approximate body organ position in snakes based upon percentage of snout to vent (cloaca) length as measured from the rostral nares (Table 8.6). *Note* this measurement does not include the tail
   b. Fractured ribs are a common finding (Hernandez-Divers & Hernandez-Divers 2001) that usually require no treatment
   c. Steatitis may be indicated by enlargement and greater density of the fat body
   d. Spondylosis/spondylitis, osseous dysplasia
2. Routine haematology and biochemistry
3. Culture and sensitivity
4. Endoscopy
5. Biopsy/necropsy
6. Ultrasonography.

Treatment/specific therapy

- *Diphyllobothrium* and *Spirometra* (sparganosis)
  - Surgical removal where feasible
  - Praziquantel at 5 mg/kg p.o., s.c. or i.m. Repeat after 2 weeks
  - Only feed prey prefrozen for at least 30 days
  - Complex life cycles
- Sarcoma
  - Attempt surgical resection
  - Chemotherapy has been attempted (Rosenthal 1994) following surgical reduction
  - Adriamycin at 1 mg/kg i.v. every 7 days for 2 weeks, then once every 2 weeks, then once every 2 weeks for a total of 6 doses of Adriamycin
  - I.v. access was maintained using a vascular port with the catheter tip into the right atrium

Table 8.6 Approximate body organ position in snakes based upon percentage of snout to vent (cloaca) length as measured from the rostral nares

Organ	(%)
Heart	22–35
Lungs	25–50
Air sac	45–85
Liver	35–60
Stomach	45–65
Spleen, pancreas and gall bladder	60–70
Small intestine	65–80
Kidneys	65–90
Colon	80–100

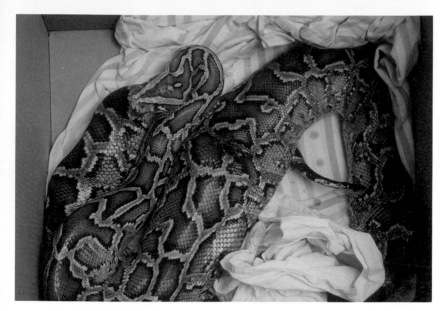

Fig. 8.8. A large Burmese python with a severe discharging abscessation of the spinal column. Radiography revealed osteolysis of the underlying vertebrae and a complete loss of continuity of the spinal column and spinal cord. This snake was paralysed caudal to the lesion.

- Other neoplasia
  - Attempt surgical resection
  - Cryosurgery
- Spondylitis/spondylosis
  - Some cases may represent a Paget's syndrome-like disease
  - Many cases actually have a spinal infection triggering osteolysis (Fig. 8.8), exostoses and bony fusion of the vertebrae
  - Consider use of antibiosis and NSAIDs, e.g. meloxicam at 50 µg/kg p.o., i.m. s.i.d.
  - Those constricting snakes with extensive fusion of the spine may be unable to prehend and feed properly and so should be considered for euthanasia
- Osseous dysplasia
  - Inherited condition. No treatment. Avoid use of parents carrying this disorder in breeding programmes
- Myopathies
  - Guarded prognosis
  - Attempt treatment with vitamin E and selenium supplementation.

Neurological disorders

Viral

- Inclusion body disease (IBD) (C-type retrovirus)
- Paramyxovirus
- Reovirus
- Lentivirus.

Bacterial

* Septicaemia
* CNS granuloma
* Encephalitis.

Fungal

* CNS granuloma
* *Cryptococcus neoformans* (see also *Systemic Disorders* and *Respiratory Tract Disorders*).

Protozoal

* *Acanthamoeba*
* *Toxoplasma*.

Nutritional

* Thiamine deficiency (esp. fish-eating snakes such as garter snakes *Thamnophis spp*)
* Biotin deficiency
* Hypoglycaemia.

Neoplasia

* Schwannoma.

Other non-infectious problems

* Organophosphate toxicity, e.g. insecticidal aerosols and diffusers
* Gout (see *Renal Disorders*)
* Liver disease (hepatic encephalopathy)
* Metabolic disease
* Trauma
* Ivermectin overdose
* Cedar shavings.

Findings on clinical examination

* Slight to marked head tremor
* Muscle tremors
* Loss of righting reflex
* 'star gazing' (Fig. 8.9)
* Aberrant behaviour
* CNS signs and/or regurgitation in pythons and boas (IBD).

Investigations

1. Radiography
2. Routine haematology and biochemistry
3. Cytology
   a. Intracytoplasmic inclusion bodies (IBD)
   b. Raised liver enzymes (hepatic encephalopathy)
4. Culture and sensitivity
   a. Blood culture (septicaemia)

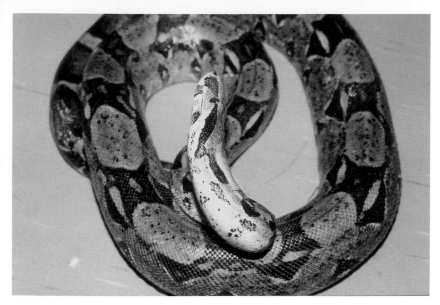

Fig. 8.9. A boa constrictor showing classic 'star-gazing' behaviour.

5. Endoscopy
6. Biopsy
   a. Liver, lung, oesophageal tonsil and other organs (IBD)
7. Ultrasonography.

Treatment/specific therapy

- Septicaemia
  - Antibiotics
  - Fluid therapy (see *Nursing Care*)
- Thiamine (vitamin B1) deficiency
  - Due to feeding fresh fish rich in thiaminase, e.g. whitebait
  - Treatment is with B1 supplementation, and is avoided by providing a dietary vitamin B1 supplement plus boiling of fish before feeding to denature the thiaminase
- Biotin deficiency
  - Seen in egg-eating snakes
  - Supplement with biotin
  - Treat symptomatically
- *Acanthamoeba* and *Toxoplasma*
  - Treatment difficult
  - Metronidazole at 100–275 mg/kg p.o. once only (only 40 mg/kg for King snakes and Indigo snakes)
  - Trimethoprim/sulphadiazine at 15 mg/kg p.o. daily
  - Potential zoonoses

- Organophosphate toxicity
  - Atropine at 0.04 mg/kg i.m.
  - Supportive treatment
- Inclusion body disease
  - No effective treatment
  - The antiretroviral combination (Trizivir GSK) which consists of abacavir (300 mg)/lamivudine (150 mg)/zidovudine (300 mg) combination given as 5.0 mg abacavir every 3rd day has been trialed unsuccessfully in a boa constrictor (Levine 2002)
  - Supportive therapy.

Ophthalmic disorders

The cornea is protected by a transparent spectacle made from fusion of upper and lower eyelids. Snakes have rods and cones but lack a fovea; some snakes possess a conus papillaris (analogous to avian pecten).

Snakes have well-developed Harderian glands; their secretions lubricate the subspectacular space. A second duct drains this space into Vomeronasal organ.

Examination of the posterior segment of the eye is difficult as the iris muscle fibres are striated and partly under voluntary control and so parasympatholytics, e.g. atropine and sympathomimetics, e.g. phenylephrine, will not work. In addition the cornea is protected by the spectacle which prevents absorption of absorption of topical non-parasympatholytic mydriatics (such as vecuronium). Consider ophthalmic examination either by using low light levels or general anaesthesia.

Bacterial

- Subspectacular abscess
- Keratitis
- Panophthalmitis.

Fungal

- Subspectacular abscess
- Keratitis
- Panophthalmitis.

Neoplasia

Other non-infectious problems

- Trauma
- Retained spectacle
- Avulsion of the spectacle (usually iatrogenic)
- Occlusion of nasolacrimal duct
- Congenital absence of nasolacrimal duct
- Stenosis due to or following inflammation
- Congenital abnormalities
- Cyclopia
- Microphthalmia – often associated with head abnormalities
- Anophthalmia
- Exposure to excessive low temperature during hibernation (cataracts)
- Lenticular cataract.

Findings on clinical examination

- Permanent opacity of the spectacle due to one or more retained spectacles (Fig. 8.10). Associated retained skin may be visible on the head
- Space beneath spectacle distended with *clear* fluid (occlusion of nasolacrimal duct)
- Subspectacular abscess
- The eye appears *opaque* and the spectacle may be bulge due to increased pressure in the corneo-spectacular space. This condition may be unilateral or bilateral. This condition can be associated with retained spectacle (dysecdysis – see *Skin Disorders*) or stomatitis (subspectacular abscess; see also *Gastrointestinal Tract Disorders*)
- Hypopyon
- Uveitis
- Cataracts
- Retinal degeneration
- Panophthalmitis.

Investigations

1. Ophthalmic examination
   a. Assess whether eye is able to rotate beneath the spectacle during rotation of the head, i.e. that there are no corneo-spectacular adhesions
   b. Space beneath spectacle distended with *clear* fluid (occlusion of nasolacrimal duct)
   c. Subspectacular abscess: the eye appears *opaque* and the spectacle may bulge due to increased pressure in the corneo-spectacular space. This condition may be unilateral or bilateral.

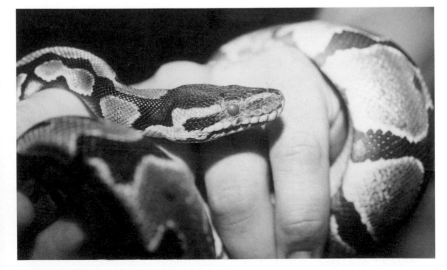

Fig. 8.10. Retained spectacle in a young Royal python.

2. Radiography
3. Routine haematology and biochemistry
4. Culture and sensitivity
5. Biopsy/necropsy
6. Ultrasonography.

Treatment/specific therapy

- Retained spectacle. This is often associated with:
  - Low humidity
  - Anorexia
  - Dermatologic conditions including snake mites (see *Skin Disorders*)
  - If the spectacle over the cornea is retained, then gentle rubbing whilst applying slight pressure with a damp cotton bud should eventually cause some rucking of the spectacle and allow its removal
  - Do not pull with forceps as you risk avulsing the cornea with consequent loss of the use of that eye. If very adherent the spectacle can be loosened by application of 10% acetylcysteine
- Subspectacular abscess
  - Treatment involves surgical incision into the spectacle to allow an assessment for any corneal lesions
  - All debris should be flushed from the corneal surface, and if possible the nasolacrimal duct cannulated and flushed
  - Topical ophthalmic antibiotic or antimycotic preparations should be used (see *Skin Disorders*)
  - Attend to any underlying conditions, e.g. stomatitis
  - A new spectacle should form at the next skin shed. To prevent dessication, consider attempting to suture contact lens in place
- Nasolacrimal duct occlusion
  - Treatment is similar to subspectacular abscess
  - Conjunctivoralostomy can be attempted in large snakes by passing a curved 18 gauge needle from the inferior conjunctival fornix into the roof of the mouth such that it emerges between the palatine and maxillary teeth. A 0.025 inch silastic tubing, threaded through the needle and secured at each end with sutures, may work in some cases
- Avulsion of the spectacle
  - Often the eye is so badly damaged that enucleation is required
  - Otherwise treat as for repair of subspectacular abscess
- Congenital defects
  - No treatment
  - Consider incubation parameters (temperature, humidity, etc.) as well as genetic factors when considering cause.

Endocrine disorders

Little studied in reptiles.

Neoplasia

- Thyroid neoplasia (especially garter snakes *Thamnophis spp*).

Other non-infectious problems

- Hyperthyroidism (see 'Dysecdysis', in *Skin Disorders*).

Findings on clinical examination

- Swollen cervical region (thyroid neoplasia)(Fig. 8.11)
- Excessive repetitive skin shedding.

Investigations

1. Radiography
2. Routine haematology and biochemistry
   a. Blood T4 levels (Table 8.7)
3. Culture and sensitivity

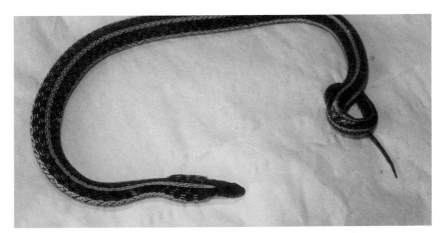

Fig. 8.11. A garter snake with a cervical swelling; surgical resection revealed a thyroid carcinoma.

Table 8.7 Blood T4 levels

Species	T4 concentration (nmol/L)	
	Range	Mean
Cornsnakes *Elaphe guttata*	0.45–6.06	2.75
Ball python *Python regius*	0.93–4.79	2.58
Milk snakes *Lampropeltis triangulum*	0.27–2.94	1.88
Boa *Boa constrictor*	0.24–3.98	2.50

Adapted from Greenacre et al (2001).

4. Endoscopy
5. Biopsy
6. Ultrasonography.

Treatment/specific therapy

- Thyroid neoplasia
  - Surgical resection. Often metastasize
- Hyperthyroidism (see *Skin Disorders*).

Renal disorders

Bacterial

- Bacterial kidney disease/abscessation.

Fungal

- Mycetoma (e.g. *Aspergillus spp*).

Parasitic

- Flukes (esp. in King snakes, indigos, boas, tropical rat snakes and bushmasters)
- Aberrant *Strongyloides spp* infestation (Veazey et al 1994).

Neoplasia

- Renal adenocarcinoma (Gravendyck et al 1997)
- Renal cell carcinoma (may metastasize to lungs and liver).

Other non-infectious problems

- Gout
- Iatrogenic drug toxicity, especially nephrotoxic drugs including the aminoglycosides.

Findings on clinical examination

- Anorexia
- Lethargy
- Weight loss
- Polydipsia/polyuria
- Marked swelling of caudal third of coelom (renomegaly, renal neoplasia, extreme renal gout)
- Anuria
- Oedema
- Pale mucous membranes
- Mortalities.

Investigations

1. Radiography
   a. Renomegaly

2. Routine haematology and biochemistry
   a. No good single test. Snakes with renal disease may show hyperuricaemia, hyperuraemia, hyperphosphataemia, hyperkalaemia, hyponatrimia and hyper- or hypoproteinaemia
3. Urinalysis
   a. Renal casts
   b. Inflammatory cells
4. Faecal examination (see *Gastrointestinal Tract Disorders*)
5. Culture and sensitivity
6. Endoscopy
   a. Abnormalities in shape, colour or size of kidneys
   b. Flukes in cloaca (and faeces)
7. Biopsy/necropsy
   a. Flukes in kidneys (also on postmortem). Can cause an interstitial nephritis and other renal abnormalities
   b. Ureteritis and nephritis caused by *Strongyloides spp*
   c. Mycetoma
8. Ultrasonography
   a. Hyper- or hypoechoic, focal or multifocal changes; alteration of size.

Treatment/specific therapy

- Flukes
  - Praziquantel at 5 mg/kg p.o., s.c. or i.m. Repeat after 2 weeks
  - Freeze food items, e.g. frogs, fish for 3 days prior to feeding to eliminate intermediate stages
- Aberrant *Strongyloides* infestation – see *Gastrointestinal Tract Disorders*
- Bacterial renal disease
  - Antibiotics (beware nephrotoxic medications)
  - Fluid therapy
- Mycetoma
  - Poor prognosis. Attempt antifungal therapy (see *Systemic Disorders*) as well as general renal supportive therapy
- Gout
  - Fluid therapy
  - Allopurinol at 10 mg/kg s.i.d. *Note* this will only prevent subsequent uric acid deposition
  - Very guarded prognosis
  - May be linked with renal disease, chronic dehydration, use of nephrotoxic drugs).

Reproductive disorders

Snakes can be either oviparous (egg-laying) or viviparous (live-bearing). Typical oviparous snakes include the colubrids and pythons. Typical viviparous snakes include the boas and garter snakes (*Thamnophis spp*).

Non-infectious problems
- Dystocia
- Preovulatory ovarian stasis (POOS)

- Egg stasis (post-ovulatory)
- Ectopic pregnancy (viviparous species)
- Prolapsed hemipene.

Findings on clinical examination

- Eggs often palpable in the caudal third of the coelom
- Straining
- Poor condition
- Obesity
- Dehydration
- Presence of some eggs or young
- One or two large, swollen often spikey structures hanging from the cloaca (prolapsed hemipenes).

Investigations

1. Radiography
   a. Snake eggs are generally poorly calcified and so appear as rounded soft-tissue opacities in the caudal coelomic cavity
   b. Fetal skeletons may be visible in advanced gestation in live-bearing snakes, e.g. boas
   c. The hemipenes of some species are calcified and can be identified radiographically
2. Routine haematology and biochemistry
3. Culture and sensitivity
4. Endoscopy
5. Biopsy
6. Ultrasonography
   a. Useful for POOS and identifying young in live-bearing snakes.

Treatment/specific therapy

- Dystocia
  - Provision of correct environment including appropriate temperature, humidity and nesting chamber may induce normal egg-laying or birth
  - Medical induction
    - There is a small window of opportunity for the effective use of oxytocin; best used within 48–72 h of obvious nesting or straining seen (Stahl 2000)
    - Use oxytocin at 5–20 IU/kg oxytocin, starting at the lower dose; repeat 2–3 times at 6–12 h intervals
    - Argipressin at 0.01–1.0 µg/kg (more potent than oxytocin in reptiles)
    - Digital manipulation. In some cases eggs can be manipulated out of the cloaca. This should be done under GA as it is a very delicate procedure, and there is a significant risk of trauma
  - Percutaneous ovocentesis. Performed under anaesthesia with sterile 20 gauge needle. Beware of yolk leaking into coelomic cavity, aspiration of the viscera or their contents, both of which will trigger a serositis. Allow snake to pass

collapsed eggs. If the eggs have been present for several days then the yolk may be solid and resistant to aspiration
- Salpingotomy. Easier than above. May require multiple incisions to remove all eggs
- Ovariosalpingectomy. Make a paramedian incision along the junction between the ventral scales and the body wall to avoid incising into the ventral midline and the underlying ventral vena cava
- Consider ovariosalpingectomy for non-breeding females to prevent future problems
- Ectopic pregnancy
  - Surgery
- Prolapse of hemipene
  - Attempt replacement (with lubrication) and purse-string suture around cloaca
  - If severely swollen topical glycerine or concentrated sucrose solution may reduce the swelling enough to allow reduction
  - Badly damaged, infected or paralysed hemipenes should be resected. Providing the snake still has one functional hemipene it can still breed.

Neonatal disorders

Non-infectious problems
- Prolapse of the umbilicus
- Congenital deformities
- Dead in shell (mid to late embryonic deaths).

Findings on clinical examination

- Bulging of tissue at the umbilicus of new born or newly hatched snakes. Bulge may contain coelomic lining, yolk sac remnant and coelomic fat.

Investigations

1. Radiography
2. Routine haematology and biochemistry
3. Culture and sensitivity
4. Endoscopy
5. Biopsy/necropsy
6. Ultrasonography.

Treatment/specific therapy

- Prolapsed umbilicus
  - Clean and replace prolapse. Suture in place
  - May require surgical resection of yolk sac remnant
  - This is particularly prevalent in hatchlings with incomplete yolk sac resorption, where the yolk sac membranes adhere to dry surfaces or to the inside of the shell (especially if the humidity is too low). Keep hatchlings with pronounced

egg sacs in moist, clean surroundings until resorption takes place. Do not attempt to separate the hatchling from the egg but increase humidity and/or remove the hatchling plus egg to a warm, humid environment to allow natural separation
- Dead in shell. Can be due to a variety of conditions. Consider:
  - Nutritional status of parents, especially the female
  - Incubation parameters (temperature, humidity, hygiene, oxygen levels, CO_2 levels)
  - Bacterial and fungal infection
- Congenital abnormalities
  - Hereditary conditions
  - Incorrect incubation parameters.

References

Abou-Madi N, Jacobson E R, Buergelt C D et al 1994 Disseminated undifferentiated sarcoma in an Indian rock python (Python morulus morulus). J Zoo Wildl Med 25(1):143–149

Gravendyck M, Marschang R E, Schröder-Gravendyck A S et al 1997 Renal adenocarcinoma in a reticulated python (Python reticulatis). Vet Rec 140:374–375

Greenacre C B, Young D W, Behrend E N et al 2001 Validation of a novel high-sensitivity radioimmunoassay procedure for measurement of total thyroxine concentration in psittacine birds and snakes. Am J Vet Res 62(11):1750–1754

Hernandez-Divers S, Hernandez-Divers S 2001 Diagnostic imaging of reptiles. In Practice 23:370–391

Jacobson E, Origgi F, Heard D et al 2002 An outbreak of Chlamydiosis in Emerald tree boas Corallus caninus. Proc Assoc Reptil Amphib Vet 47–48

Kenny M J, Shaw S E, Hillyard P D et al 2004 Ectoparasite and haemoparasite risks associated with imported exotic reptiles. Vet Rec 154:434–435

Levine B S 2002 Use of nucleoside reverse transcriptase inhibitors in a boa constrictor (Boa c. constrictor) with boid inclusion body disease. Proc Assoc Reptil Amphib Vet 59–61

Mehlhorn H, Schmahl G, Frese M et al 2005a Effects of a combination of emodepside and praziquantel on parasites of reptiles and rodents. Parasitol Res 97:S64–S69

Mehlhorn H, Schmahl G, Mevissen I 2005b Efficacy of a combination of imidacloprid and moxidectin against parasites of reptiles and rodents: case reports. Parasitol Res 97:S97–S101

Pees M C, Kiefer I, Ludewig E W et al 2007 Computed tomography of the lungs of Indian pythons (Python molurus) Am J Vet Res 68:428–434

Raiti R, Garner M M, Wojcieszyn J 2002 Lymphocytic leukemia and Multicentric T-cell lymphoma in a diamond python, Morelia spilota spilota. J Herp Med and Surg 12(1):26–29

Reavil D R, Helmer P, Scmidt R E 2003 Reovirus outbreak in Arizona mountain king snakes (Lampropeltis pyromelana pyromelana). Proc Assoc Reptil Amphib Vet 58–59

Rosenthal K. 1994 Chemotherapeutic treatment of a sarcoma in a corn snake. Proc Assoc Reptil Amphib Vet 46

Soldati G, Lu Z H, Vaughan L et al 2004 Detection of Mycobacteria and Chlamydiae in granulomatous inflammation of reptiles: A retrospective study. Vet Pathol 41:388–397

Stahl S 2000 Reptile obstetrics. In: Exotic Animal Medicine and Surgery, BSAVA Continuing Education Course, 3 November–5 November

Valentinuzzi M E, Hoff H E, Geddes L A 1969a Electrocardiogram of the snake: Observations on the electrical activity of the snake heart. J Electrocardiol 2(1):39–50

Valentinuzzi M E, Hoff H E, Geddes L A 1969b Electrocardiogram of the snake: Effect of the location of the electrodes and cardiac vectors. J Electrocardiol 2(3):245–252

Valentinuzzi M E, Hoff H E, Geddes L A 1969c Electrocardiogram of the snake: Intervals and durations. J Electrocardiol 2(4):343–352

Veazey R S, Stewart T B, Snider T G 1994 Ureteritis and nephritis in a Burmese python (Python morulus bivittatus) due to Strongyloides sp. infection. J Zoo Wildl Med 25(1):119–122

CHAPTER 9

Tortoises and turtles

Chelonia, such as tortoises and their semi-aquatic relatives, terrapins (or turtles) are becoming very popular as pets, especially in Europe where there is a long history of keeping the Mediterranean *Testudo* species as house and garden pets. Although CITES II listed, this trade is being fuelled by the increasing availability of captive-bred specimens, especially from Eastern Europe.

Table 9.1 Commonly encountered tortoises and turtles: Key facts

Species	Notes	Common disorders
The Mediterranean *Testudo* species including the southern European Herman's *tortoise* (*T. hermanni*), members of the north African spur-thighed complex (*T. graeca*) and the Horsfield's tortoise (*T. horsfeldi*)	These are small to moderately large species; most can be safely hibernated but see *Hibernation* for more details. Diet should primarily be leafy greens with added calcium supplementation. No animal protein should be given	Metabolic bone disease (MBD), chelonian herpes virus (CHV), ascarids
African spur-thighed tortoise *Geochelone sulcata*	This species from sub-Saharan Africa is a potential monster that can weigh up to 50–80 kg. They require tropical heat with relatively low humidity. Diet as for *Testudo spp*	Metabolic bone disease (MBD), chelonian herpes virus
The leopard tortoise (*G. pardalis*)	Another sub-Saharan African species. Requires tropical temperatures and a *Testudo*-like diet	Metabolic bone disease (MBD)
Red-footed tortoises (*G. carbonaria*)	Tropical South America. They need tropical temperatures, high humidity (70%) and a diet with more fruit that *Testudo spp* with a small amount of animal protein	Metabolic bone disease (MBD)

Table 9.1 Commonly encountered tortoises and turtles: Key facts—cont'd

Species	Notes	Common disorders
Red-eared slider (*Trachemys picta elegans*)	Less common in the European pet trade following several scares over Salmonella and concerns over alien releases. It is semi-aquatic and requires a dry, warm haul-out area on which to bask. They are carnivorous as hatchlings and feed on commercially available insect larvae, e.g. bloodworms; graduating up to sea foods such as prawns, fish, mussels and cockles plus calcium supplement. Commercial pelleted foods are available	Metabolic bone disease (MBD), hypovitaminosis A
Box turtles (*Terrapene spp*).	Omnivorous, requiring slugs, snails, earthworms, waxworms, mealworms, fruit, green leafed vegetables and mushrooms	Metabolic bone disease (MBD), tympanic scale abscesses

Captive care

As with lizards, the long-term welfare of captive chelonia is intimately dependant upon their environment and they must be provided with appropriate temperatures, full spectrum diet and correct nutrition including a calcium supplement (see *Lizards* for more detail). This especially applies to hatchlings of the *Testudo spp*, where a vivarium is mandatory despite the relative hardiness of the adults.

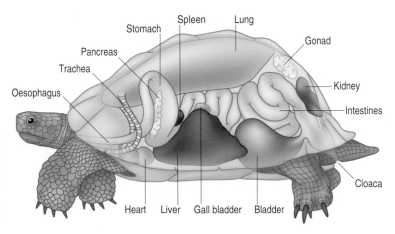

Fig. 9.1. Internal anatomy of a tortoise (lateral).

Importance of lighting

Light in the spectrum of 290–315 nm (ultraviolet-B, UVB) is required for endogenous vitamin D_3 production; ultraviolet-A (UVA) spectrum (320–400 nm) has been shown to have a beneficial influence upon normal behaviour.

Endogenous vitamin D_3 production in reptiles is a many-step process that involves not only exposure to UVB, but also thermal isomerization and modification in the liver and kidneys. Therefore, correct environmental temperatures and healthy organs are required for normal vitamin D_3 synthesis.

Dietary supplementation with vitamin D_3 alone is not sufficient for chelonia. In addition dietary calcium supplementation is essential for all captive chelonia. The commercially available leafy greens and vegetables usually offered to tortoises are inherently low in calcium but high in phosphates. Evidence suggests that in the wild tortoise select high calcium foods. A Ca:P ratio of 3.5:1 is recommended.

Consultation and handling

Most terrestrial chelonia can be safely handled without fear of being bitten, but take care with larger terrapins, or potentially dangerous species such as snapping turtles. These should be held at the rear of the carapace, and in the case of snappers, at the base of the tail.

Start the examination at the head, as this is likely to be withdrawn into the shell precluding further examination. Grasp the head behind the back of the skull and draw it out to its fullest extent. With most tortoises the mouth can now be opened and examined using the tip of a finger as a gag. With terrapins and similar a gag must be used. The rest of the body can then be examined systematically. Useful auscultation of the lung fields can sometimes be achieved by placing a damp towel over the carapace on to which the stethoscope is placed.

Weight: length measurement as an indicator of health in mediterranean tortoises

For Herman's tortoise (*T. hermanii*) and the spur-thigh complex (*T. graeca*), an indication of health can be gained by the following (Peter Heathcote, pers. comm.). This is achieved by the following actions:

1. Weigh the tortoise (in grams).
2. Measure the straight length of the carapace (cm) – *note* that this straight length of the carapace is a linear measurement from the most rostral point of the carapace to the most caudal. It is not a measurement over the dome of the carapace.
3. The weight of the tortoise (g) is then divided by the (straight length of the carapace^3), i.e. tortoise weight (g)/straight length of the carapace (cm)^3
4. The resultant number is compared with the straight length of the carapace:
   a. Straight length of carapace >15 cm; normal ratio 0.21–0.23
   b. Straight length of carapace <15 cm; normal ratio 0.23–0.25.
5. Tortoises with a ratio of 0.17 or less are considered critical.
6. Examples for tortoises with a high ratio are obesity (hepatic lipidosis), gravid (multiple eggs, averaging around 10 g each) or fluid retentive.

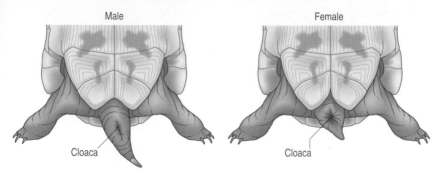

Fig. 9.2. Sexing of *Chelonia*.

Sexing

As a general rule, males have longer tails, a slit-like opening to the cloaca and a degree of concavity to the plastron, although this varies from species to species (Fig. 9.2). Chelonia have temperature-dependant sex determination and it is likely that variations in temperature at thermally-sensitive stages of embryonic development may produce a range of such secondary sexual characteristics, meaning that in some cases sexing is not an exact science.

Male red eared sliders have elongated claws on their front feet that are used to 'tickle' the nose of the female during courtship.

Microchipping

- Subcutaneously in the left hind leg (intramuscularly in thin-skinned species) and subcutaneously in the tarsal area in giant species. *Note* that haemorrhage is common with accidental intramuscular injection in smaller chelonia
- Skin closure is achieved either by suture or with tissue glue.

Blood sampling

Optimum site for collection in most chelonia is the jugular vein or brachial vein. Collection from the dorsal coccygeal vein and the subcarapacial jugular anastomosis are readily contaminated with lymph.

Note that EDTA destroys chelonian RBCs. Take sample into heparin and make a smear immediately. EDTA is, however, good for WBC preservation.

Nursing care

Provide appropriate environment including provision of:
1. Optimal temperature (basking lights, heat mats, etc., to allow thermoregulation). Use of max–min thermometers will assist in monitoring temperature ranges incumbent reptiles are exposed to

2. Full-spectrum lighting (provision of UV-A and UV-B)
3. Humidity
4. Ventilation
5. Easily cleaned accommodation; use paper substrate and disposable/sterilizable hides and other vivarium furniture (see 'Fig. 7.3'd, in *Lizards*)
6. Keep individually, to minimize intra-specific stress and competition for resources.

Large terrestrial chelonia often appear to have difficulty with transparent barriers and may spend a considerable amount of time attempting to walk through, over or under glass vivarium sides and doors. Blanking off these sides with tape or paint may reduce this behaviour.

With semi-aquatic chelonia such as terrapins, for general care they should be provided with a dry haul-out area which has an overhanging heat source to allow thorough drying of the carapace and sufficient water such that the terrapin can rest with its hind feet on the bottom and its nostrils above the surface. A weak terrapin is at risk of drowning. In some cases a terrapin may need to be 'dry-docked' for a period of time. Where possible, this can entail only short periods in a deeper bath. This can be combined with feeding as healthy terrapins will often prefer to feed submerged. Alternatively, serious attention to and monitoring of its fluid status should be undertaking if access to water is felt inappropriate (see *Fluid Therapy* below).

Fluid therapy

See 'Fluid therapy', in *Lizards*.

The assessment of dehydration in chelonia can be difficult visually. An obvious sign in chelonia is sunken eyes, so it is better to monitor PCV. This varies with species, but should be around 26–32 L/L.

Fluids administration

1. Daily bathing in shallow, warm water is often beneficial; it encourages many chelonia to drink as well as defaecate and urinate. Many chelonia can absorb fluids across the cloacal lining.
2. Stomach tubing is often feasible in small to medium-sized chelonia (Fig. 9.3). Large chelonia are often physically too strong to hold for stomach tubing (Fig. 9.4).
3. Oesophagostomy tubes are often very useful for medium to long-term fluid and nutritional management.
4. All parenteral fluids should be warmed to around 26°C.
5. In chelonia, fluid can be given into the epicoelomic space by passing a 1–1.5-inch needle through the pectoral musculature such that the needle is inserted dorsal to and parallel with the plastron, but is beneath the pectoral girdle. The needle is directed towards the contralateral hind leg.
6. Another site is by intraosseous catheter into the vertical plastro-carapacial bridge.
7. Whole blood transfusions can be undertaken using blood obtained from the same or related species.
8. Oxyglobin at 10 mL/kg once only has been used successfully.

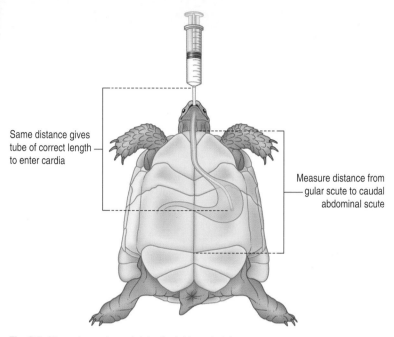

Fig. 9.3. Measuring a stomach tube for tubing a tortoise.

Same distance gives tube of correct length to enter cardia

Measure distance from gular scute to caudal abdominal scute

Nutritional support

Liquidized normal diet or proprietary support diets can be used, given either by stomach tube or by oesophagostomy tube.

Analgesia (see 'Analgesia', in *Lizards*).

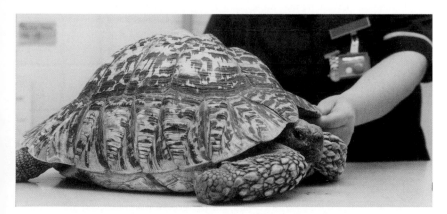

Fig. 9.4. Large terrestrial *Chelonia* such as this leopard tortoise are physically very strong.

Anaesthesia

For general notes, see 'Anaesthesia', in *Lizards*.

Induction and maintenance of anaesthesia in chelonia

1. Propofol at 12–15 mg/kg i.v. delivered into the jugular vein, the subcarapacial jugular anastomosis or the dorsal coccygeal vein
2. Alfaxalone at 2.0 mg/kg i.v as above. Can be maintained either with further top-ups at 2.0 mg/kg or by gaseous anaesthesia
3. With prolonged IPPV the lungs may become permanently expanded so regular deflation by flexion and compression of all four legs in towards the shell should be undertaken
4. In chelonia, ultrasound can be used to monitor heartbeat by placing the ultrasound head into the clavicular fossa
5. Otherwise as for *Lizards*.

Skin disorders

The structure of chelonian skin of the legs, tail, neck and head is as in other reptiles. However, the chelonian shell is unique – in most species there are 54 epidermal scales covering 59 dermal bony plates. The epidermal and dermal seams rarely overlap, possibly giving increased strength to the shell structure. These epidermal scales are often referred to as *scutes* or *shields*. Even here, the skin still has epidermal and dermal components.

The scute epidermis consists of:

1. Horny material containing both pigmented and non-pigmented material. This layer contains a mixture of α- and β-type keratin
2. Pseudostratified columnar epithelium. Occasional melanophores may be seen
3. Dermis overlies the dermal bone
4. In the seam between the scutes the epidermal cell layers are three to four cells thick and it is here that differentiation into keratin-producing cells occurs, and so new horny tissue is produced. Unlike in other reptiles, the keratin is usually retained, thereby producing the typical rings on the scutes
5. Cellular proliferation and keratinization are continuous.

chelonia generally shed their skin in a piecemeal and uncoordinated fashion. Semi-aquatic chelonia will often shed the older outer scutes.

In some species such as the spur-thighed tortoise (*Testudo graeca*) there is hinge between the abdominal and femoral scutes of the plastron, while in others, e.g. the Russian tortoise (*T. horsfieldii*), there is not. Box turtles, e.g. the Eastern box *Terrapene carolina*, also have a hinged plastron that enables them to withdraw both the head and all four limbs within the shell, protecting them with the trapdoor-like plastron.

Following injury, exposed carapacial or plastral bone, if allowed to dry out, dies off superficially; new scutes are formed beneath the exposed bone such that eventually this outer layer is shed.

Differential diagnoses for skin disorders

Abnormal skin shedding (dysecdysis)

* In terrapins a form of dysecdysis is seen where there is a failure of the outer layers of the carapacial scutes to shed and air becomes trapped beneath these producing silvery patches. This may occur if the terrapin is unable haul out and bask properly, to dry out their shell.

Pruritus

* Ectoparasites
* Dermatitis.

Erosions, ulceration and shell deficits

* Trauma
  * Often secondary to damage from another tortoise. Some males, especially the Turkish spur-thigh tortoise (*Testudo ibera*), are very aggressive to conspecific and heterospecific males
* Bacterial infection
* Keratinolytic bacteria from soil in the shell
* Other bacteria, e.g. *Aeromonas spp* in damp conditions
* *Benekea chitinovora* (terrapins)
* Septicaemia (opportunistic species)
* Septicaemic cutaneous ulcerative disease (SCUD)(especially softshell turtles). Often due to *Citrobacter freundii* or *Pseudomonas spp*. Other G −ves may also cause this condition in aquatic chelonia
* Mycobacteria (see *Systemic Disorders*)
* Fungal infections
* 'Dry' lesions in terrestrial chelonia are often due to soil-derived keratinolytic mycotic infections such as *Geotrichum candidum* and *Scolecobasidium humicola*
* *Fusarium incarnatum* (Gopher tortoises *Gopherus berlandieri*) (Rose et al 2001)
* *Microsporum spp, Mucor spp,* (ulcerative epidermitis in softshell *Trionyx spp*)
* Chromomycosis, e.g. *Scolecobasidium humicola, Cladosporium herbarum, Phialophora spp, Hormodendrum spp, Curvularia spp, Fonsecaea spp, Rhinocladiella spp and Drechslera spp*
* Saprolegnia can infect freshwater aquatic chelonia, often secondarily invading wounds and lesions. Appears as a cotton wool-like covering while submerged that collapses on removal from the water
* *Paecilomyces lilacinus* (Lafortune et al 2005)
* Iatrogenic hypervitaminosis A (a necrotic dermatitis leading to a full-thickness skin sloughing)
* Burns
* Spirochid flukes (terrapins)
* Renal failure (loss of scutes often accompanied by excess exudation and ascites)
* Shell fractures, see *Musculoskeletal Disorders*
* Dog or other predator attack
* Rat or rodent attack (gnawed lesions on the legs, especially the lateral surfaces of the front legs) (Fig.9.5).

Nodules and non-healing wounds

* Abscess
* Granuloma (bacterial including mycobacteria, fungal)

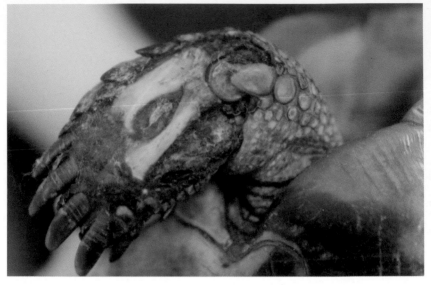

Fig. 9.5. Rat damage in a Mediterranean spur-thighed tortoise. The elbow joint has been exposed.

- *Cistudinomyia* (*Sarcophaga*) *cistudinis,* esp. in the axillial and femoral fossae of box turtles (*Terrapene spp*)
- Gas bubble disease in aquatic chelonia (rare)
- Spirochid flukes (terrapins)
- Subepidermal mites
- Dermal papillomatosis (side-neck turtles – *Platemys spp*)
- Chelonia herpes virus (CHV) (see also *Respiratory Tract Disorders*)
- Pox-like virus in *Testudo hermanni.*

Changes in pigmentation
- Erythema (septicaemia)
- Burns
- Liver disease (and other possible aetiologies for coagulation abnormalities)
- Haemoprotozoans
- Renal failure (often accompanied by excess exudate and loss of scutes)
- Algal growths (aquatic chelonia)
- Scar tissue (depigmented)
- *Fusarium semitectum* is a cause of whitish skin blemishes in *Gopherus berlandieri*
- Failure of the scutes to be able to dry out (semi-aquatic chelonia).

Ectoparasites
- Myiasis (fly strike; maggots)
- *Calliphora vicina*
- *Lucillia ampullacea, L. coeruleiviridis*
- *Cistudinomyia* (*Sarcophaga*) *cistudinis*
- Bot fly larvae
- Ticks, e.g. *Ambylomma sparsum, A. marmoreum*

- Subepidermal mites (African spurred tortoise *Geochelone sulcata*) (Nicasio et al 2002)
- Spirochid flukes (terrapins)
- Spiruruids
- Leeches (wild caught or feral freshwater chelonia)
- Barnacles (*Balanus spp*) recorded on diamondback terrapins (*Malaclemys terrapin*) (Werner 2003).

Burns

Neoplasia

Shell deformities

- Excessive protein intake
- Metabolic bone disease (nutritional osteodystrophy)
- Old shell lesions, e.g. traumatic injuries
- Dyskeratosis. Cause unknown, but may be linked to systemic disease (Homer et al 2001).

Findings on clinical examination

- Reddened, thickened areas of skin suggest an underlying infection. These may be moist
- Loss of dermal structures such as toenails
- Overgrowth of dermal structures such as the toenails, beak and scutes
- Partial or complete loss of scutes
- Silvery patches on the scutes of semi-aquatic chelonia. Many of these such as red-eared terrapins (*Chrysema scripta elegans*) do routinely shed scutes. Failure to do so results in air trapped beneath loosened scutes
- Exposure of underlying bone
- Flaking and fissuring of the keratin scutes
- Inflammation and exudate accompanied by separation of the scutes from the underlying bone can be indicative of severe septicaemia or renal disease
- Pruritus. The reptile may scratch against objects. The body plan of chelonia means that they are rarely able to scratch themselves in any meaningful manner, nor can they self-mutilate
- Spirochid eggs cause vascular occlusion, causing focal and coalescing areas of ulcerative necrosis of the carapace and plastron
- Obvious parasites
- Penetrating injuries through scutes into underlying bone. May reach into coelomic cavity or lungs (dog bites)
- Live maggots on or around open wounds; swellings under the skin (myiasis)
- Exfoliation of skin of head and neck associated with necrotic stomatitis (CHV)
- Papular lesions around the eyes (*T. hermanni*) – pox-like virus.

Investigations

1. Radiography
2. Sterile swabs taken for bacterial or fungal culture
3. Impression smears or other samples taken for staining and cytology

4. Blood samples for general haematology and biochemistry
5. Biopsy of suspect lesions
   a. Dracunculid larvae may be present in the skin (Spirurids). Adults lie in coelomic cavity
6. Discuss environmental management with owner:
   a. Are calcium and vitamin D3 supplements offered routinely?
   b. Is full-spectrum lighting provided?
   c. Are fluorescent tubes changed at the correct frequency (usually every 6 months)?
   d. Are high-protein foods being offered?
7. Endoscopy
8. Ultrasonography.

Management

1. Any shell lesions should be investigated further by debridement around the lesion to remove fissures that could harbour persistent infections. This is potentially a very painful procedure and if large areas are to be debrided then general anaesthesia should be considered
2. Small-to-medium lesions can be managed with the application of topical iodine and/or topical antimicrobials
3. Larger lesions may require dressing:
   a. For terrestrial chelonia, application of a topical amorphous hydrogel dressing, e.g. IntraSite Gel (Smith and Nephew Healthcare Ltd.) topically with a covering of a non-adhesive dressing promotes granulation and coverage of the underlying bone
   b. For aquatic chelonia applying Orabase (Squibb) or bone wax can be used to achieve a relatively watertight protective seal
4. Consider fluid therapy if large areas of underlying bone are newly exposed and exuding
5. Attempted covering of exposed bone with products such as methylmethacrylate or fibreglass should be delayed until all signs of infection have resolved
6. Those chelonia on a high-protein diet may require burring back of excessively long toenails and upper and lower beak
7. Long-term dry-docking of aquatic chelonia is contraindicated as dehydration and anorexia are common sequelae.

Treatment/specific therapy

- Ticks and maggots
  - These should be physically or surgically removed. Permethrin-based formulations are safe, although those products with synergists such as piperonyl butoxide should be avoided if possible. Fipronil may not affect a 10% kill of *Amblyomma* ticks (Burridge et al 2002). *Do not use ivermectin as this is toxic to chelonia*
  - *Note* that ticks are vectors for *Babesia/Hepatozoon* and *Ehrlichia*-like organisms
  - *Note* that the tick *Amblyoma marmoreum* can transmit Heartwater (*Cowdria ruminatium*) to domestic and native wildlife. This and other ectoparasites may act as vectors for other diseases.

- Bacterial and fungal infections
  - SCUD in freshwater terrapins is caused by *Citrobacter freundii* and other G −ve bacteria. Often linked to high levels of environmental bacterial contamination so this should be addressed
  - Antibiotics or antifungals as required
- Saprolegniosis. Salt solutions as low as 10 parts per thousand (ppt) (mg/100 mL) will inhibit infections
- *Paecilomyces lilacinus* in the freshwater aquatic fly river turtle *Carettochelys insculpta* was controlled (Lafortune 2005) with:
  - Permanent salt bath at 5 ppt (0.5%) for 14 days then increased to 7 ppt
  - Malachite green and formalin dips (0.15 mg/L of 0.038% malachite green and 4.26% formaldehyde) for 15 min b.i.d. for 33 days
  - Itraconazole at 10 mg/kg p.o. every 48 h for 20 days
- Spirochid flukes: praziquantel at 10 mg/kg
- Address any dietary or environmental deficiencies
- Dog attack
  - Covering antibiotics
  - Non-penetrating injuries – clean with topical iodine solution
  - Dress any penetrating injuries with non-adhesive dressings. Only once any secondary infection cleared should the lesion be sealed with synthetic polymers such as polymethylmethacrylate or fibreglass
- Rat or rodent attack
  - Often during or shortly after hibernation when tortoises are sluggish
  - Commonly affects the lateral (outer) surfaces of the front legs, which are drawn across in front of the head for protection. Other limbs and the shell may be damaged as well
  - The radius and ulna may be exposed, as may the elbow joint
  - Clean and debride any devitalized tissue
  - Application of topical amorphous hydrogel dressings, e.g. IntraSite Gel (Smith and Nephew Healthcare Ltd.) will encourage secondary healing. A non-adhesive dressing should be applied
  - Healing can take many months before re-epithelialization occurs to a sufficient extent
  - If the elbow joint is exposed:
    - Strap up the leg so that the tortoise cannot weight-bear on that leg
    - Provide support by the attachment of a prop (e.g. half billiard ball; toy wheel) to the plastron of that quadrant
    - In severe cases, one leg can be amputated at mid-humeral or mid-femoral level
- Neoplasia
  - Rarely diagnosed, or at least reported in the literature
  - Chemotherapy in reptiles is in its infancy and most tumours are managed surgically. Accessible cutaneous tumours can be treated by injecting cisplatin directly into the tissue mass on a weekly basis as a debulking exercise
  - Radiation has been used to treat an acute lymphoblastic leukaemia in a sungazer lizard (*Cordylus giganteus*)
  - Surgical laser has been used in the treatment of a dermal melanoma in a green iguana.

Respiratory tract disorders

Differential diagnoses for nasal tract disorders

Runny nose syndrome (RNS) is a poorly understood clinical syndrome. Linked with chelonian herpes virus, *Mycoplasma agassizii* and various bacteria. No single pathogenic agent as yet established.

Viral

- Chelonian herpes virus (CHV). A significant cause of RNS. Other commonly associated signs are stomatitis (with diphtheritic membranes on tongue, oropharynx and naso-pharynx. Dysphagia and hypersalivation may be seen. Less often there will be cervical oedema, diarrhoea and central nervous signs including hind limb paresis
- Iridovirus. Can present similarly to CHV, especially with stomatitis and glossitis. May cause hepatitis
- Virus X. An as yet unidentified virus or group of viruses isolated from *Testudo* and *Geochelone spp* that are linked to rhinitis, diphtheroid-necrotizing stomatitis/pharyngitis, pneumonia, enteritis and ascites (Marshang & Ruemenapf 2002).

Bacterial

- Often opportunistic bacterial infections. Consider occult abscessation
- Mycobacteria (see *Systemic Disorders*)
- Mycoplasmosis
- *M. agassizii* identified as a cause of RNS in gopher tortoises.

Fungal

- No definitive nasal fungal pathogens have been isolated, but a variety of fungi, regarded as commensals or secondary invaders, have been described in Sulawesi tortoises (*Indotestudo forstenii*) (Innis et al 2003).

Protozoal

- Intranuclear coccidiosis. Undescribed protozoan found in the mucosal lining of the nares, conjunctiva and Eustachian tubes. May occur elsewhere, e.g. in renal and colonic mucosal epithelial cells. Linked, along with *Mycoplasma agassizii*, with severe necrotizing sinusitis (Innis et al 2003).

Nutritional

- Hypovitaminosis A (see *Nutritional Disorders*).

Neoplasia

Other non-infectious problems

- Poor husbandry (including nutrition) plus exposure to suboptimal temperatures.

Findings on clinical examination

- Clear, serous to gelatinous or mucopurulent nasal discharge
- Necrosis of external nares, including the nasal septum that may extend several millimetres caudally. The vomer and palatine bones may be severely damaged, and oronasal fistulae may develop

- Occasionally accompanied by pharyngeal and tongue lesions
- Other, systemic clinical signs may be seen depending upon aetiology
- Aquatic and semi-aquatic chelonia may swim with one side held lower than the other (pneumonia – asymmetrical or unilateral pulmonary consolidation).

Investigations

1. Examination of discharge – wet smear plus staining for cytology and Gram staining.
2. Culture and sensitivity of discharge sample
   a. Submit mucus sample for mycoplasma PCR, isolation or electron microscopy
   b. Submit mucus sample for virus isolation
3. Radiography
4. Routine haematology and biochemistry
5. Mycoplasma serology
6. CHV serology
7. Endoscopy
8. Biopsy/necropsy
   a. Histopathology for intranuclear coccidiosis
9. Ultrasonography.

Management

1. Covering systemic and/or topical antibiosis. Consider nebulization
2. Topical iodine application to any areas of ulceration or exposed bone
3. Flushing of the nares. This should be attempted from both directions, with saline or an antibiotic ointment
   a. With a syringe placed flush with the external nares such that any mucus or accumulated material is displaced caudally into the mouth, from where it can be remove
   b. Retrograde flushing can be achieved by placing antibiotic ointment on to the roof of the mouth at the nasopharynx, and displacing the antibiotic up and into the nasal cavity by compression with a cotton bud
4. Surgical debridement may be required of any necrotic bone
5. Supportive treatment – may require placement of an oesophagostomy tube to bypass the buccal cavity.

Treatment/specific therapy

- Chelonian herpes virus (CHV)
  - Acyclovir at 80 mg/kg s.i.d. for cases of herpesvirus. Efficacy appears variable
- Other viral infections – supportive treatment only
- Non-specific bacterial infections – appropriate antibiotics
- Mycoplasmosis
  - Enrofloxacin at 5–10 mg/kg s.i.d.
  - Doxycycline at 2.5–10 mg/kg p.o. s.i.d. or b.i.d. or 50 mg/kg i.m. (loading dose) followed by 25 mg/kg every 3 days
  - Tylosin at 5 mg/kg i.m. or p.o. s.i.d.
  - Clarithromycin at 15 mg/kg p.o. every 2–3 days.

- Intranuclear coccidiosis
  - Potentiated sulphonamides (patient must be well hydrated)
  - Toltrazuril at 7.5 mg/kg p.o. s.i.d. for 2 days. Repeat after 12 days.

Lower respiratory tract disorders

Respiratory anatomy

The glottis is located at the base of the muscular, fleshy tongue relatively caudal in the oropharynx. The trachea has complete cartilaginous rings. It bifurcates into two bronchi a relatively short distance along the neck and each of the two bronchi enter a lung dorsally. The lungs occupy dorsal section of shell and are adhered to the overlying dermal bones of the carapace. The lungs are paired and sac-like with the gas exchanging alveoli situated at the periphery of these organs. The lack of a functional diaphragm allows inflammatory exudates to accumulate in the dependant portions of the lungs.

Common respiratory signs

Differential diagnoses of dyspnoea:
1. Chelonia are unable to cough so respiratory disease is likely to present as a dyspnoea
2. Pneumonia
3. Severe stomatitis/pharyngitis
4. Tracheal obstruction
5. Coelomic mass
6. Overheating.

Differential diagnoses of respiratory noise:
1. Runny nose syndrome
2. Nasal foreign body
3. Tracheal obstruction/foreign body
4. Oesophageal obstruction/foreign body
5. Pneumonia.

Differential diagnoses for respiratory disorders

Viral

- Chelonian herpes virus
- Iridovirus
- Virus X.

Bacterial

- Various, especially environmental contaminants including *Pseudomonas*
- Mycobacteria (see *Systemic Disorders*).

Fungal

- Mycotic pneumonia
- Often secondary to suboptimal temperatures or prolonged antibiotic use
- Many species described including *Candida albicans* and *Paecilomyces*.

Parasitic

- Migrant ascarids (often *Sulcascaris* or *Angusaticaecum*), both in the trachea and the lungs
- Trematodes (aquatic chelonia – fish, amphibians and crustaceans can act as intermediate hosts).

Nutritional

- Hypovitaminosis A predisposes to secondary lung infections.

Neoplasia

- Metastases

Other non-infectious problems

- Obstruction. Accumulations of mucus and inflammatory material from lower respiratory tract disease can act as obstructions
- Drowning (typically terrestrial tortoises found in garden pond)
- Hyperthermia (overheating). Collapsed and may be salivating copiously.

Findings on clinical examination

- Clearly audible respiratory sounds. May be quite moist in nature.
- Dyspnoea. Exaggerated respiratory movements
- Discharge in mouth or at glottis
- Aquatic chelonia may consistently list to one side whilst swimming due to asymmetric consolidation in lungs
- Aquatic chelonia may be reluctant to enter water.

Investigations

1. Radiography.
    a. Lateral and cranio–caudal views more use than dorso-ventral to detect areas of consolidation
    b. Compression of the lung fields may indicate an extrapulmonary lesion, e.g. obesity, hepatomegaly
    c. Lung lesions can be accessed for swabbing, biopsy, etc., by carapacial osteotomy once position is ascertained by radiography
2. Culture and sensitivity
3. Tracheal wash. Staining of collected material and/or submission for culture and sensitivity
4. Endoscopy
5. Routine haematology and biochemistry
6. Endoscopy
7. Biopsy/necropsy
8. Ultrasonography.

Management

- Systemic antibiosis plus any specific medication
- Nebulization may be effective if there is little build up of inflammatory material
- Direct application to lesions via carapacial osteotomy.

Treatment/specific therapy

- Viral infections – supportive treatment only
- CHV (see 'Differential diagnoses for nasal tract disorders', in *Respiratory Tract Disorders*)
- Hypovitaminosis A
  - Vitamin A supplementation (see *Nutritional Disorders*)
- Bacterial pneumonia
  - As discussed under 'Management', above
- Mycotic pneumonia
  - Difficult to treat. Use antimycotics within framework suggested under 'Management', above
  - Ketoconazole at 10–30 mg/kg p.o. s.i.d.
  - Itraconazole 5 mg/kg p.o. e.o.d.
  - Griseofulvin 20–40 mg/kg p.o. every 3 days
- Ascarids
  - Fenbendazole at 50–100 mg/kg. Repeat every 2 weeks if necessary. *Note* that fenbendazole is metabolized to oxfendazole by the liver
  - Oxfendazole at 68 mg/kg. Repeat every 2 weeks if necessary
  - Topical emodepside plus praziquantel preparations (Profender, Bayer) at 56 µL/100 g body weight (Mehlhorn et al 2005)
  - Prevention: routine worming every 6 months (pre and post-hibernation for Mediterranean and other species where applicable), plus disposal of faeces as soon as observed
- Trematodes
  - Praziquantel at 10 mg/kg p.o. i.m. Repeat after 2 weeks
- Drowning
  - Vigorously pump water out of the lungs by holding the tortoise vertically with head downwards and repetitively flexing the limbs into the inguinal and femoral fossae, thereby compressing the lungs
  - Place in a high oxygen atmosphere
  - Furosemide at 5 mg/kg i.m. b.i.d. to encourage a diuresis
- Hyperthermia
  - Place into cool water
  - Dexamethasone at 30–150 µg/kg i.m., i.v. i.o. may be given.

Ear disorders

Differential diagnoses for tympanic scale (aural) abscess

Bacterial

- Ascending infection from the pharynx up the Eustachian tube so often reflects normal buccal flora. Often G −ve opportunistic bacteria especially *Proteus vulgaris*, *E. coli* and *Aeromonas hydrophila* (Willer et al 2003)
- Mycoplasmosis.

Fungal

- Yeasts.

Parasitic

- Ascarid (*Angusticaecum spp*) described in Mediterranean spur-thighed tortoise *Testudo graeca* (Cutler 2004).

Nutritional

- Possibly related to hypovitaminosis A.

Neoplasia

Other non-infectious problems

- Poor husbandry and suboptimal temperatures
- Exposure to organochlorine pesticides.

Findings on clinical examination

- Commoner in box turtles than other terrestrial chelonia
- Swollen tympanic scale – can be unilateral or bilateral (Fig. 9.6)
- A plug of purulent material may be visible in the pharynx at the site of the Eustachian tube.

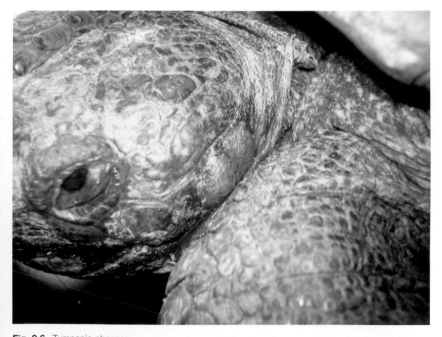

Fig. 9.6. Tympanic abscess.

Investigations

1. Investigate oropharynx – if ascarid present, is likely to be visible
2. Routine culture and sensitivity of purulent material
3. Cytology
4. Radiography
5. Endoscopy
6. Routine haematology and biochemistry
7. Endoscopy
8. Biopsy/necropsy
9. Ultrasonography.

Management

1. Remove any ascarid present via the pharynx if possible
2. Either under GA or local anaesthetic, incise through tympanic scale
3. Remove purulent material and flush. Check that Eustachian tube is patent by monitoring pharyngeal ostium
4. Tympanic scale can be sutured, but often left to heal by second intention thereby allowing repeated flushing.

Treatment/specific therapy

- Bacterial infections – appropriate antibiosis
- Yeasts
  - Nystatin at 100 000 units/kg p.o. daily for 10 days
- Ascarids
  - Fenbendazole at 50–100 mg/kg. Repeat every 2 weeks if necessary. *Note* that fenbendazole is metabolized to oxfendazole by the liver
  - Oxfendazole at 68 mg/kg. Repeat every 2 weeks if necessary
  - Topical emodepside plus praziquantel preparations (Profender, Bayer) at 56 µL/100 g body weight (Mehlhorn et al 2005)
  - Prevention: routine worming every 6 months (pre and post-hibernation for Mediterranean and other species where applicable
- Hypovitaminosis A, see *Nutritional Disorders.*

Gastrointestinal tract disorders

Disorders of the oral cavity

Viral

- Chelonian herpes virus stomatitis (see also 'Runny nose syndrome', in *Respiratory Tract Disorders*)
- Papillomavirus.

Bacterial

- Stomatitis (see also 'Runny nose syndrome', in *Respiratory Tract Disorders*).

Fungal

● Stomatitis.

Parasitic

● Monogenetic trematodes (in semi-aquatic chelonia *Chrysemys*, *Trachemys* and *Chelodina spp*).

Nutritional

● Oak leaf toxicity (see *Urinary Disorders*).

Neoplasia

Other non-infectious problems

● Fractured jaw especially at mandibular symphysis
● Overheating
● Overgrown beak.

Findings on clinical examination

● Inflammation of the oral and pharyngeal membranes progressing to ulcerative lesions involving the palatine area and the trachea. A diphtheritic membrane may be present (CHV, bacterial and fungal stomatitis, oak leaf toxicity)
● Difficulty with prehension or processing of food
● Obvious lesion on lower jaw (fractured mandible). Not always visible, however
● Loss of rostral lower jaw, including the intermandibular joint (sequel to bilateral mandibular fractures and/or osteomyelitis)
● Asymmetry of skull, swelling of one or both mandibles (metabolic bone disease – see *Musculoskeletal Disorders*, abscess/osteomyelitis, fracture, neoplasia)
● Icterus (see *Hepatic Disorders; Cardiovascular Disorders*). In some *Testudo* species, e.g. *T cyrenacea*, the mucous membranes are naturally very yellow in appearance
● Cyanosis
● Excessive ptyalism (overheating, stomatitis).

Investigations

1. Radiography
   a. Consider if risk of underlying osteomyelitis
   b. Likely to require GA to get head into suitable position for radiography
2. Routine haematology and biochemistry
3. Culture and sensitivity
4. PCR for CHV
5. Cytology
   a. Intranuclear inclusions (CHV), fungal hyphae
   b. Gram stain (bacteria, yeasts)
   c. MZN (mycobacteria)
6. Endoscopy
7. Biopsy
8. Ultrasonography.

Treatment/specific therapy

- Fractured jaw
  - Can be due to traumatic handling (e.g. during stomach tubing), pathological (e.g. infection, metabolic bone disease)
  - Placement of an oesophagostomy tube will help with fluid and nutritional support during recovery
  - Surgical repair difficult in smaller chelonia – pins traversing the intermandibular space can interfere with tongue mobility
  - Many terrestrial chelonia can manage surprisingly well following the loss of the intermandibular joint providing food is prepared in smaller pieces for them
- Bacterial and fungal stomatitis
  - Topical antibiotics/antifungals plus topical povidone-iodine daily
  - Surgical debridement of necrotic tissue may be necessary, followed by systemic and topical treatment
- Monogenetic trematodes
  - Usually seen in wild-caught piscivorous aquatic and semi-aquatic chelonia
  - Probably non-pathogenic
  - Praziquantel at 10 mg/kg p.o. i.m. Repeat after 2 weeks
- Overgrown beak. Can be associated with:
  - Malocclusion following a jaw fracture (can be iatrogenic while stomach tubing)
  - Excessive protein intake, often accompanied by relative lack of dietary calcium (i.e. Metabolic bone disease – see *Musculoskeletal Disorders*). In this case, there are often associated skull and shell deformities
  - Burr back the beak into more appropriate shape.

Differential diagnoses for gastrointestinal disorders

Chelonia, like birds, will often produce both faecal and urinary components of their excretions at the same time, mixed to some extent inside the proctodeum of the cloaca. In herbivorous chelonia, the faeces should be well formed. Loose faeces suggest gastrointestinal disease, a low-fibre diet, excess fruit intake or anxiety.

In all terrestrial chelonia the bladder is large and acts as a significant organ for water storage. Urination during handling as a sign of anxiety is not uncommon. The urine often consists of a combination of a mucilaginous portion stained white or yellow with urate crystals, and a clear watery portion. The urate portion may not be present every time.

Viral

- Reovirus.

Bacterial

- Salmonellosis (chelonia can act as asymptomatic reservoirs)
- *Campylobacter fetus*
- *Vibrio spp*
- *Clostridium spp.* Can be linked to long-term antibiosis.

Fungal

- Mycotic enteritis.

Protozoal

- Cilates, e.g. *Balantidium spp, Nyctotherus spp*
- Flagellates, e.g. *Trichomonas, Trichomonas*
- *Entamoeba invadens* (usually asymptomatic in chelonia, but can cause enterocolitis and myositis (Philbey 2006)
- *Cryptosporidium spp*
- *Caryospora spp*
- *Eimeria spp.*

Parasitic

- Nematodes
  - Ascarids : *Angusticaecum* and *Sulcascaris*
  - Oxyurids: *Tachygonetria spp, Alaeuris spp., Mehdiella spp, Thaparia spp*
  - Acanthocephalans (especially aquatic and semi-aquatic chelonia)
  - Hookworms: *Camallanus spp, Spineoxys spp* (freshwater chelonia)
- Cestodes
  - *Ophiotaenia spp, Glossocercus spp, Bancroftiella spp* (freshwater chelonia)
  - Flukes.

Nutritional

- Dysbiosis (lack of fibre, too much fruit in diet, long-term antibiosis)
- Poisoning
  - Oak leaf
  - Azaleas, rhododendrons, *Pieris spp* (Pizzi et al 2005) and other members of the *Ericaceae* (see *Cardiovascular Disorders*)
  - Heavy metal, e.g. lead, zinc (see *Systemic Disorders*).

Neoplasia

Other non-infectious problems

- Green, well-formed faeces. Normal if fed mostly on pelleted foods
- Constipation
- Foreign body
- Gastric dilatation
- Cloacal prolapse
  - Cloacitis
  - Cloacoliths
  - Intestinal foreign body
  - Intussusception
  - Extra-intestinal mass, e.g. renal neoplasm, bladder stone
  - Dystocia
  - Hypocalcaemia/metabolic bone disease
  - Parasitism.

- Diarrhoea – voluminous, runny faces. May be foul smelling (flagellates, dysbiosis)
- Green, well-formed faeces (pelleted food)
- Regurgitation (and gastritis)
- Dehydration (sunken eyes)

- Lethargy
- Lack of faeces (foreign body, bladder stone, renal neoplasia, intussusception)
- Ulceration of the oral mucous membranes
- Petechial haemorrhages (hookworms)
- Oedematous swelling at cloaca (cloacal prolapse – differentiate from phallus in male)
- Death.

Investigations

1. Microscopy (Fig. 9.7)
   a. Fresh faecal sample – 'wet prep' (Table 9.2)
2. Radiography
   a. Contrast studies
   b. Barium sulphate suspension at 5 mL/kg by gavage in the leopard tortoise (*Geochelone pardalis*) (Table 9.3)
   c. Recommended timing for radiography following barium gavage is zero, 10 min, 2, 6, 12, 24 and 72 h
   d. Water-soluble iodine-based contrast media such as Gastrografin (at 1 mL per 130 g in Herman's tortoise *Testudo hermanni* (Table 9.4)
   e. Hernandez-Divers & Hernandez-Divers (2001) suggest similar results with the non-ionic iodine-based contrast medium iohexol at 7.5–10 mL/kg by gavage, with recommended timing for radiography following iohexol gavage given as 0, 20, 40, 60, 120 and 240 min at 30°C
   f. Colonic contrast studies can be performed by retrograde introduction of the contrast media via a catheter into the colon via the cloaca
   g. Foreign body. Small pieces of gravel or stone can be normal; large numbers suggest a gut stasis, obstruction or pica
   h. Ileus – common with dysbiosis
3. Routine haematology and biochemistry
4. Culture and sensitivity
5. Endoscopy

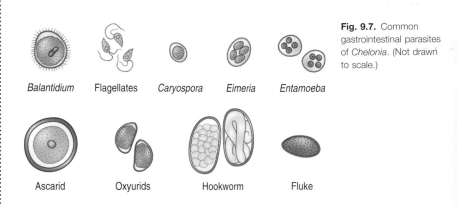

Fig. 9.7. Common gastrointestinal parasites of *Chelonia*. (Not drawn to scale.)

Balantidium   Flagellates   *Caryospora*   Eimeria   Entamoeba

Ascarid   Oxyurids   Hookworm   Fluke

Table 9.2 Faecal parasites

Faecal parasite	Comments
Ascarid eggs (*Angusticaecum, Sulcascaris*)	Typical ascarid eggs
Hookworm eggs	Thin-walled, oval eggs
Strongyle eggs: *Tachygonetria spp*	Thin-walled, often D-shaped eggs
Fluke eggs	Thin-shelled, often with single operculum. Orange or deep yellow colour. Miracidium may be visible
Flagellates	Numerous motile pear- to circular-shaped protozoa approximately 8 × 5 μm
Balantidium spp, Nyctotherus spp	Large, motile ciliates
Cryptosporidium	Oocysts may be visible using phase contrast microscopy after floatation. Otherwise consider MZN staining
Eimeria oocysts	Elongate
Caryospora	Circular – 1 sporocyst
Amoebiasis (see also *Liver Disorders*). Common species of enteric amoeba below	Cysts are approx 11–20 μm. Trophozoites (amoeboid form) have a single nucleus and average 16 μm when fixed. The distinguishing features of speciate cysts below
Entamoeba	Multinucleate cysts; nuclear endosomes measure up to nucleus diameter
Acanthamoeba	Large cysts. Single nucleus containing endosome over one half diameter. Irregular outline
Hartmannella	As above but regular outline
Endolimax	Multinucleate; nuclear endosomes same diameter as nucleus, each of which has a dark-staining rim

Table 9.3 Barium sulphate suspension at 5 mL/kg by gavage in the leopard tortoise (*Geochelone pardalis*)

Position of barium sulphate	Time following administration
Complete gastric emptying	5–9 h
Entry to small intestine	0.2–1 h
Entry to large intestine	5–8 h
Exit from colon	144–166 h
Still present in GIT	8 days

Adapted from Taylor et al (1996).

Table 9.4 Water soluble iodine-based contrast media such as Gastrografin (at 1 mL/130 g in Herman's tortoise *Testudo hermanni*

Body temperature (°C)	Average total gut transit time (h)
15.2	8–24
21.5	3–8
30.6	1.5–4

Adapted from Meyer (1998).

6. Biopsy
   a. Larvae encapsulated in gut wall (acanthocephalans) or other tissues, e.g. skin (Spirurids – see *Skin Disorders*)
   b. Amoebiasis
7. Ultrasonography.

Management

- Fluid therapy (see *Nursing Care*)
- Covering antibiosis.

Treatment/specific therapy

- Salmonellosis
  - Probably best considered as a normal constituent of chelonian cloacal/gut microflora
  - Rarely pathogenic to chelonia
  - Excretion likely to increase during times of stress, e.g. movement, illness
  - Treatment usually not appropriate as unlikely to be effective long term and may encourage resistance
  - Recommendations for prevention of salmonellosis from captive reptiles issued by the Center for Disease Control in the USA. These are:
    - Pregnant women, children <5 years of age and persons with impaired immune system function (e.g. AIDS) should not have contact with reptiles
    - Because of the risk if becoming infected with Salmonella from a reptile, even without direct contact, households with pregnant women, children <5 years of age or persons with impaired immune system function should not keep reptiles. Reptiles are not appropriate pets for childcare centres
    - All persons should wash hands with soap immediately after any contact with a reptile or reptile cage
    - Reptiles should be kept out of food preparation areas such as kitchens
    - Kitchen sinks should not be used to wash food or water bowls, cages or vivaria used for reptiles, or to bath reptiles. Any sink used for these purposes should be disinfected after use
- Mycotic enteritis
  - Nystatin at 100 000 units/kg p.o. daily for 10 days
  - Ketoconazole at 10–30 mg/kg p.o. s.i.d.
  - Itraconazole 5 mg/kg p.o. e.o.d.

- Amoebiasis
  - Metronidazole
    - 100–257 mg/kg body weight. Repeat after 2 weeks if necessary
    - 20 mg/kg e.o.d. until eradication
  - Chloroquine
    - 125 mg/kg p.o. every 48 h for 3 treatments
    - 50 mg/kg i.m. every 7 days for 3 weeks
  - Iodoquinol/diiodohydroxyquin 50 mg/kg p.o. s.i.d. for 21 days. *Note* possibly toxic to black rat snakes.
  - Paromomycin
    - 300–360 mg/kg e.o.d. for 14 days
    - 25–100 mg/kg daily for 4 weeks
- Caryospora
  - Sulphadimethoxine at 50 mg/kg daily for 3 days; stop for 3 days then repeat 3 day course
- *Cryptosporidium*
  - Direct life cycle; infection by exposure to water containing infective oocysts
  - There is no recognized effective treatment
  - Try metronidazole at 100–275 mg/kg p.o. once only
  - Nitazoxanide at 5 mg/kg s.i.d.
  - Paromomycin at 300–800 mg/kg p.o. s.i.d. for 10 days
  - Oocysts (*C. parvum*) in water can be viable after 7 months at 15°C
  - Disinfect by exposing to water above 64°C for >2 min
  - *Cryptosporidium* oocysts are very resistant to chlorine or iodine
- Ascarids, hookworms and oxyurids
  - Fenbendazole at 50–100 mg/kg. Repeat every 2 weeks if necessary. *Note* that fenbendazole is metabolized to oxfendazole by the liver
  - Oxfendazole at 68 mg/kg. Repeat every 2 weeks if necessary
  - Topical emodepside plus praziquantel preparations (Profender, Bayer) at 56 μL/100 g body weight (Mehlhorn et al 2005)
  - Prevention: routine worming every six months (pre and post-hibernation for Mediterranean and other species where applicable), plus disposal of faeces as soon as observed
    Note that *Oxyuris* worms usually have a direct life cycle
  - Hookworms have a direct life cycle; infective larvae can penetrate the skin or infect via the contaminated food and water
- Flukes and cestodes
  - Praziquantel at 10 mg/kg. i.m. p.o.
- Ciliates
  - Usually part of normal gut fauna. Large numbers may indicate gut dysbiosis. Sensitive to metronidazole
- Flagellates
  - Metronidazole
    - 100–257 mg/kg body weight. Repeat after 2 weeks if necessary
    - 20 mg/kg e.o.d. until eradicated
  - Dysbiosis
    - High-fibre diets; reduce fruit intake. Fluid and nutritional support
    - Antimicrobials often not necessary unless suspect bacterial or mycotic overgrowth

- Gastric dilatation
  - Pass stomach tube to release gas
  - Tube activated charcoal or simethicone
  - Typically linked to an excess intake of fermentable carbohydrate; may be linked with abnormal gut motility or obstruction
- Cloacal prolapse
  - Prevent dessication and trauma by wrapping in non-adhesive protective film-wrap or equivalent
  - Topical sugar may reduce oedema by osmosis
  - Replace and purse-string suture around cloaca for several weeks
  - Limit feeding to reduce straining during defaecation
  - If repeatedly prolapses consider cloacopexy
  - Attend to underlying aetiologies, e.g. uroliths
- Oak and other poisoning
  - If diagnosed antemortem attempt removal of oak leaves from stomach either by endoscopy or via a coleotomy
  - Supportive therapy, especially fluids due to renal effects
  - Foreign body
  - If in stomach may be accessible with endoscopy
  - Use of lubricants such as liquid paraffin should be judicious as this may complicate subsequent therapy
  - Surgical enterotomy
- Intussusception
  - Surgical enterectomy.

Nutritional disorders

- Metabolic bone disease (MBD) (see also *Musculoskeletal Disorders*)
- Hypovitaminosis A
  - Especially in young semi-aquatic chelonia, e.g. red-eared sliders (*Trachemys scripta elegans*)
  - A variety of ocular lesions including swollen eyelids due to squamous metaplasia of the orbital glands and their ducts. A whitish cellular mass may develop behind the lower lid. Terrestrial chelonia may appear 'bespectacled'
  - Squamous metaplasia also affects the renal tubules, causing kidney damage
  - Affected chelonia are often anorexic, as they cannot see to locate food
  - Treatment is with vitamin A given i.m. at 1 000–5 000 IU weekly for 4 weeks, and the addition of dietary vitamin A supplements
  - Ensure diet contains natural sources of vitamin a precursors, especially with red, orange and yellow vegetables, e.g. sweet peppers, plus leafy greens
- Poisoning with azaleas, rhododendrons, and other members of the *Ericaceae* (see *Cardiovascular and Haematological Disorders*)
- Hepatic lipidosis (see *Hepatic Disorders*)
- Dysbiosis
  - Excess fermentable carbohydrate intake usually combined with insufficient fibre (too much fruit) (see *Gastrointestinal Tract Disorders*)

Hepatic disorders

Viral

- Chelonian herpesvirus (CHV).

Bacterial

- Abscessation
- *Salmonella typhimurium* (González Candela et al 2005)
- Mycobacteriosis (granulomas – may be multifocal).

Fungal

Protozoal

- Amoebiasis.

Nutritional

- Hepatic lipidosis
- Chronic debilitation
- Cholecystolithiasis (gallstones).

Neoplasia

Findings on clinical examination

- Malaise
- Listlessness
- Anorexia
- Weight loss
- Jaundice (icterus). Note that some *Testudo spp*, e.g. *T. cyrenacia*, naturally have yellowish oral mucous membranes
- Greenish faeces
- Diarrhoea
- Death.

Investigations

1. Microscopy
   a. Faecal examination: cysts and trophozoites may be present (amoebiasis)
2. Radiography
3. Routine haematology and biochemistry
4. Culture and sensitivity
5. Endoscopy
6. Biopsy/necropsy
   a. Granulomatous hepatitis (bacterial, fungal infection)
   b. Amoebiasis
   c. ZN staining and PCR for mycobacteria
7. Ultrasonography.

Management

- Milk thistle (*Silybum marianum*) is hepatoprotectant. Dose at 4–15 mg/kg b.i.d. or t.i.d.
- For ascites try furosemide at 2–5 mg/kg s.i.d. if ascitic
- Lactulose 0.05 mL/100 g p.o. s.i.d.

Treatment/specific therapy

- Mycobacteriosis – see *Systemic Disorders*
- Amoebiasis
  - Metronidazole 20 mg/kg e.o.d. until eradication
  - Chloroquine
    - 125 mg/kg p.o. every 48 h for three treatments
    - 50 mg/kg i.m. every 7 days for 3 weeks
  - Iodoquinol/diiodohydroxyquin 50 mg/kg p.o. s.i.d. for 21 days. *Note* possibly toxic to black rat snakes
  - Paromomycin
    - 300–360 mg/kg e.o.d. for 14 days
    - 25–100 mg/kg daily for 4 weeks
- Cholecystolithiasis and cholecystitis
  - Consider NSAIDs, e.g. meloxicam at 0.2 mg/kg once daily or every other day (in the green iguana, see Hernandez-Divers 2006) and covering antibiosis
  - Surgery to remove gallstones may be feasible
  - Linked to high dietary levels of processed dog and cat food (excessive protein, lipid, vitamin A and D_3 intake)
  - Feed a more appropriate herbivorous diet.

Pancreatic disorders

Diabetes mellitus (see *Endocrine Disorders*).

Cardiovascular and haematological disorders

Cardiovascular anatomy

Three-chambered heart consisting of two atria and one ventricle. A series of muscular ridges plus the timing of ventricular contraction tend to functionally divide the ventricle into two (the *cavum venosum,* the *cavum pulmonale* and the *cavum arteriosum*), thereby separating systemic from pulmonary blood flow.

The renal portal system (RPV). The RPV is large vessel arising near the confluence of the epigastric and external iliac veins. It drains into the kidney. Blood returning from the tail, hind legs and other closely situated structures may pass through these vessels, or may bypass and enter the systemic circulation direct. This appears to depend upon various factors such as hydration status and core body temperature. May be more significant for drugs excreted by tubular secretion than by glomerular filtration.

Differential diagnosis for cardiovascular disorders

Viral

- Iridovirus (epicarditis but associated with other more typical iridovirus signs).

Bacterial

- Endocarditis.

Fungal

Protozoal

- *Haemogregarina spp*
- *Haemoproteus spp*
- *Plasmodium spp*
- *Pirhaemocyton* (may actually be iridoviral inclusions).

Parasitic

- Spirochid flukes, both adults and eggs.

Nutritional

- Excessive calcium intake
- Excessive vitamin D3 intake
- Ingestion of azaleas, rhododendrons and other members of the *Ericaceae* (contain several toxins including cardiac glycosides).

Neoplasia

Other non-infectious problems

- Metastatic mineralization
- Amyloidosis
- Renal disease
- Myocardial disease
- Hyperkalaemia
- Pericardial effusion
- Visceral gout (uric acid in pericardial sac), see *Urinary Disorders*.

Findings on clinical examination

- Anorexia
- Oedema
- Weakness
- Weight loss
- Areas of cutaneous mineralization (with metastatic mineralization)
- Spirochid fluke parasitism in freshwater turtles associated with subcutaneous oedema, blood-tinged coelomic fluid, hepatic, pancreatic and splenic necrosis. Many organs can be affected due to microgranulomas triggered by the fluke eggs.

Investigations

1. Radiography
   a. May be useful to diagnose metastatic mineralization but unlikely to be useful for radiographic evaluation of the heart

2. Routine haematology and biochemistry
3. Cytology (blood smear)
   a. *Haemogregarina spp*
4. Blood culture and sensitivity
5. Endoscopy
6. Ultrasonography may be useful in large chelonia (Redrobe & Scudamore 2000)
7. Electrocardiography. Potentially useful but few normal values established
   a. Normal ECG values in anesthetized red-eared slider (*Trachemys scripta elegans*) using a three electrode, lead II trace, after Holz & Holz (1995). Some comparative values from conscious terrapins (from Kaplan & Shwartz (1963), cited in Holz & Holz 1995) are given for comparison (Table 9.5)
   b. Note that the QRS complex was always in the form of a large R wave – no Q or S wave deflections were visible
   c. Azalea toxicity: paroxysmal tachycardia, atrial fibrillation, premature ventricular beats, extra systoles, ectopic ventricular contractions (Frye & Williams 1995)
   d. Atrial fibrillation and first-degree heart block may be an indicator of calcium deficiency.

Management

- The usual cardiac drugs are largely untried and, therefore, treatment with these is speculative, although still worth attempting
- Diuretics, e.g. furosemide at 5 mg/kg i.m. b.i.d. to encourage a diuresis.

Table 9.5 Normal ECG values in anaesthetised red-eared slider (*Trachemys scripta elegans*) using a three electrode, lead II trace, with comparative values from conscious terrapins

Variable	Normal ECG values[a]	Comparative values[b]
Body weight (kg)	0.45–1.81	
Heart rate (beats/min)	25 (16–37)	34
P, duration (s)	0.12 (0.04)	0.09
P, amplitude (mV)	0.030 (0.017)	
PR interval	0.51	0.41
QRS duration (s)	0.15 (0.02)	0.11
R, amplitude (mV)	0.254 (0.067)	
T, amplitude (mV)	0.068	
R–R interval (s)	2.38	
QT interval, (s)	1.41 (0.38)	
ST interval (s)	1.05 (0.24)	0.81

[a]From Holz & Holz (1995).
[b]From Kaplan & Shwartz (1963), cited in Holz & Holz (1995).

Treatment/specific therapy

- Haemoparasites
  - Loading dose of chloroquine phosphate (5 mg/kg p.o.) and primaquine phosphate (0.5 mg/kg p.o.)
  - Continue with chloroquine at 2.5 mg/kg p.o. once weekly and primaquine at 0.5 mg/kg once weekly for 12–16 weeks
- Flukes – praziquantel
- Azalea poisoning
  - Atropine sulphate at 0.04 mg/kg i.v.
  - After 2 min, calcium gluconate at 2 mg/kg by slow i.v. injection over the next 5 min
  - Once ECG normal, consider gastric lavage
  - Supportive treatment
- Hypocalcaemia – see *Musculoskeletal Disorders*.

Systemic disorders

Viral

- Chelonian herpes virus (CHV)
- Papilloma-like virus (see Drury et al 1998).

Bacterial

- Mycobacteria (see below)
- *Chlamydophila pneumoniae*
- Chlamydia-like organisms (possibly *Parachlamydia acanthamoeba*, *Simkania negevensis*) (Soldati et al 2004)
- Spirochaetes.

Fungal

- *Exophiala spp.*

Protozoal

- Intranuclear coccidiosis.

Nutritional

- Hypocalcaemia (including metabolic bone disease).

Neoplasia

Other non-infectious problems

- Ivermectin toxicity
- Anaemia
- Gout (renal, visceral and articular) See *Urinary Disorders*
- Hypoglycaemia (including post-hibernational anorexia)
- Cardiac disease (see *Cardiovascular and Haematological Disorders*)
- Heavy metal, e.g. lead, zinc.

Findings on clinical examination

- Weakness
- Emaciation and weight loss
- Anorexia
- Ocular and nasal discharge, stomatitis, with or without bouts of paralysis (CHV)
- Lethargy, anorexia, paralysis following ivermectin administration (ivermectin toxicity)
- Oedema.

Investigations

1. Radiography
   a. Heavy metal poisoning
2. Routine haematology and biochemistry
   a. Serum lead and zinc. Consider blood sampling other in-contact chelonia to establish normal ranges)
3. Serology and PCR for CHV
4. PCR for CHV
5. ZN staining and PCR for mycobacteria
6. Immunohistochemistry and PCR for *Chlamydophila* and *Chlamydia*-like organisms (Soldati et al 2004)
7. Culture and sensitivity
8. Endoscopy
9. Ultrasonography
10. Biopsy/necropsy
    a. Single or multiple granulomas (mycobacteria, fungi, *Chlamydophila pneumoniae*, Chlamydia-like organisms)
    b. Eosinophilic intranuclear protozoan-like organisms typically in the renal epithelial cells hepatocytes, pancreatic acinar cells and intestinal epithelial cells (Jacobson et al 1994).

Management

- See *Nursing Care.*

Treatment/specific therapy

- Chelonian herpes virus
  - No effective treatment but consider acyclovir at 80 mg/kg s.i.d. Efficacy appears variable
  - Supportive treatment only (but see *Respiratory Tract Disorders*)
- Bacterial infections
  - Appropriate antibiosis
  - General nursing care
- Mycobacteriosis
  - Potential zoonosis. Consider euthanasia.
  - No successful treatment for mycobacteriosis in reptiles reported

- Intranuclear coccidiosis
  - Potentiated sulphonamides at 30 mg/kg s.i.d.
- Ivermectin toxicity
  - i.v. fluids at 5 mL/kg per h for up to 3 h then 5–10 mg/kg per day
  - Methylprednisolone 1 mg/kg i.v. s.i.d.
  - May require continued support for many weeks (see Divers et al 1999)
- Heavy metal poisoning
  - Remove metallic foreign bodies via endoscope if possible
  - Sodium calcium edetate at 35 mg/kg by slow i.v. daily for 2 weeks.

Musculoskeletal disorders

Bacterial

- Osteomyelitis
- *Corynebacterium aquaticum* (see Philbey et al 2006).

Fungal

Protozoal

- Amoebiasis.

Nutritional

- Metabolic bone disease (MBD). Actually a complex of disorders including:
  - Dietary calcium deficiency
  - Dietary calcium/phosphorus imbalance
  - Protein excess
  - Hypovitaminosis D_3
    - Lack of exposure to ultraviolet light
    - Incorrect environmental temperatures
    - Lack of dietary vitamin D_3
  - Protein deficiency
  - Liver, kidney and intestinal disease
  - Multiple factors may be involved
  - Metastatic calcification of smooth muscle of various organs including cardiovascular system, pulmonary system, gut and urogenital system. Typically linked to excess dietary vitamin D_3 intake, e.g. over supplementation, feeding with dog and cat food.

Neoplasia

Other non-infectious problems

- Metabolic bone disease (hepatic, renal and intestinal disease, see also 'Nutritional', above)
- Fractures of the shell or limbs (usually traumatic)
- Joint dislocations (traumatic)
- Degenerative joint disease due to:
  - Obesity
  - Articular gout (see *Urinary Disorders*)
  - Trauma

- Septic arthritis
- Osteochondritis
- Coxofemoral arthritis (Philbey et al 2006)
- Lawn mower trauma.

Findings on clinical examination

- Soft shell (*note* that in terrestrial chelonia, the shell should be hard by 12 months of age), flattened shell, doming of scutes (MBD)
- Weakness – unable to support its own weight, hind legs articulated backwards as if sliding rather than held beneath the body (MBD)
- Beak abnormalities including overgrowth
- Soft mandibles (MBD)
- Claw abnormalities including overgrowth (MBD)
- Limb swellings (fractures, dislocations, osteomyelitis, myositis, septic or aseptic arthritis)
- Vague signs of ill-health (anorexia, lack of movement, lethargy).

Investigations

1. Radiography
   a. Reduced bone density, cortical thinning, thickening of limb bones and shell (fibrous osteodystrophy)
   b. Fractures (shell, limbs)
   c. Lytic bone lesions (osteomyelitis)
   d. Areas of abnormal calcification (metastatic calcification)
2. Routine haematology and biochemistry
   a. Blood vitamin D_3 (25-hydroxycholecalciferol) levels; also total calcium, ionized calcium, phosphate)
   b. Acierno et al 2006 measured 25-hydroxyvitamin D_3 in red-eared sliders (*Trachemys scripta elegans*) (Table 9.6)

Table 9.6 25-hydroxyvitamin D_3 in red-eared sliders (*Trachemys scripta elegans*)

Red-eared slider turtles (*Trachemys scripta elegans*)	25-hydroxyvitamin D_3 concentrations (nmol/L)	
	Mean	SD
Supplemental UV radiation	71.7	46.9
No provision of supplemental UV radiation	31.4	13.2

Adapted from Acierno et al (2006).

3. Culture and sensitivity
4. Cytology (FNA)
5. Endoscopy

6. Biopsy/necropsy
   a. Amoebiasis
7. Ultrasonography
8. ECG – atrial fibrillation (see *Cardiovascular and Haematological Disorders*).

Management

* Close attention should be paid to environmental parameters, especially exposure to UV lighting, temperature and dietary supplementation.

Treatment/specific therapy

* Amoebiasis (see *Gastrointestinal Tract Disorders*)
* Metabolic bone disease
  * Usually due to secondary nutritional hyperparathyroidism linked with either failure to provide sufficient calcium supplementation or exposure to UV-B
  * Parenteral calcium gluconate or lactate at 1.0–2.5 mg/kg daily
  * Oral vitamin D_3 at 1–4 IU/kg daily
  * Dietary calcium supplementation
  * Exposure to full spectrum lighting as a UV-B source
  * Calcitonin at 1.5 IU/kg s.c. s.i.d. if is normocalcaemic
* Metastatic calcification
  * No effective treatment
  * Reduce hypercalcaemia by:
    * Calcitonin at 1.5 IU/kg s.c. s.i.d.
    * Fluid therapy at 15 mL/kg Hartman's solution intracoelomic until normocalcaemic
  * Although often linked to excessive vitamin D3 supplementation, many cases may be due to low levels of calcitrol, commonly secondary to renal disease. This leads to toxic levels of PTH production with associated abnormal tissue mineralization and further renal damage
* Osteochondritis
  * Arthrotomy and surgical removal of any loose bone fragments
  * NSAID therapy, e.g. meloxicam at 0.2 mg/kg once daily or every other day (in the green iguana, see Hernandez-Divers 2006)
* Joint dislocations
  * Reduce surgically if possible and immobilize as described for long bone fractures, below
* Abscessation and osteomyelitis, myositis
  * Appropriate antibiosis
  * Consider amputation if damage is extensive
* Fractures
  * Long bone fractures – stabilization by confining the flexed limb into its fossa with strong adhesive tape may be sufficient to allow callus formation and healing. Otherwise surgical reduction and internal/external fixation
  * Shell fractures may require surgical plating. Shell deficits will require bridging with fibreglass or methylmethacrylate
* Lawn mower trauma

- Tortoises in long grass can be damaged during mowing, especially by 'hover-mowers'
- Injuries usually include injuries to the dorsal carapace, often with exposure of the lungs
- Because the lungs in tortoises are naturally rigid (attached to the inner surface of the carapace) then respiration is usually not compromised
- Flush the lungs with sterile saline to remove any debris and treat as for *Respiratory Tract Disorders*
- As with other shell traumas (see *Skin Disorders*) do not place a permanent covering, e.g. methylmethacrylate, over the deficit until any infection has resolved.

Neurological disorders

Viral
- Chelonian herpes virus (CHV).

Bacterial
- Septicaemia
- Granuloma/meningitis
- Intracranial/extracranial abscess (vestibular syndrome).

Fungal
- Granuloma/meningitis.

Protozoal

Parasitic
- Myiasis (aberrant) (Sales et al 2003).

Nutritional
- Hypocalcaemia (see 'MBD', in *Musculoskeletal Disorders*).

Neoplasia
- Central nervous system neoplasia
- Other non-infectious problems
- Ivermectin toxicity.
- CNS gout (uric acid deposition) (see *Urinary Disorders*)
- Heavy metal poisoning.

Findings on clinical examination

- Weakness
- Hind-limb weakness. Especially common in old female Herman's tortoises. Often of unknown aetiology but consider CHV or CNS gout
- Lethargy, anorexia, paralysis following ivermectin administration (ivermectin toxicity)
- Vestibular syndrome (head tilt, circling to one side)
- Anorexia.

Investigations

1. Radiography
   a. Skull
   b. Subtle spinal lesions unlikely to be seen on radiography
   c. Metallic objects in gut, especially nails, lead shot, etc.
2. MRI scan
3. Routine haematology and biochemistry
4. Blood lead or zinc levels
5. Culture and sensitivity
6. Endoscopy
7. Ultrasonography.

Treatment/specific therapy

- Hypocalcaemia (see 'MBD', in *Musculoskeletal Disorders*)
- Ivermectin toxicity (see *Systemic Disorders*)
- Aberrant myiasis
  - No safe systemic insecticidal preparation. Necrosis of dead larva may release toxins
- Vestibular syndrome
  - Consider surgical removal or debridement if due to a contributing abscess, if feasible
- Heavy metal toxicity
  - Remove metallic foreign body if possible
  - NaCa edetate at 35 mg/kg i.m. s.i.d. until clinically normal (see Chitty 2003).

Ophthalmic disorders

Chelonia have both rods and cones but lack a fovea. Instead they have an area centralis or area temporalis: sections of retina sensitive to detail, edges or movement. There is no conus papillaris. Chelonia have both lachrymal and Harderian glands.

For examination of the posterior segment of the eye is difficult as the iris muscle fibres are striated and partly under voluntary control. Therefore, parasympatholytics, e.g. atropine and sympathomimetics, e.g. phenylephrine, will not work. Consider examination by:
1. Using low light levels
2. General anaesthesia
3. Non-parasympatholytic mydriatics such as vecuronium.

Viral

- Chelonia herpes virus
- Pox-like virus.

Bacterial

- Secondary infection
- Eyelid granuloma (mycobacteriosis)
- *Pasteurella*.

Fungal

- Keratitis (Fig. 9.8)
- *Exophiala spp.*

Parasitic

- Nematode larvae (red-eared slider *Trachemys scripta elegans*)
- Microfilariae.

Nutritional

- Hypovitaminosis A (especially semi-aquatic chelonia) (Fig. 9.9).

Neoplasia

Other non-infectious problems

- Ageing (cataracts)
- Sub-zero temperatures (cataracts, vitreal haze)
- Nutritional deficiencies (cataracts)
- Trauma
- Poor water quality (aquatic chelonia esp. snapping turtle *Chelydra serpentina*)
- Exposure to ultraviolet-C (incorrect UV lighting)
- Congenital defects
- Cyclopia
- Microphthalmia

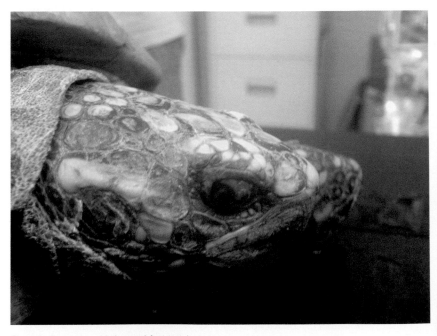

Fig. 9.8. Fungal keratitis in a red-foot tortoise.

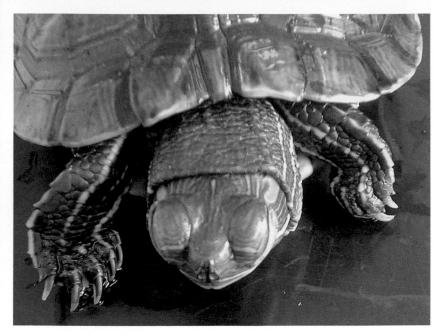

Fig. 9.9. Hypovitaminosis A in a hatchling red-eared slider.

* Anophthalmia
* Arcus senilis
* Chronic hypertrophy of the nictitating membrane
* Coagulative keratopathy.

Findings on clinical examination

* Conjunctivitis
* Blepharitis
* Ocular discharge
* Corneal ulceration
* Deep ulceration followed by perforation and iris collapse
* Hypopyon
* Uveitis
* Keratitis
* Cataracts
* Grossly swollen eyelids; unable to open one or both eyes (hypovitaminosis A, infection)
* In terrestrial chelonia, the eyelid lesions give a semblance of spectacles
* A whitish cellular mass may develop behind the lower lid
* Anorexia (cannot see to locate food)
  Note renal disease may be concurrent with hypovitaminosis A (see *Urinary Disorders*)

- Nematode larvae within the choroid (red-eared slider *Trachemys scripta elegans*)
- Obvious worm in the anterior chamber (microfilariae)
- Panophthalmitis
- Ocular signs possibly accompanied by stomatitis and rhinitis (chelonian herpes virus)
- Yellow papular lesions of the eyelids in *Testudo hermanni* (pox-like virus).

Investigations

1. Ophthalmic examination
2. Radiography
3. Routine haematology and biochemistry
4. Culture and sensitivity
5. Endoscopy
6. Biopsy/necropsy
   a. ZN staining and PCR for mycobacteria
7. Water quality testing for aquatic chelonia (esp. pH, ammonia, nitrites, nitrates, temperature)
8. Ultrasonography
9. Reassess lighting (exposure to UV-C).

Management

1. Many non-specific ocular lesions respond well to vitamin a supplementation at 1000–5000 IU i.m. weekly for 4 weeks, and the addition of dietary vitamin A supplements
2. Enucleation may be required for severely damaged or infected eyes.

Treatment/specific therapy

- Hypovitaminosis A (see *Nutritional Disorders*)
- Eyelid granuloma
  - Topical treatment
  - Consider resection
- Fungal keratitis
  - Topical antimycotics, e.g. clotrimazole
  - Systemic antimycosis may be required
- Congenital defects
  - No treatment
  - Consider incubation parameters (temperature, humidity, etc.) as well as genetic factors when considering cause
- Cataracts
  - Phacoemulsification (see Kelly et al 2005)
  - Lens extraction
- Arcus senilis. Age related. No treatment
- Chronic hypertrophy of the nictitating membrane
  - Lavage of the conjunctival space
  - Topical application of ophthalmic corticosteroid preparation

- Coagulative keratopathy
  - Topical ophthalmic ointment containing proteolytic enzyme
  - May occur post-hibernation
- Poor water quality
  - Identify abnormality and correct (see *Tropical Freshwater Fish*)
- Microfilariae and helminths
  - Fenbendazole at 50–100 mg/kg. Repeat every 2 weeks if necessary
  - Do not use ivermectin (see *Systemic Disorders*)
- Exposure to UV-C
  - Provision of incorrect lighting, e.g. UV-sterilization tubes, blacklights for tanning beds instead of the correct full-spectrum lighting
  - Correct lighting; provision of a darkened area during the initial recovery period may be beneficial
  - Supportive treatment as may be anorexic due to compromised vision.

Urinary disorders

Bacterial

- Cystitis
- Pyelonephritis.

Fungal

- Cystitis
- Pyelonephritis.

Protozoal

- Hexamita
- *Myxidium spp* (Myxozoa) (crowned river turtle *Hardella thurjii*; see Garner et al 2003).

Parasitic

- Monogenetic trematodes (in semi-aquatic chelonia *Chrysemys*, *Trachemys* and *Chelodina spp*).

Nutritional

- Hypovitaminosis A (squamous metaplasia of the renal tubules)
- Oak leaf toxicity (see *Gastrointestinal Tract Disorders*).

Neoplasia

Other non-infectious problems

- Bladder calculi/stones
- Gout (renal)
- Iatrogenic (nephrotoxic drugs, e.g. aminoglycosides)
- Pelvic obstruction (foreign body, coxofemoral arthritis – see *Musculoskeletal Disorders*, retained eggs)
- Interstitial nephropathy
- Tubulonephropathy
- Glomerulonephropathy.

Findings on clinical examination

- Anorexia
- Lethargy
- Weight loss
- Polydipsia/polyuria
- Polyuria
- Urinary tenesmus
- Yellow urates (denotes prolonged retention)
- Anuria
- Oedema
- Hind-limb weakness (see also *Neurological Disorders*)
- Pale mucous membranes
- Ocular disease, especially in semi-aquatic chelonia (hypovitaminosis A)
- Mortalities.

Investigations

1. Radiography
   a. Soft-tissue mineralization; increased soft-tissue or mineral density in renal region
   b. Uroliths. *Note* that the bladder is voluminous in chelonia and bladder stones may appear further cranial and more lateral than expected
   c. Pneumocystography may help to differentiate eggs in the bladder from eggs in the reproductive tract (see *Reproductive Disorders*).

Pneumocystography in larger chelonia

1. Catheterize the urethra.
2. Flush out the bladder contents.
3. Infuse 10–20 mL/kg of air (stop if resistance encountered).
4. 2–5 mL of iohexol to produce a double contrast pneumocystogram.

(Hernandez-Divers & Hernandez-Divers 2001)

Intravenous urography

1. Fast chelonian for 2–3 days.
2. Maintain at 30°C.
3. Place i.v. catheter into right jugular vein.
4. Use suitable urography medium – inject 800–1200 mg iodine into the jugular vein.
5. Lateral and DV radiographs taken at 0, 1, 3, 5, 15, 30 and 60 min.
6. As an adjunct, inject medium into dorsal coccygeal tail vein. Radiographs taken after 30 s.

(Hernandez-Divers & Hernandez-Divers 2001)

2. Routine haematology and biochemistry
   a. Blood uric acid levels, urea, creatinine, calcium and phosphorus
3. Urinalysis including cytology
   a. Renal casts
   b. Inflammatory cells
   c. Centrifuged urine (supernatant)
4. Detectable levels of AP, AST, ALT, urea, calcium, CK, creatinine, glucose, LDH, magnesium, ammonia, phosphorus, total bilirubin total protein and uric acid
5. Parameters raised with renal disease: AST, urea, calcium, CK, creatinine, glucose, LDH, ammonia and phosphorus. Uric acid may be significantly raised or lowered than normal (Koelle & Hoffman 2002)
6. Culture and sensitivity
7. Endoscopy
8. Biopsy/necropsy
9. Ultrasonography.

Management

● Fluid therapy (see *Nursing Care*).

Treatment/specific therapy

● Bacterial pyelonephritis and cystitis
  ● Appropriate antibiosis
● Fungal pyelonephritis and cystitis
  ● Appropriate mycosis (see *Respiratory Tract Disorders*)
● Myxozoans
  ● No effective treatment
● Flukes
  ● Probably non-pathogenic
  ● Praziquantel at 10 mg/kg
● Hexamitiasis
  ● Cause of renal tubular damage
  ● Metronidazole
    ● 100–257 mg/kg body weight. Repeat after 2 weeks if necessary
    ● 20 mg/kg e.o.d. until eradicated
  ● Dimetridazole at 40 mg/kg p.o. for 5 days
● Gout
  ● Fluid therapy
  ● Allopurinol at 10 mg/kg s.i.d. *Note* that this will only prevent subsequent uric acid deposition
  ● Very guarded prognosis
● Uroliths/bladder calculi
  ● Adults – surgical cystotomy; note that the chelonian bladder is very thin and difficulty can be experienced during closure. One method is by marsupialization of bladder to body wall at inguinal fossa
  ● Hatchling/small chelonia. Success can be achieved by long-term treatment with allopurinol at 10 mg/kg s.i.d. indefinitely; this helps prevent enlargement of the stone such that in time the growing chelonian may be able to pass the calculus.

Endocrine disorders

Thyroid activity in chelonia can be affected by temperature; low temperatures (10°C for 15 days) inhibit thyroid activity while high temperatures (32–34°C) stimulate thyroid activity in soft-shelled turtle *Lissemys punctata punctata* (Sengupta et al 2003).

Nutritional

- Thymic hyperplasia (goitre associated with iodine deficiency).

Neoplasia

- Multicentric lymphoblastic lymphoma (thyroid).

Other non-infectious problems

- Thymic hyperplasia (not diet related; possibly antigenic stimulation)
- Diabetes mellitus.

Findings on clinical examination

- Marked swelling ventral neck (goitre)
- Polydipsia, polyuria, inappetence (diabetes mellitus).

Investigations

1. Radiography
2. Routine haematology and biochemistry
   a. Hyperglycaemia, normal renal parameters (diabetes mellitus) (differentiate from stress hyperglycaemia)
   b. Serum insulin
   c. Serum glucagon (may be more important in glucose regulation than insulin)
   d. Serum thyroxine levels (consider sampling conspecifics to establish normal ranges)
   e. Normal $T3_{(total)}$ <0.0154 nmol/L
   f. Normal $T4_{(total)}$ = 0.05–0.1 nmol/L
   g. However, Hulbert (2000) cites $T4_{(total)}$ values for growing red eared sliders *Trachemys scripta* of 80–145.0 nM/L
   h. *Note* that thymic hyperplasia can occur with normal T3 and T4 levels (Fleming et al 2004)
3. Culture and sensitivity
4. Endoscopy
5. Biopsy/necropsy
6. Ultrasonography.

Treatment/specific therapy

- Thymic hyperplasia (nutritional)
  - Supplement with iodine
  - Sodium or potassium iodide solution at 0.25–0.5 mg/kg i.v. or p.o. every 7 days
  - Lugols iodine solution at 0.5–2.0 mg/kg p.o. every 7 days

- Other dietary supplements high in iodine include kelp tablets
- Usually associated with feeding high volumes of Brassicas (cabbage family), which contain goitrogens which antagonize thyroid function
- Volcanic island herbivores, e.g. Galapagos tortoises especially predisposed
- Thymic hyperplasia (non-nutritional)
  - Investigate other, non-nutritional, causes
- Diabetes mellitus
  - Rare but very guarded prognosis
  - Commercial insulin unlikely to work – reptilian insulin is different to mammalian
  - Attempt feeding high-fibre, low-carbohydrate diet to allow natural modulation of glucose uptake.

Hibernation associated disorders

Many species of chelonia undergo a seasonal period of dormancy. Typically this is a period of hibernation (brumation) to survive times of low temperatures and poor food resources, but occasionally it may be to survive times of high temperatures or drought (aestivation).

Commonly kept species suitable for hibernation

1. Mediterranean species that are safe to hibernate include *Testudo ibera*, *T. whitei*, *T. marginata*, *T. hermanii* and *T. horsfieldi*. Of the *T. g. graeca* group the Moroccan and Algerian races are safe to hibernate
2. North American gopher tortoise *Gopherus agassizi*
3. Northern populations of the ornate box turtle (*Terrapene ornata*) and eastern box turtle (*T. carolina*)
4. Some populations of Bell's hinge-back tortoise (*Kinixys belliana*) will aestivate during periods of drought
5. Painted terrapins (Chrysemys spp) and some sliders (*Trachemys spp*), e.g. red-eared sliders (*T. scripta elegans*).

Commonly kept species that should not be hibernated

1. Mediterranean species: Egyptian tortoise (*Testudo kleinmanni*) and the Tunisian tortoise (*T nabulensis.*). The Libyan race of *T. g. graeca* should either not be hibernated, or only allowed to do so for a relatively short time, such as 6–8 weeks
2. Indian star tortoise (*Geochelone elegans*), red-foot tortoise (*G. carbonaria*), yellow-foot tortoise (*G. denticulata*), leopard tortoise (*G. pardalis*) and African spur-thigh tortoise (*G. sulcata*)
3. Serrated hinged-back tortoise (*Kinixys erosa*) and Homes' hinge-backed tortoise (*K. homeana*)
4. Vietnamese leaf turtle (*Geoemyda spengleri*)
5. Keeled box turtle (*Pyxidea mouhoti*).

Hibernation triggered by environmental stimuli

1. Reducing ambient temperatures
2. Reducing photoperiod
3. Reducing light intensity.

Testudo spp during hibernation lose around 0.2–0.4 g/day so expect a loss of around 1% of body weight per month. Water is lost via respiration, so PCV rises from 0.28–0.29 L/L to 0.34–0.38 L/L while urea levels rise from <10 mmol/L to <103 mmol/L.

The ideal temperature for hibernation is around 5–6°C, while re-emergence is initiated by temperatures rising consistently above 10°C. At this time, there is a major rise in blood glucose from liver glycogen stores to fuel initial foraging. *Testudo spp* will eat when blood glucose is at least 3.2 mmol/L. As a general rule, a post-hibernational tortoise:

1. Must drink or absorb water across the cloacal lining within 10 days to produce a reduction in blood urea levels and PCV
2. Must eat within 3–4 weeks.

Post-hibernational anorexia

Typically, this is due to inadequate preparation the previous summer and autumn, with poor/inappropriate nutrition, but it can also be due to unsuitable hibernation facilities or concurrent disease, e.g. stomatitis, CHV. Such tortoises will have utilized entire fat reserves, exhausted fat-soluble vitamins supplies and are forced to breakdown muscle and other tissues as a protein source to provide an alternative energy and amino acid source.

Findings on clinical examination

- Cataracts and vitreal haze (see *Ophthalmic Disorders*)
- Frost-bite
  - Covering antibiotics
  - Application of a topical amorphous hydrogel dressing, e.g. IntraSite Gel (Smith and Nephew Healthcare Ltd.) topically to lesions
  - Systemic NSAIDs, e.g. meloxicam.

Investigation

1. Radiography
2. Routine haematology and biochemistry
   a. As minimum assess PCV, glucose and urea
      Note that LDH and CK levels are likely to be naturally higher in hibernating chelonia (see Birkedal & Gesser 2004)
3. Culture and sensitivity
4. Endoscopy
5. Ultrasonography
6. Assessment of hibernation environment.

Treatment

- Fluid therapy (see *Nursing Care*)
- Vitamin supplementation
- Feeding by stomach tube or via pharyngostomy tube. Supplement with probiotics

- Hospitalize in vivarium: summer temperatures (preferred body temperature for *Testudo spp* is around 30°C) and 12–14 h of full-spectrum lighting
- Treat any concurrent disease

Note that treatment can be prolonged

Reproductive disorders

Nutritional

- Poor plane of nutrition
- Hypocalcaemia (see *Musculoskeletal Disorders*).

Neoplasia

- Obstructive dystocia.

Other non-infectious problems

- Fractured egg
- Egg yolk serositis
- Dystocia
  - Preovulatory ovarian stasis (POOS)
  - Egg stasis (post-ovulatory)
- Egg retention in the urinary bladder
- Prolapse of the phallus.

Findings on clinical examination

- Restlessness – may be extreme
- Digging
- Abnormally low clutch of eggs
- Anorexia
- Depression
- Egg may be palpable on cloacal examination
- Swollen reddish or grayish structure hanging from the vent (prolapsed phallus – differentiate from cloacal prolapse) (Fig. 9.10).

Investigations

1. Radiography
   a. Post-ovulatory eggs are heavily shelled and are readily demonstrable on radiography
   b. Radiography of dystocic chelonia allows:
      i. Assessment of total number of eggs present
      ii. Any abnormal or fractured eggs
      iii. Any egg-pelvic disproportion
      iv. Presence of eggs in the bladder (occasionally following attempted oxytocin induction). These eggs typically have thick, uneven walls due to uric acid deposition
      v. Some underlying causes, e.g. MBD (active or historical), bladder calculi or foreign bodies that may be causing an obstruction
2. Cytology – coelomic tap (yolk serositis)

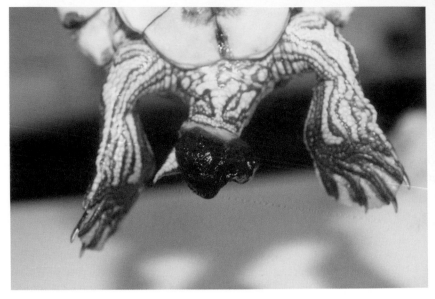

Fig. 9.10. Prolapsed phallus in a red-eared slider.

3. Routine haematology and biochemistry
4. Culture and sensitivity
5. Endoscopy
6. Biopsy/necropsy
7. Ultrasonography
   a. Place probe into inguinal fossa to pick up ova in preovulatory ovarian stasis
   b. Eggs in the bladder.

Treatment/specific therapy

- Dystocia
  - Provision of correct environment including appropriate temperature, humidity and nesting chamber may induce normal egg-laying. Supplement with calcium, e.g. calcium gluconate at 1 mL/kg p.o. b.i.d.
  - May be linked with stress
  - Medical induction
    - Calcium at 100 mg/kg every 6–12 h
    - 1–10 IU/kg oxytocin given 1 h after last calcium. Unlike in snakes there appears to be a wide 'window' of many weeks where oxytocin is effective for induction
    - Repeat over 2–3 cycles if the reptile is otherwise healthy
    - If some eggs still retained after 48 h, consider surgery
    - Argipressin at 0.01–1.0 µg/kg (more potent than oxytocin in reptiles)
  - Salpingotomy
  - Plastral coeliotomy

- Pre-femoral coeliotomy
  - Ovariosalpingectomy (as for *salpingotomy*)
- Egg retention in the urinary bladder
  - Cystotomy: temporary marsupialization of the bladder via the inguinal fossa
- Fractured egg
  - Risk of egg yolk serositis and trauma from sharp shell fragments
  - Consider either endoscopic or surgical retrieval
- Egg yolk serositis.
  - Coeliotomy followed by extensive lavage and removal of any egg fragments; surgical repair of oviduct or salpingectomy if necessary
- Prolapsed phallus
  - If fresh and relatively non-traumatized, replace and retain with a purse-string suture
  - If badly damaged or if purse-string unsuccessful consider resection. This will only interfere with reproduction, not with urination.

Paediatric and neonatal disorders

Bacterial

- Systemic infections.

Fungal

Protozoal

Parasitic

- Nematodes (see *Gastrointestinal Tract Disorders*).

Nutritional

- Metabolic bone disease
- Uroliths (Fig. 9.11).

Other non-infectious problems

- Prolapse of the umbilicus
- Congenital abnormalities.

Findings on clinical examination

- Lethargy
- Loss of appetite
- Cryptic behaviour (hiding)
- Bulging of tissue at the umbilicus of new born or newly hatched chelonia. Bulge may contain coelomic lining, yolk sac remnant and coelomic fat
- Oedema.

Investigations

1. Radiography
2. Routine haematology and biochemistry
   a. Serum calcium and ionized calcium

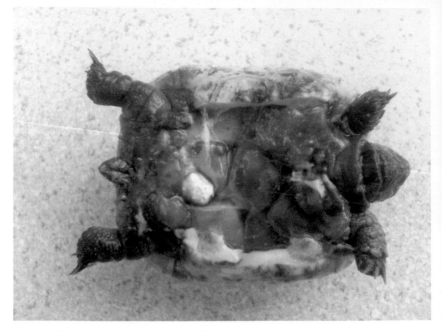

Fig. 9.11. Bladder urolith in a hatchling spur-thighed tortoise (plastron removed).

3. Culture and sensitivity
4. Endoscopy
5. Biopsy/necropsy
6. Ultrasonography.

Treatment/specific therapy

- Systemic infections
  - Difficult to diagnose in hatchlings as small size precludes adequate sampling
  - Covering antibiosis often gives a good clinical response
- Metabolic bone disease – see *Musculoskeletal Disorders*
    Note that hatchling chelonia are naturally soft and somewhat flexible
  - MBD is often accompanied by hypovitaminosis A (especially semi-aquatic chelonia) and other signs of disease, e.g. anorexia, lethargy
  - May be delayed if calcium status of female was good; signs only once calcium reserves utilized
  - If very early onset may be due to poor calcification of egg, a reflection of poor calcium status of the mother
- Prolapsed umbilicus
  - Clean and replace prolapse. Suture in place
  - May require surgical resection of yolk sac remnant
  - This is particularly prevalent in hatchlings with incomplete yolk sac resorption, where the yolk sac membranes adhere to dry surfaces or to the inside of the shell

(especially if the humidity is too low). Keep hatchlings with pronounced egg sacs in moist, clean surroundings until resorption takes place. Do not attempt to separate the hatchling from the egg but increase humidity and/or remove the hatchling plus egg to a warm, humid environment to allow natural separation

- Oedema
  - Occasionally seen in hatchling *Testudo spp*
  - Swollen body
  - Soft shell
  - On postmortem the carcass is oedematous; uroliths may be present
  - Unknown aetiology
- Uroliths
  - See *Urinary Disorders* for treatment
  - Can occur individually or in groups
  - May be linked to poor environmental conditions, e.g. marginal chronic dehydration
  - In some cases hatchlings may have inherited susceptibility (clutch mates under different husbandry regimes developed uroliths (personal observation)).

Husbandry related disorders

- Water quality
  - Poor water quality, especially high ammonia levels, can cause skin and ophthalmic disorders and mortalities in young semi-aquatic chelonia. (See *Freshwater Tropical Fish* for details on Management.)
- Metabolic bone disease (see *Musculoskeletal Disorders*)
- Post-hibernational anorexia (see *Hibernation Associated Disorders*).

References

Acierno M J, Mitchell M A, Roundtree M K et al 2006 Effects of ultraviolet radiation on 25-hydroxyvitamin D3 synthesis in red-eared slider turtles (Trachemys scripta elegans). Am J Vet Res 67:2046–2049

Birkedal R, Gesser H 2004 Effects of hibernation on mitochondrial regulation and metabolic capacities in myocardium of painted turtle (Chrysemys picta). Comp Biochem Physiol 139(Part A):285–291

Burridge M J, Peter T F, Allan S A et al 2002 Evaluation of safety and efficacy of acaricides for control of the African tortoise tick (Amblyomma marmoreum) on leopard tortoises (Geochelone pardalis) J Zoo Wildl Med 33:52–57

Chitty J R 2003 Lead toxicosis in a Greek tortoise (Testudo graeca). Proc Assoc Reptil Amphib Vet 101:16

Cutler S L 2004. Nematode-associated Aural Abscess in a Mediterranean Tortoise, Testudo graeca. J Herp Med and Surg 14(3):4–5

Divers S J, Lawton M P C, Stoakes L C 1999 Anthelminthic treatment of Chelonians. Vet Rec Nov 20:620

Drury S E N, Gough R E, McArthur S et al 1998 Detection of herpesvirus-like and papilloma-like particles associated with diseases of tortoises. Vet Rec 143:639

Fleming G J, Heard D J, Uhl E W et al 2004 Thymic hyperplasia in subadult Galapagos tortoises, Geochelone nigra. J Rept Med Surg 14(1):24–27

Frye F L, Williams D L 1995 Self-assessment colour review of reptiles and amphibians. Manson, London, p 30

Garner M M, Raiti P, Bartholomew J L et al 2003 Renal myxozoanosis in two crowned river turtles (Hardella thurjii, Emydidae). Proc Assoc Reptil Amphib Vet 93–95

González Candela M, Martín Atance P, Seva J et al 2005 Granulomatous hepatitis caused by Salmonella typhimurium in a spur-thighed tortoise (Testudo graeca). Vet Rec 157:236–237

Hernandez-Divers S J 2006 Single-dose oral and intravenous pharmacokinetics of meloxicam in the green iguana (Iguana iguana). Br Vet Zoo Soc Proc, May

Hernandez-Divers S, Hernandez-Divers S 2001 Diagnostic imaging of reptiles. In Practice 23:370–391

Holz R M, Holz P 1995 Electrocardiography in anaesthetised red-eared sliders (Trachemys scripta elegans). Res Vet Sci 58:67–69

Homer B L, Li C, Berry K H et al 2001 Soluble scute proteins of healthy and ill desert tortoises (Gopherus agassizii) Am J Vet Res 62(1):104–110

Hulbert A J 2000 Thyroid hormones and their effects: a new perspective. Biol Rev 75:519–631

Innis C J, Garner M, Tabaka C et al 2003 Clinical and histopathology findings in Sulawesi tortoises (Indotestudo forstenni) with necrotizing sinusitis and rhinitis. Proc ARAV

Jacobson E R, Schumacher J, Telford S R Jr et al 1994 Intranuclear coccidiosis in radiated tortoises (Geochelone radiata). J Zoo Wildl Med 25(1):95–102

Kelly T R, Walton W, Nadelstein B et al 2005 Phacoemulsification of bilateral cataracts in a loggerhead sea turtle (Caretta caretta). Vet Rec 156:774–777

Koelle P, Hoffman R 2002 Urinalysis in European tortoises. Part II. Proc Assoc Rept Amphib Vet 115–117

Lafortune M, Wellehan J F X, Terrell S P et al 2005 Shell and systemic Hyalohyphomycosis in Fly River turtles, Carettochelys insculpta, caused by Paecilomyces lilacinus. J Herp Med Surg 15(2):15–19

Marshang R E, Ruemenapf T H 2002 Virus 'X'; characterizing a new viral pathogen in tortoises. Proc ARAV

Mehlhorn H, Schmahl G, Frese M et al 2005 Effects of a combination of emodepside and praziquantel on parasites of reptiles and rodents. Parasitol Res 97:S64–S69

Meyer J 1998 Gastrografin as a gastrointestinal contrast agent in the Greek tortoise (Testudo hermanni). J Zoo Wildl Med 29(2):183–189

Nicasio J, Campillo B, Frye F L 2002 Preliminary report of subepidermal mite infestation in an African Spurred tortoise, Geochelone sulcata. Proc ARAV 17

Philbey A W 2006 Amoebic enterocolitis and acute myonecrosis in leopard tortoises (Geochelone pardalis). Vet Rec 158:567–569

Philbey A W, Lawrie A M, Taylor D J et al 2006 Lower urinary tract obstruction in a Mediterranean spur-thighed tortoise (Testudo graeca) with coxofemoral arthritis). Vet Rec 159:492–495

Pizzi R, Goodman G, Gunn-Moore D et al 2005 Pieris japonica intoxication in an African spurred tortoise (Geochelone sulcata). Vet Rec 156:487–488

Redrobe S P, Scudamore C L 2000 Ultrasonographic diagnosis of pericardial effusion and atrial dilation in a spur-thighed tortoise (Testudo graeca). Vet Rec 146:183–185

Rose F L, Koke J, Koehn R 2001 Identification of the aetiological agent for necrotizing scute disease in the Texas tortoise. J Wildl Dis 37:223–228

Sales M J, Ferrer D, Castellà J et al 2003 Myiasis in two Hermann's tortoises (Testudo hermanni). Vet Rec 153:600–601

Sengupta A, Ray P P, Chaudri-Sengupta S et al 2003 Thyroidal modulation following hypo- and hyperthermia in the soft-shelled turtle Lissemys punctata punctata Bonnoterre. Eur J Morphol 41(5):149–154

Soldati G, Lu Z H, Vaughan L et al 2004 Detection of mycobacteria and Chlamydiae in granulomatous inflammation of reptiles: A retrospective study. Vet Pathol 41:388–397

Taylor S K, Citino S B, Zdziarski J M et al 1996 Radiographic anatomy and barium sulphate transit time of the gastrointestinal tract of the leopard tortoise (Testudo pardalis). J Zoo Wildl Med 27(2):180–186

Werner R E 2003 Parasites in the Diamondback terrapin, Malaclemys terrapin: A review. J Herp Med and Surg 13(4):5–9

Willer C J, Lewbart G A, Lemons C 2003 Aural abscesses in Wild eastern Box turtles, (Terrapene carolina Carolina), from North Carolina: Aerobic Bacterial Isolates and distribution of Lesions. J Herp Med Surg 13(2):4–9

10

Amphibians

• •

Amphibians are a popular group of pets amongst herpetologists and some aquarists. Popular species include a number of Anurids (frogs and toads) and some Urodeles (salamanders and newts).

Table 10.1 Popular species of amphibians: Key facts

Species	Notes	Common disorders
Horned frogs (*Ceratophrys spp*)	From South America, these sit-and-wait predatory frogs grow large and have a strong bite	Aeromonas infections, gout, corneal lipidosis
Poison-arrow frogs (*Dendrobates spp*)	South American. Skin toxins are based on plant alkaloids ingested by native prey insects. Captive bred and long-term captives usually safe to handle with appropriate precautions	Bacterial and fungal infections
White's tree frogs *Littoria caerulea*	A large Australian tree frog requiring high temperatures (26–32°C daytime; 20–24°C nighttime) and a comparatively low humidity (50–60%)	Bacterial and fungal infections
African clawed toad *Xenopus laevis* (in both wild and albino forms)	Totally aquatic. Extremely popular	Bacterial and fungal infections. Poor water quality
Axolotl *Ambystoma mexicanum*	A neotenous salamander originating from Mexico. Keep cool (15–20°C)	Poor water quality, ingestion of foreign bodies, bite injuries from other axolotls
Caecilians, such as *Typhlonectes compressicauda*	These aquatic and moist subterranean worm-like amphibia are occasionally available in aquarium outlets	Fungal skin infections, poor water quality

Consultation and handling

Handle amphibians with damp hands and/or smooth latex gloves to protect the delicate skin and mucous covering. Amphibia can be very unpredictable and are excellent at leaping from the unsuspecting grasp of the veterinarian, therefore beware of potentially traumatic falls to the floor. Wrapping them in very damp, thin paper towels enables some control; areas of interest are accessed by gently tearing through the paper.

Large frogs such as horned frogs (*Ceratophrys spp*) and African giant frogs (*Pyxicephalus adspersus*) can inflict a painful bite and are likely to do so. Handle these by gently grasping them around the waist. Large marine toads (*Bufo marinus*) may eject toxins from their parotid glands if severely stressed. Wild-caught poison-arrow frogs can produce potentially very toxic skin secretions which are manufactured from prey; captive-bred frogs usually do not produce such toxins but caution is advised.

Most amphibia have very thin, moist skins, which allow significant absorption of topical medications. This should be borne in mind if using topical preparations designed for mammalian species but these can be used advantageously, as therapeutic levels of active medications may be able to be achieved following topical application of injectable drugs, e.g. antibiotics.

Nursing care

Provide appropriate environment including provision of:
1. Optimal temperature (basking lights where appropriate, heat mats etc. to allow thermoregulation). Use of max–min thermometers will assist in monitoring temperature ranges to which incumbent amphibia are exposed
2. Full-spectrum lighting appears to be relatively unimportant for the majority of amphibia; if in doubt, use a light with a minimal (2%) UV output
3. Humidity is crucially important. A relative humidity of 80% or higher is generally recommended
4. Ventilation. Important, but may need to be sacrificed somewhat to maintain high humidity levels
5. Easily cleaned accommodation; use paper substrate and disposable/sterilizable hides and other vivarium furniture
6. Keep individually to minimize intra-specific stress and competition for resources.

Fluid therapy

Dehydrated amphibians show increased tackiness of the skin mucous covering, tightening of the skin, sunken eyes and weight loss. Dehydration can also affect cutaneous gaseous exchange leading to hypercapnia and acidosis.

Dehydrated terrestrial amphibia should be placed in a shallow bath of clean, dechlorinated and well-oxygenated water.

Fluid therapy for amphibia

1. Intracoelomic fluids should be slightly hypotonic:
   a. 1:2 sodium chloride 0.9%:glucose 5%
   b. 1:2 Hartmann's solution:glucose 5%
   c. 9:1 saline:sterile water (Wright 1995).
2. Do not exceed 25 mL/kg as an initial dose.

Nutritional support

Offer commercially available live food if possible. If anorexic:
1. Place whole prey items into mouth
2. Consider use of stomach tube; initially use commercially available 'critical care' products for reptiles (usually containing amino-acids, vitamins and electrolytes) and graduate to available high-energy formulations available for domestic dogs and cats.

Analgesia

Morphine. Intracoelomic at 10–100 mg/kg in frogs.

Anaesthesia

Terrestrial amphibians have several respiratory surfaces, which can complicate the control of anaesthesia. These include the lungs, skin and buccal lining. Aquatic amphibia respire largely through gills.

When inducing terrestrial amphibia in a water bath always guard against the possibility of drowning. Once anaesthetized, large amphibia can be intubated and maintained as for reptiles with isoflurane, but maintenance can be difficult due to alternative respiratory surfaces.

Transcutaneous anaesthetic techniques in amphibians

1. Isoflurane at 4–5% bubbled into water and administered according to the amphibian's response, *or* place animal in damp towels in induction chamber.
2. Mix 3.0 mL of liquid isoflurane + 1.5 mL of water + 3.5 mL KY jelly:
   a. Apply this mixture to animal's dorsum at roughly 0.025–0.035 mL/g body weight depending on species. Use a lower dose for frogs and newts, higher for toads.
   b. Once the solution has been applied, place the animal in a small sealed container until induction has occurred (around 5–15 min). When righting and withdrawal reflexes lost, wipe the dermis free of anaesthetic. Should give 45–80 min of surgical time.
3. Fish anaesthetics can be used, such as MS222 (see *Goldfish and Koi*).

Parenteral anaesthesia for amphibians

Propofol at 10 mg/kg i.v. in all large species; for salamanders use ventral tail vein, for frogs and toads use abdominal vein or heart or at 25–35 mg/kg intracoelomically (tiger salamander).

Skin disorders

The amphibian skin is thin and covered with a layer of mucous, which acts as an anti-bacterial and antifungal barrier. It is highly porous to medications and toxins; many treatments can be administered topically to achieve systemic effects. Normal flora are G −ve, such as *Aeromonas spp*, *Pseudomonas spp*, *Proteus spp* and *E. coli*. However, these can also be pathogenic and so results may require a degree of interpretation.

Hypovitaminosis A may contribute to secondary skin infections, e.g. chytridiomy-cosis, possibly by reducing cutaneous mucous production (see also 'Hypovitaminosis A', in *Gastrointestinal Disorders*).

Pruritus

* Trombiculid mites (terrestrial forms)
* Poor water quality, especially high ammonia levels, can cause skin irritation in both adults and tadpoles
* Environmental tobacco smoke.

Erosions and ulceration

* Traumatic wounds, e.g. bites
* Bacterial (see also 'Changes in pigmentation', below)
* Iridovirus (ranavirus including ranavirus III; see *Systemic Disorders*)
* Mycobacteriosis
* Cutaneous capillariasis: *Pseudocapillaroides xenopi* (African clawed toads)
* Fungal infections include *Batrachochytrium dendrobatidis* (chytridiomycosis) and *Basidiobolus ranarum*
* Microsporidia
* Trombiculids in terrestrial amphibia (erythematous vesicles).

Nodules and non-healing wounds

* Trematodes (*Clinostomum attenuatum*).

Changes in pigmentation

* Erythema and ulceration ('red leg')
* Environmental pathogens (*Aeromonas spp*, *Pseudomonas spp*)
* Environmental irritants
* Iridovirus (ranavirus)
* Chlamydophila in *Xenopus laevis*
* Chromomycosis
* *Saprolegnia* (aquatic amphibia). Cotton-wool-like growth on the skin
* Trombiculids in terrestrial amphibia (erythematous vesicles)

- Whitish patches on caecilians (fungal infection, water too hard, poor water quality)
- Environmental toxins (see also *Systemic Disorders*)
- Chlorhexidine
- Povidone iodine
- Chlorine
- Quaternary ammonium compounds
- Ammonium.

Ectoparasites

- Aquatic adult and larval amphibians
- *Oodinium pillularis*
- Ciliated protozoa
- Crustacea
- Argulus (large, disc-shaped crustacean)
- Copepods
- Leeches
- Trombiculids
- *Bufolucilia spp* (toadfly) (see *Respiratory Disorders*).

Neoplasia

- Haemangioma.

Findings on clinical examination

- Inflammation and ulceration (see 'Erosions and ulceration' and 'Changes in pigmentation', above). Septicaemic infections may be accompanied by systemic signs such as inappetence, lethargy, convulsions, swelling of the body (either with fluid or gas) and obvious eye abnormalities
- Wasting (often despite an apparently good appetite), ulceration, swellings either at the skin or deeper (Mycobacteriosis).
- Greying of the skin (excess mucous production) over the skin and gills. Respiratory impairment. Debilitation and death (Ectoparasites, including *Oodinium pillularis*)
- Dark, raised nodules in the skin, debilitation and weight loss (Chromomycosis – see also *Systemic Disorders*)
- Skin sloughing, splayed leg (chytridiomycosis)
- Inactivity
- Anorexia
- Damage and deformity to the head, especially the nares, in toads (*Bufolucilia*)
- Raised mass (granuloma, neoplasia).

Investigations

1. Skin scrapings
   a. *Oodinium:* can be quite large, up to 1.0 mm diameter, oval shaped with a very dark appearance because of chloroplasts. Not usually mobile
   b. *Pseudocapillaroides xenopi*: eggs and worms visible
   c. Copepods
   d. Trombiculid mites
2. Radiography

3. Routine haematology and biochemistry
4. Culture and sensitivity
5. Endoscopy
6. Biopsy/necropsy
7. Ultrasonography.
8. Water quality testing.

Management

1. Fluid therapy – see *Nursing Care*
2. Wound management
   a. Debride and clean by flushing with sterile saline
   b. Iodine compounds and chlorhexidine are potentially toxic
   c. Wounds (and haemostasis achieved) should be sealed either by suturing or with cyanoacrylate.

Treatment/specific therapy

- Trauma – see 'Wound management', above
- *Aeromonas* and *Pseudomonas*
  - Appropriate antibiosis
  - Often secondary to immunocompromise from poor environmental conditions, e.g. inappropriate temperature, poor nutrition
- *Chlamydophila*
  - Appropriate antibiosis, e.g. doxycycline at 10–50 mg/kg p.o. s.i.d.
- Mycobacteriosis
  - Treatment is rarely effective and so euthanasia should be considered
- *Saprolegnia*
  - Removing visible hyphae by swabbing the affected area with a 10% povidone-iodine solution s.i.d.
  - Salt water baths (10–25 mg sea salt per litre) s.i.d. for 10–30 min
  - Often secondary to poor water quality and high biological contamination of water
- *Basidiobolus ranarum*
  - Benkalkonium chloride dips, at 2 mg/100 mL water for 30 min every 48 h for 3 treatments
- Chromomycosis
  - No effective treatment. Consider euthanasia
- Chytridiomycosis
  - Larval stages lack keratinized skin so less susceptible to infection, so heavy mortalities may follow metamorphosis (post metamorphic death syndrome, PMDS). Can be carried on mouthparts of larvae
  - Very virulent; consider euthanasia
  - Some cases respond to itraconazole baths. Create 0.01% itraconazole solution (dilute a 10 mg/mL itraconazole suspension in 0.6% saline) and undertake 5 min baths in this solution daily for 11 days
    Note that chlorhexidine is potentially toxic to amphibia
- *Oodinium* and ciliated protozoa.
  - Try a proprietary *Oodinium* (velvet) treatment formulated for aquarium fish

- Metronidazole at 10–14 mg/L for up to 24 h daily for 10 days
- Quinine hydrochloride at 10–20 mg/L indefinitely. Some amphibia may be sensitive to this
- The encysted stage is relatively resistant to chemical attack
- Antibiotic cover should be considered, as secondary infections are common at the areas where the skin is damaged
- Eliminate the parasite from a show aquarium by removing all amphibians (and fish), reducing or cutting out the light levels and raising the temperature to 30–32°C for 3 weeks
- *Microsporidia*
  - Chloramphenicol sodium succinate (5–10 mg/kg intracoelomic) plus topical oxytetracycline and polymyxin B s.i.d.
- *Pseudocapillaroides xenopi*
  - Fenbendazole at 50–100 mg/kg p.o.
  - Thiabendazole at 50–100 mg/kg p.o.
  - Levamisole (100–300 mg/L) bath for 1 h once weekly for up to 12 weeks
- Leeches
  - Individual removal
- Copepods
  - Hypertonic bath (10–25 g NaCl (not table salt)) for 5–30 min
  - Treat with lufenuron at 0.088 mg/L as a single dose
- *Argulus* (Fish louse)
  - Individual removal of parasites
  - Treat with lufenuron at 0.088 mg/L as a single dose.
  - A potassium permanganate bath at 10 p.p.m. (mg/L) for 5–60 min can be used to rid both individual amphibia and plants of this parasite
- Trombiculids
  - Physical removal of mites with damp cotton-bud
  - Topical ivermectin: Dilute 1:50 in Hartman's solution and apply topically to dorsal surface
- *Bufolucilia* (toadfly)
  - Physical removal of parasites if possible
  - Flush the nares and oropharynx with ivermectin or levamisole
  - Covering antibiosis.

Respiratory tract disorders

Amphibians respire through a variety of organs – namely the lungs, buccopharyngeal lining, skin and gills (larval amphibia). In terrestrial amphibia dehydration may affect gaseous exchange at the skin leading to hypercapnia and acidosis.

Bacterial

- Pneumonia.

Fungal

- Pneumonia.

Protozoal

- Oodinium and other aquatic protozoa (larval amphibian, see *Respiratory Disorders* in *Tropical Freshwater Fish*).

Parasitic

- *Rhabdias spp*
- Trematodes (wide variety – see *Systemic Disorders*).

Neoplasia

Other non-infectious problems

- Acute pulmonary emphysema
- Poor water quality, especially larval amphibians. High ammonia and nitrite levels may predispose to gill damage and secondary bacterial and fungal infections.

Findings on clinical examination

- Increased respiratory rate (especially larval amphibia)
- Open mouthed breathing
- 'Wet' or unusual respiratory noises
- Discharge around the glottis or inside the proximal trachea
- Occluded nostrils
- Sudden death.

Investigations

1. Microscopy
2. Faecal examination
3. Embryonated eggs or rhabditiform larvae (*Rhabdias spp*)
4. Transillumination of very small or transparent amphibia
   a. May see large adult worms in lungs
5. Radiography
6. Routine haematology and biochemistry
7. Culture and sensitivity
8. Endoscopy
9. Biopsy
10. Ultrasonography
11. Water-quality testing.

Management

1. For aquatic amphibia, transfer to a shallow container and increase aeration to maximally oxygenate water
2. For terrestrial amphibia, transfer to a high oxygen environment. *Note* that high air flow rates may increase the risk of dehydration from moisture loss across the skin.

Treatment/specific therapy

- Pneumonia
- Appropriate antimicrobials
- *Oodinium*

- Proprietary fish treatments
- Metronidazole at 50 mg/L for up to 24 h daily for 10 days
- Quinine hydrochloride at 10–20 mg/L indefinitely. Some amphibia may be sensitive
- The encysted stage is relatively resistant to chemical attack
- Can colonize the intestines of fish and possibly larval amphibia, where again it can be protected from medications
- Antibiotic cover should be considered as secondary infections are common at the areas where the skin is damaged
- Eliminate the parasite from a show vivaria/aquaria by removing all amphibia, reducing or cutting out the light levels and raising the temperature to 30–32°C for 3 weeks
- Rhabdias
  - Ivermectin
    - Dilute 1:50 in Hartman's solution and apply topically to dorsal surface
    - 10 g/L bath for 1 h weekly for up to 12 weeks
  - Levamisole (100–300 mg/L) bath for 1 h once weekly for up to 12 weeks
  - Fenbendazole at 50–100 mg/kg p.o.
- Acute pulmonary emphysema
  - Repetitive aspiration of coelomic air until pulmonary lesion seals
  - Covering antibiosis.

Gastrointestinal tract disorders

Bacterial

- Enteritis (rarely encountered).

Fungal

- Enteritis (rarely encountered).

Protozoal

- *Entamoeba ranarum*
- Ciliates.

Parasitic

- *Strongyloides spp*
- A variety of nematode species may be detected
- Acanthocephalans
- Cestodes (wide variety – see *Systemic Disorders*)
- Trematodes (wide variety – see *Systemic Disorders*).

Nutritional

- Short-tongue syndrome of frogs (suspected hypovitaminosis A).

Neoplasia

- Myxoma (esp. tree frogs).

Other non-infectious problems

- Gastric impaction (esp. large frogs, e.g. horned frogs *Ceratophrys spp*). May be the result of gastric overload, i.e. offered too large food item
- Gastric prolapse
- Intestinal foreign body
- Cloacal prolapse (especially tree frogs).

Findings on clinical examination

- Diarrhoea, blood in faeces, wasting, loss of appetite (*Entamoeba*)
- Firm swelling from lining of oral cavity; if large can affect frog's ability to feed (myxoma)
- Inability to catch prey
- Weight loss
- Swollen, often gassy coelom (gastric impaction)
- Anorexia
- Inactivity
- Cloacal prolapse (intestinal parasitism, enteritis, toxins).

Investigations

1. Faecal examination
   a. Entamoeba: multinucleate cysts; nuclear endosomes measure up to nucleus diameter
   b. Ciliated protozoa
2. Radiography
3. Routine haematology and biochemistry
4. Culture and sensitivity
5. Endoscopy
6. Biopsy/necropsy
   a. Squamous metaplasia of the mucous-secreting glands of the tongue (short tongue syndrome)
   b. Hepatic retinol levels in suspected hypovitaminosis A (Table 10.2)
7. Ultrasonography
8. Water quality testing.

Table 10.2 Hepatic retinol levels in suspected hypovitaminosis A

Species	'Short tongue syndrome' affected Wyoming toad *Bufo baxteri* (*n* = 6)	Healthy Wyoming toad *Bufo baxteri* (*n* = 3)	Healthy southern toad *Bufo terrestris* (*n* = 4)	Healthy American toad *Bufo americanus* (*n* = 2)
Hepatic retinol (µg/g)	0.004–7.3	81–138	96–243	418–569

Adapted from Pessier et al (2002).

Management

- See *Nursing Care.*

Treatment/specific therapy

- *Entamoeba ranarum*
  - Metronidazole at 10–14 mg/L
- Ciliated protozoa
  - These are usually considered normal gut commensals
  - If high numbers and amphibia showing consistent clinical signs treat as for *Entamoeba*
- *Strongyloides spp*
  - Ivermectin
    - Dilute 1:50 in Hartman's solution and apply topically to dorsal surface
    - 10 g/L bath for 1 h weekly for up to 12 weeks
  - Levamisole (100–300 mg/L) bath for 1 h once weekly for up to 12 weeks
- Nematodes and acanthocephalans
  - As for *Strongyloides spp* above
  - Fenbendazole 50–100 mg/kg p.o. Repeat after 2 weeks as necessary
- Acanthocephalans require intermediate arthropod host so can be self-limiting
- Myxoma
  - Surgical resection
  - Radiosurgery
  - Likely to recur but grow very slowly
- Short-tongue syndrome
  - Supplement with vitamin A
    Note that commercial injectable vitamin A preparations are too concentrated for amphibia
  - 2 IU/g every 72 h i.m. or 1 IU/g orally or topically s.i.d.
  - May require hand-feeding as prey-capturing adhesive qualities of the tongue significantly reduced
- Gastric impaction
  - Removal of impaction contents by gastric lavage, endoscopic retrieval or gastroenterotomy
  - Broad-spectrum covering antibiotics
- Gastric prolapse
  - Appears as a fleshy structure above the tongue
  - Can be a normal activity in some frogs
  - Can be pathologic – often linked to starvation or increased intracoleomic pressure
  - Gently replace stomach and fill with liquid food to maintain position
  - Often fatal
- Intestinal foreign body
  - Laxatives often beneficial due to short GI tract
  - May require enterotomy
- Cloacal prolapse
  - Investigate possible underlying aetiologies, e.g. endoparasites.
  - Surgical replacement often poorly tolerated
  - Prognosis is guarded.

Nutritional disorders

- Hypocalcaemia (metabolic bone disease – see *Musculoskeletal Disorders*)
- Hypervitaminosis D_3 accompanied by hypercalcaemia (see *Systemic Disorders*)
- Hypovitaminosis A (see also *Gastrointestinal Disorders* and *Ophthalmic Disorders*)
- Obesity (especially horned frogs *Ceratophrys spp*)
  - Manage by switching to a low-energy diet, e.g. substituting more invertebrate prey for mammalian plus supplement with vitamin E especially
- Lipid keratopathy (see *Ophthalmic Disorders*).

Hepatic disorders

Bacterial

- *Aeromonas spp, Pseudomonas spp*
- Mycobacteria.

Fungal

Protozoal

- Amoebiasis.

Parasitic

Neoplasia

- Cholangiocellular carcinoma.

Findings on clinical examination

- Ascites (see *Systemic Disorders*)
- Anasarca.

Investigations

1. Radiography
2. Routine haematology and biochemistry
3. Culture and sensitivity
4. Endoscopy
   a. Multifocal abscessation (mycobacteriosis)
5. Biopsy/necropsy
6. Ultrasonography
7. Water quality testing.

Management

- Milk thistle (*Silybum marianum*) is hepatoprotectant. Dose at 4–15 mg/kg b.i.d. or t.i.d.
- Aspirate excess fluid from the coelom if ascitic

- Furosemide at 2.5 mg/kg i.m. b.i.d.
- For aquatic and semi-aquatic amphibia attempt to correct osmotic imbalance by keeping in either salt solution (0.55–1.0%) or magnesium sulphate solution.

Treatment/specific therapy

- Bacterial hepatitis
  - Appropriate antibiosis
- Mycobacteriosis
  - Potential zoonosis
  - Consider euthanasia as treatment often unrewarding (but see *Systemic Disorders* in *Tropical Freshwater Fish*)
- Hepatic amoebiasis
  - Metronidazole at 100 mg/kg p.o. every 14 days (Wright 1995).

Cardiovascular and haematological disorders

Amphibians have a well-developed lymphatic system with a significant exchange rate with the vascular system (up to 10 mL/h in the frog). Lymph is circulated with a varying number of lymph hearts. Cardiac and/or lymph heart disease and insufficiency is likely to lead to fluid accumulation in the coelom and lymphatics, presenting as an ascites or anasarca-like condition.

Bacterial
- Endocarditis.

Fungal

Protozoal
- Trypanosomes.

Parasitic
- Microfilaria (see *Systemic Disorders*).

Dietary

Neoplasia

Other non-infectious problems
- Cardiomyopathy
- Lymph heart insufficiency.

Findings on clinical examination

- Oedema, ascites (may be gross and present with swollen coelom, or confined to one or more limbs)
- Anorexia
- Mortalities.

424

Investigations

1. Radiography
2. Routine haematology and biochemistry
3. Culture and sensitivity
4. Endoscopy
5. Biopsy
6. Ultrasonography
7. Electrocardiogram
8. Water-quality testing.

Management

1. Fluid accumulation causes a reduction in circulating fluid volume, tissue hypoxia and lung compression
2. Aspirate excess fluid from the coelom
3. Furosemide at 2.5 mg/kg i.m. b.i.d.
4. For aquatic and semi-aquatic amphibia attempt to correct osmotic imbalance by keeping in either salt solution (0.55–1.0%) or magnesium sulphate solution
5. Treat any underlying specific causes.

Treatment/specific therapy

- Bacterial and fungal disorders
  - Appropriate antimicrobials
- Trypanosomes
  - Bath in quinine sulphate (30 mg/L) for 1 h daily.

Systemic disorders

Viral

- Ranavirus type III (iridovirus) (tadpole oedema disease) (see also *Renal and Urinary Disorders*)
- Bohle iridovirus (in Australian amphibia).

Bacterial

- *Aeromonas spp; Pseudomonas spp*
- *Flavobacterium spp.*
- *Mycobacteriosis*, esp. *M. marinum, M. chelonae, M. ranae, M. xenopi, M. fortuitum*, and rarely *M. avium* complex (*M. intracellulare* and *M. a. avium*).

Fungal

- Chromomycosis (see also *Skin Disorders*), e.g. *Veronea botryosa* (Mayer et al 2000)
- *Batrachochytrium dendrobatidis* (chytridiomycosis)
- *Mucor amphibiorum.*

Parasitic

* Microfilaria
* Cestodes (wide variety – see *Systemic Disorders*)
* Trematodes (wide variety – see *Systemic Disorders*).

Nutritional

* Hypervitaminosis D_3/hypercalcaemia (see *Nutritional Disorders*)
* Hypocalcaemia (see *Musculoskeletal Disorders*).

Neoplasia

* Fibrosarcoma
* Thymoma (Jacobson et al 2004)
* Gonadal neoplasia.

Other non-infectious problems

* Acute pulmonary emphysema (see *Respiratory Disorders*)
* Renal disease
* Cardiovascular disease
* Failure of lymph hearts
* Intestinal disease (gaseous bloating) (see *Gastrointestinal Disorders*)
* Keeping in very soft water (inducing osmotic imbalance)
* Thermal shock (Green et al 2003)
* Environmental toxins
* Chlorhexidine
* Povidone iodine
* Chlorine toxicity (tadpoles, aquatic amphibia)
* Quaternary ammonium compounds
* Ammonium
* Heavy metal, esp. zinc, lead or copper (see also *Neurological Disorders*).

Findings on clinical examination

* Weight loss
* Anorexia
* Unwilling/unable to move
* Splayed legs, skin sloughing (chytridiomycosis). High mortalities following meta-morphosis (post metamorphic death syndrome)
* Swollen coelom (Ascites, anasarca, lymphodema, septicaemia, renal disease, acute pulmonary emphysema, hypervitaminosis D_3)
* Septicaemic infections may be indicated by signs typical of 'red leg' (see *Skin Disorders*), such as inflammation, ulceration, inappetence, lethargy, convulsions, coelomic swelling and obvious eye abnormalities
* Dark, raised nodules in the skin, debilitation and weight loss (chromomycosis)
* Increased mucous production, erythema, agitation, lethargy, dyspnea, convulsions, paralysis diarrhoea and death following exposure to chlorhexidine (chlorhexidine toxicity)
* Mortalities.

Investigations

1. Radiography
2. Routine haematology and biochemistry
   a. Cold-adapted amphibia show an increased RBC, haemoglobin concentration, heterophilia, lymphopaenia and eosinopaenia
3. Culture and sensitivity
4. Endoscopy
   a. Microfilaria free in coelomic cavity
5. Biopsy/necropsy
   a. Microfilaria in vasculature or encysted in a variety of tissues and organs
   b. A wide variety of trematodes and cestodes at different developmental stages may be encountered in a variety of tissues
6. Ultrasonography
7. Water-quality testing.

Management

1. Ascites and anasarca
   a. Fluid accumulation causes a reduction in circulating fluid volume, tissue hypoxia and lung compression
   b. Aspirate excess fluid from the coelom
   c. Furosemide at 2.5 mg/kg i.m. b.i.d.
   d. For aquatic and semi-aquatic amphibia attempt to correct osmotic imbalance by keeping in either salt solution (0.55–1.0%) or magnesium sulphate solution
   e. Treat any underlying specific causes.

Treatment/specific therapy

- Bacterial infections (*Aeromonas, Pseudomonas, Flavobacterium*)
  - Appropriate antibiosis
- Mycobacteriosis
  - Potential zoonosis so consider euthanasia
- Hypervitaminosis D_3/hypercalcaemia
  - Metastatic calcification in many organs, e.g. heart, liver, kidneys leads to marked ascites
  - Treat symptomatically
  - Investigate possible causes of dietary imbalance
- Chromomycosis
  - Treatment often ineffective
  - Some apparent success with fluconazole (Mayer et al 2000)
  - Consider euthanasia
- Chytridiomycosis
  - Larval stages lack keratinized skin so less susceptible to infection, so heavy mortalities may follow metamorphosis (post metamorphic death syndrome – PMDS). Can be carried on mouthparts of larvae
  - Very virulent; consider euthanasia

- Microfilaria
  - Ivermectin
    - Dilute 1:50 in Hartman's solution and apply topically to dorsal surface
    - 10 g/L bath for 1 h weekly for up to 12 weeks
  - Mortalities may occur following treatment
- Trematodes and cestodes
  - Praziquantel at 10 mg/L bath for 3 h as a single dose or 8–24 mg/kg p.o., s.c. daily for 14 days
- Thermal shock
  - Usually diagnosed postmortem
  - History of sudden temperature change – either to a markedly low or high temperature
  - If identified soon enough return to clean, well-oxygenated water close to previous temperature
  - Supportive treatment
- Environmental toxins
  - Bathe amphibian in clean water
  - Supportive therapy, e.g. parenteral fluids
- Ammonia toxicity
  - If due to poor water quality undertake partial water changes to dilute the ammonia levels
  - Adding zeolite will absorb large quantities of ammonia
  - Longer-term control may include addition of commercially available *Nitrosomonas* bacterial cultures or equivalent
- Chlorine toxicity
  - Place in aged water
  - Avoid either by use of aged water or commercial dechlorinators as used for aquarium fish.

Musculoskeletal disorders

Bacterial

- Bacterial osteomyelitis
- Mycobacteriosis.

Fungal

- Mycotic osteomyelitis
- Chromomycosis.

Protozoal

- *Pleistophora* (*Microsporidia*).

Parasitic

- *Ribeiroia ondatrae* (trematode).

Nutritional

- Metabolic bone disease (MBD) (especially at time of metamorphosis).

Neoplasia

Other non-infectious problems
* Gout (articular and periarticular) especially in horned frogs (*Ceratophrys spp*)
* Trauma (fractures).

Findings on clinical examination

* Swellings (abscess, gout, fracture)
* Any limb or spinal swelling, fracture or paralysis should be considered as a possible sign of a pathologic fracture
* Soft mandibles, fore-shortening of the maxillae, swollen mid-shaft of long bones, kyphosis/scoliosis, weakness, inability to support own bodyweight (MBD)
* Muscle weakness, inability to support body or hunt/locate food
* Muscle fasciculations and other neurological signs
* Kyphosis (microsporidial myositis)
* Supernumerary limbs, limb abnormalities (*Ribeiroia ondatrae*, trematode).

Investigations

1. Radiography
2. Cytology
   a. Fine needle aspirate
   b. Gout tophi
3. Routine haematology and biochemistry
4. Culture and sensitivity
5. Endoscopy
6. Biopsy
7. Ultrasonography.

Treatment/specific therapy

* Gout
  * In large amphibians, e.g. horned frogs, may be linked to excessive mammalian prey intake; these are often fed on small mice whereas their natural diet would be mostly insectivorous
  * Allopurinol at 10 mg/kg s.i.d.
* Metabolic bone disease
  * Classically a nutritional secondary hyperparathyroidism due to relative lack of calcium
  * May be especially pronounced at time of metamorphosis
  * Post-metamorphic amphibia may exhibit signs of MBD even on a good diet, as a result of a larval calcium deficit. *Note* that in many adult Urodeles and larval anurans prolactin is an important hypercalcaemic hormone as well as PTH and 1,25 hydroxy vitamin D_3
  * Daily baths in a high calcium and vitamin D_3 solution (2–3 IU/mL)
  * Oral or injectable calcium and vitamin D_3 supplementation (may be absorbed transcutaneously so can try applying to skin of back of terrestrial amphibia)
  * Supplement with dietary calcium

- Some species endemic to hard water areas may have a higher calcium requirement
- Abscessation and osteomyelitis, myositis
  - Appropriate antibiosis
  - Consider amputation if damage is extensive
- Fracture
  - Differentiate between pathologic fracture (chromomycosis, neoplasia) and traumatic with radiography
  - For compound fractures, deal with skin lesions as described under *Skin Disorders*
  - Extensive trauma to limbs is often best dealt with by amputation. Many Urodeles are able to regenerate lost limbs and tails.

Neurological disorders

Bacterial
- Septicaemia
- CNS granuloma.

Fungal
- CNS granuloma.

Neoplasia

Other non-infectious problems
- Hypoglycaemia (weakness)
- Environmental toxins (see also *Systemic Disorders*)
  - Chlorhexidine
  - Povidone iodine
  - Chlorine toxicity (tadpoles, aquatic amphibia)
  - Quaternary ammonium compounds
  - Ammonium
  - Poor water quality
  - Cleaning agents
  - Heavy metal especially zinc, lead or copper (see also *Systemic Disorders*).

Findings on clinical examination

- Abnormal behavioural signs especially in larval amphibia (poor water quality)
- Flaccid paralysis
- Disorientation
- Seizures
- Loss of righting reflex
- Mortality.

Investigations

1. Radiography
2. Routine haematology and biochemistry

   a. Blood glucose levels: in the North American bullfrog (*Rana catesbeiana*) normal resting glucose levels around 0.4 mmol/L; 1.3 mmol/L when stressed (Crawshaw 1998)

3. Culture and sensitivity
4. Endoscopy
5. Biopsy
6. Ultrasonography
7. Water quality testing.

Management

See *Nursing Care.*

Treatment/specific therapy

- Bacterial and fungal diseases
  - Appropriate antimicrobials
  - Supportive care
- Hypoglycaemia
  - Oral glucose, but see 'Cataracts', under *Ophthalmic Disorders*
- Environmental toxins (see *Systemic Disorders*)
- Heavy metal poisoning
  - Remove suspected source
  - Remove to unaffected water
  - Oxygenate or aerate water well.

Ophthalmic disorders

The amphibian eye changes during metamorphosis. At hatching, each larva has a duplex cornea with an inner cornea and a second, outer, cornea. At metamorphosis, these fuse into a single, mammalian-like cornea. Pupillary dilation is best achieved under GA with tricaine methane sulphonate (MS222). Otherwise, intracameral muscle relaxants such as vecuronium, succinyl choline or D-tubocurarine are required.

Bacterial

- Subspectacular abscess (larval amphibians)
- Keratitis and ulceration
- Uveitis.

Fungal

- Keratitis and ulceration
- Uveitis.

Protozoal

Parasitic

Nutritional

- Calcium lesions in the cornea

- Cholesterol lesions (lipid keratopathy)
- Hypovitaminosis A.

Neoplasia

Other non-infectious problems

- Corneal trauma
- Crickets and other prey insects
- Collision with environmental objects including transparent barriers.

Findings on clinical examination

- Keratitis
- Calcium and cholesterol lesions in the cornea
- Bilateral conjunctival swellings (hypovitaminosis A)
- Fluorescein positive corneal lesions (corneal ulceration)
- Buphthalmos
- Cataracts.

Investigations

1. Ophthalmic examination
2. Radiography
3. Routine haematology and biochemistry
4. Culture and sensitivity
5. Endoscopy
6. Biopsy
7. Ultrasonography
8. Water-quality testing, especially for aquatic amphibia.

Treatment/specific therapy

- Hypovitaminosis A (see *Gastrointestinal Disorders*)
- Lipid and calcium keratopathies
    - If only small part of cornea affected then monitor
    - Partial keratectomy if cornea largely affected plus topical antibiosis
    - Lipid keratopathy may be linked with:
        - Fat mobilization during oogenesis in females
        - Failure to achieve (high) preferred body temperatures
        - Diets high in mammalian fat, e.g. rodents
- Corneal ulcers and secondarily infected corneal traumas
    - Under anaesthetic swab for culture and sensitivity, clean and debride lesion
    - Apply appropriate antibiosis and allow time for absorption
    - Seal with cyanoacrylate (Bicknese & Cranfield 1995)
- Uveitis
    - Topical and systemic antibiosis
    - Enucleation. *Note* that many frogs and toads use the eyes during swallowing, so enucleation *may* affect feeding ability
    - In cases of buphthalmus, if enucleation decided against, consider tarsorrhaphy to protect cornea from desiccation

- Cataracts
  - Various aetiologies including nutritional, toxic and infectious should be considered
  - Temporary cataracts in poison-arrow frogs lined with provision of 5% dextrose as part of supportive therapy (Williams & Whitaker 1994).

Endocrine disorders

Despite extensive studies into the amphibian endocrine system, especially with regard to metamorphosis, pathology of the endocrine system is little documented. Supplementation with thyroxine is known to trigger metamorphosis in the axolotl; prolonged larval stages may reflect a hypothalamic-pituitary-thyroidal dysfunction.

Neoplasia

- Thymoma (see *Systemic Disorders* and *Renal and Urinary Disorders*).

Renal and urinary disorders

Viral

- Ranavirus type III (iridovirus) (tadpole oedema disease) (See also *Systemic Disorders*)
- Herpes virus (induces renal adenocarcinoma in leopard frogs *Rana pipiens*).

Bacterial

- Nephritis.

Fungal

- Nephritis.

Protozoal

- *Entamoeba ranarum* (renal amoebiasis)
- Myxosporea.

Parasitic

- Trematodes (wide variety – see *Systemic Disorders*).

Neoplasia

- Renal adenocarcinoma (in the leopard frog *Rana pipiens*, likely to be induced by a herpes virus
- Thymoma (see also *Systemic Disorders*).

Other non-infectious problems

- Prolapse of the urinary bladder (differentiate from cloacal or oviductal prolapse)
- Cystic calculi (tree frogs).

Findings on clinical examination

- Ascites (see also *Systemic Disorders*)
- Ascites in tadpoles (ranavirus type III) but see also *Systemic Disorders*)
- Loss of appetite, anorexia
- Weight loss
- Inactivity.

Investigations

1. Urinalysis of terrestrial amphibia
   a. Renal casts
   b. Inflammatory cells
   c. Bacteria
2. Radiography
3. Routine haematology and biochemistry
   a. Inverse calcium:phosphorus ratio, hypoproteinaemia, hypoalbuminaemia suggest renal disease (or hepatic disease)
   b. Nephrotic syndrome (may be linked with thymoma; Jacobson et al 2004)
4. Culture and sensitivity
5. Endoscopy
6. Biopsy/necropsy
   a. Haemorrhage into Bowman's capsule, necrosis of glomerular endothelial cells and tubular necrosis (ranavirus type III)
7. Ultrasonography
8. Water quality testing.

Management

- See *Nursing Care.*

Treatment/specific therapy

- Ranavirus type III
  - No effective treatment. Potentially very infectious so consider euthanasia
- Bacterial and fungal nephritis
  - Appropriate antimicrobials
- Myxosporea
  - No effective treatment available. Try fumagillin as for fish at 1 g/kg food for 10–14 days for prevention
- Renal amoebiasis
  - Metronidazole at 100 mg/kg p.o. every 14 days
- Renal neoplasia
  - Partial or unilateral nephrectomy
- Urinary bladder prolapse
  - Clean and aspirate out any urine
  - Gently replace
  - Consider cystopexy

- Surgical following a coeliotomy
- Percutaneous cystopexy. Achieved by inserting a small probe into the bladder per cloaca as a guide to identify the position of the bladder. Hold the probe against the coelomic wall while transcutaneous sutures are positioned.

Reproductive disorders

Neoplasia

Other non-infectious problems

- Oviductal prolapse
- Ovarian prolapse.

Findings on clinical examination

- Ovary or oviduct partially protruding from cloaca, usually following egg-laying.

Investigations

1. Radiography
2. Routine haematology and biochemistry
3. Culture and sensitivity
4. Endoscopy
5. Biopsy
6. Ultrasonography
7. Water quality testing.

Management

See *Nursing Care.*

Treatment/specific therapy

- Oviductal and ovarian prolapse
  - Attempt surgical resection
  - Very guarded prognosis
- Gonadal neoplasia
  - Surgical resection.

References

Bicknese E J, Cranfield M J 1995 Cyanoacrylate treatment for corneal ulcers in Kokoe-Pa poison dart frogs (Dendrobates histrionicus). Proc Assoc Reptil Amphib Vet 67–73

Crawshaw G J 1998 Amphibian emergency and critical care. Veterinary Clinics of North America: Exot Anim Pract 1(1):207–231

Green S L, Moorhead R C, Bouley D M 2003 Thermal shock in a colony of South African clawed frogs (Xenopus laevis). Vet Rec 152:336–337

Jacobson E R, Robertson D R, Lafortune M et al 2004 Renal failure and bilateral thymoma in an American bullfrog Rana catesbiana. J Herpet Med Surg 14(2):6–11

Mayer J, Martin J C, Garner M M et al 2000 Chromoblastomycosis due to a synanamorph of Veronea botryosa in a colony of White's Tree frogs (Litoria caerula). Br Vet Zoo Soc Proc Spring Meeting, 11

Pessier A P, Roberts D R, Linn M et al 2002 'Short tongue syndrome', Lingual squamous metaplasia and suspected hypovitaminosis A in captive Wyoming toads, Bufo baxteri. Proc Assoc Reptil Amphib Vet 151–153

Williams D L, Whitaker B R 1994 The amphibian eye – a clinical review. J Zoo Wildl Med 25(1):18–28

Wright K M 1995 Amphibian medicine. Proc Assoc Reptil Amphib Vet 59–64

Goldfish and koi

This chapter covers those disorders likely to be seen in goldfish and koi, which constitute the most popular section of fish-keeping. Tolerance of wide temperature ranges means that these species can be kept outside, as well as inside, in most temperate countries such as Europe and North America. However, they are also happy at more tropical temperatures and in those countries such as Singapore, Malaysia and southern China where they are kept alongside 'tropical species'. Hence, this disorders chapter should be read in conjunction with that on *Tropical Freshwater Fish*.

Fish-keeping is a huge worldwide hobby and industry. Unfortunately, veterinarians are often last to be consulted over a fish-related problem, or else they are approached purely as a source of antibiotics and other regulated medications. This is because:

1. There are a great many proprietary products available for the treatment of ornamental fish, which aquarists are able to access from their aquarium retailer without recourse to the veterinarian. Most of these products are poorly regulated and, therefore, their efficacy is often very poor in contrast to the claims made for them; a problem compounded by inadequate diagnostics by both aquarist and helpful retailer. Ectoparasitic preparations are usually sufficiently efficacious to justify their use when their safety and ease of use is also brought into consideration.
2. This ready availability of proprietary medications devalues professional input.
3. There is a low economic cost for many widely kept fish.
4. There is a historical perception that veterinarians know little about fish and fish diseases.

Consultation and handling

The key to successful fish-keeping, and a major stumbling point, is water quality. Recommended water-quality parameters for koi and goldfish are listed in Table 11.1.

Hobbyist test kits are available to measure these parameters and they give reasonable results; accurate testing requires professional equipment.

If possible, fish should be examined in their home aquarium or pond. However, if the pond is large it may pay to ask for the fish to be caught and separated before arrival, as much time can be wasted attempting to catch the fish. Ponds are rarely built with recapture in mind. Once caught, place the fish on a damp towel for examination. If necessary sedate with MS222 or benzocaine (see 'Anaesthesia', below).

Always examine the ventral surface, as lesions here may not be obvious when viewed from above. Skin scrapes should be taken from the operculae, the flank, and around the base of the fins. Examine the gills and oral cavity.

Table 11.1 Recommended water quality parameters for koi and goldfish

Parameter	Value
Temperature (°C)	10–30 (preferred range = 22–28 for Koi)
pH	6.0–8.4 (preferred 7.0–8.0)
Hardness (CaCO$_3$) (mg/L)	100–250
Conductivity (mS/cm)	180–480
Ammonia (total) (mg/L)	<0.02
Nitrite (mg/L)	<0.2
Nitrate (above ambient tapwater levels) (mg/L)	<40
Oxygen (mg/L)	5.0–8.0
Chlorine (mg/L)	0.002

Adapted from Jepson (2001).

Blood sampling

This is best done under anaesthesia (see below). Blood can be drawn using a well-heparinized syringe from the ventral tail vein, which runs midline just below the caudal vertebrae. In small fish this can be accessed via the ventral midline while in larger fish, a lateral approach is often better. This same approach can be used for intravenous injections.

For the internal anatomy of a goldfish, see Figure 11.1.

Nursing care

Provision of optimal water quality is essential to maximize recovery. A separate hospital aquarium or vat can be used but the water quality in this facility should be as good as in a main display (Fig. 11.2). The water should be filtered, but because of

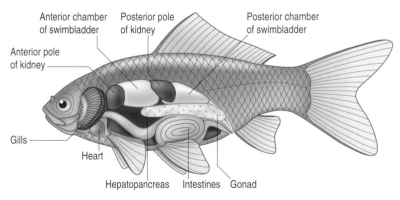

Fig. 11.1. Internal anatomy of goldfish. *Note* that goldfish and koi do not possess a true stomach. Adhesions between the internal organs are normal and not the result of coelomitis.

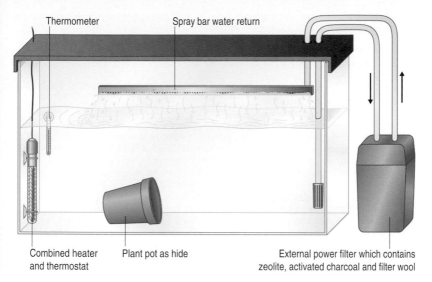

Thermometer   Spray bar water return

Combined heater   Plant pot as hide   External power filter which contains
and thermostat   zeolite, activated charcoal and filter wool

Fig. 11.2. Clinical aquarium setup.

the use of medications such as antibiotics, biological filtration cannot be used. After each patient, the aquarium or vat should be dismantled and cleaned out with an iodine-based disinfectant.

Reliance is placed upon physical and chemical methods of water purification. Zeolite will absorb ammonia excreted by the fish, while activated charcoal will adsorb many harmful chemicals from the water. If salt is used, a small protein skimmer would be of great benefit. Ozonizers and ultraviolet sterilization are also useful adjuncts. Keep decorations to a minimum, giving just sufficient for nervous fish to hide behind. All materials used should be readily cleanable, such as plastic – and avoid live plants and bogwood where possible, as these can act as disease reservoirs. Temperature can be maintained at the optimum using commercial aquarium heaters. For koi and goldfish, a temperature of 18–25°C should be considered. Keeping fish in a permanent 5 g/L solution of salt (use aquarium or sea salt, not table or rock salt) will reduce the osmotic load on a sick koi or goldfish.

Antibiotics can be administered either by:
1. Injection. Optimum site is either immediately in front or behind the dorsal fin in the midline
2. In feed (but note that many sick fish are inappetent)
3. Bath (may damage biological filtration)
4. Gavage.

Analgesia

Butorphanol at 0.05–0.5 mg/kg i.m.

Anaesthesia

There are a number of anaesthetic preparations and protocols described, but the author has found tricaine methane sulphonate and benzocaine to be the most useful.

Suitable anaesthetic agents

1. Tricaine methane sulphonate (MS-222)
   a. This is a benzocaine derivative with a sulphonate radical giving it water solubility (and increased acidity). It is absorbed and primarily excreted across the gill epithelium. Hypoxia can be a problem
   b. Tricaine methane sulphonate can be added directly to water in incremental doses but fish may show mild signs of distress due to a rapid fall in pH. As a rough guide, sedation is achieved at 20–50 mg/L and anaesthesia at 50–100 mg/L
   c. To avoid this, dissolve in saturated solution of $NaHCO_3$ to form a buffered stock solution of 10 g/L (10 000 p.p.m.). *Note* that this is unstable in light
   d. Recovery from short procedures is rapid (<10 min) but following lengthy operations it can be prolonged (<6 h), especially in large fish.
2. Benzocaine
   a. Must be dissolved in ethanol or acetone (stock solution of 100 g/L). Unstable in light. The author finds it less reliable than tricaine methane sulphonate, possibly due to effects of solute.

Anaesthetic protocol for fish anaesthesia

Induction

1. During anaesthesia, the water quality should be optimal for that species.
2. There is a risk of hypoxia due to respiratory depression, therefore aerate/oxygenate the water well.
3. Fish are ectotherms, therefore higher temperatures speed up induction and recovery, but water at higher temperatures holds less oxygen.
4. Food withheld for one feeding cycle – regurgitation can clog gill rakers and foul water.
5. Handle fish carefully with wet hands to avoid damage to mucous layers.
6. Before induction prepare two supplies of well oxygenated water of the same suitable water quality – one with anaesthetic solution and one without.
7. Induction is either by addition of the anaesthetic to the bath with the fish already in situ, or fish is placed into a bath containing the anaesthetic solution.

Maintenance

1. Fish can be maintained out of water for prolonged periods of time for surgery providing the gills are constantly bathed in oxygenated water. The simplest method is for an assistant to constantly and gently syringe water into the mouth such that it flows over the gills and out beneath the operculae. Water is selected from either the anaesthetic-containing or anaesthetic-free container as required.
2. For more advanced anaesthetic techniques, the fish can be placed over a water reservoir, with water continuously pumped from this reservoir and introduced into the oral cavity via a tube. The water exiting the operculae flows back into the reservoir below.
3. Anaesthesia is usually maintained at a concentration of tricaine methane sulphonate at 50–100 mg/L.
4. If performing multiple anaesthetics beware build up of ammonia and proteinaceous material from sloughed mucous.
5. During recovery, water flow over gills should be in physiologically normal direction as reversal short circuits normal counter current gaseous exchange mechanism.

Skin disorders

Skin structure

The skin is a large and complex organ that is constantly in contact with the immediate environment of the fish. Its functions include an osmotic barrier, disease barrier, protection, intra-specific signaling and camouflage. Histologically it consists of:
1. Cuticle. A thin mucopolysaccharide layer containing mucous, sloughed cells and antibodies
2. Epidermis. Stratified squamous epithelium plus mucous secreting cells
3. Dermis
   a. Stratum spongiosum. This contains chromatophores
   b. Scales (flat plates of bone) are also present in this layer
   c. Stratum compactum. This is a dense, collagenous tissue
4. Hypodermis. Loosely arranged, often vascular and may contain adipose tissue. Attaches integument to underlying muscle.

Note that the scales of fish are dermal structures (not epidermal thickenings as seen in reptiles), therefore the loss of scale involves damage to the overlying epidermis and a potential breach in the fishes' immune and osmotic barrier.

Differential diagnoses for skin disorders

Pruritus

- Scratching against surfaces. Sometimes termed 'flashing' or 'flicking'
- Ectoparasites
- Poor water quality.

Erosions and ulceration including fin rot

- Bacterial disease, typically *Aeromonas spp*, Cytophagic-like bacteria, *Flavobacterium spp*. Also mycobacteriosis (see *Musculoskeletal Disorders*). With *Cytophaga psychrophila* infection is often on the dorsal fin spreading towards the base where a large ulcer forms – this is sometime referred to as 'saddle-back' disease (Figs 11.3, 11.4)
- Fungal disease, such as *Fusarium spp* (see also *Ophthalmic Disorders*)
- Protozoa (*Trichodina, Epistylis*), *Thelohanellus hovorkai* (Yokohama et al 1999)
- Large ectoparasites, e.g. *Argulus, Learnea*
- Trauma with secondary bacterial infections. Often damage to skin and/or loss of eyes and fins. May occur due to predator attack, e.g. heron, raccoon, cat or during handling or spawning
- Sunburn. Will affect only the white or unpigmented areas of the dorsal surface.

Nodules and non-healing wounds

- Nuptial tubercles (normal in sexually mature goldfish and other cyprinids; usually confined to the operculae and leading rays of the pectoral fins. In some fancy goldfish, those on the fins can be very large and nodular, resembling neoplasia)
- Obvious discrete pin-head white spots (*Ichthyophthirius multifilis*). White spot disease. Also often breathing difficulties, irritation. Fins clamped
- Candle-wax masses on skin and fins on cyprinids, especially carp/koi. Retarded growth in young koi. Carp pox (cyprinid herpesvirus 1; CHV-1). *Note* may cause mass mortalities in young (2-week-old) carp (Sano et al 1991) (see *Systemic Disorders*)
- *Dermocystidium koi* (see also *Musculoskeletal Disorders*)

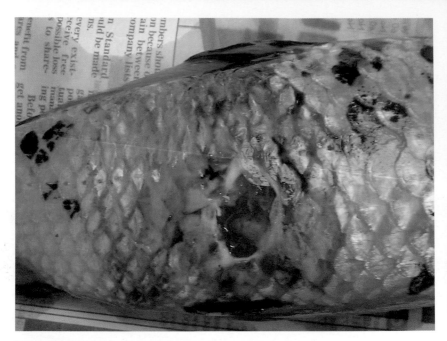

Fig. 11.3. Bacterial ulceration in a koi.

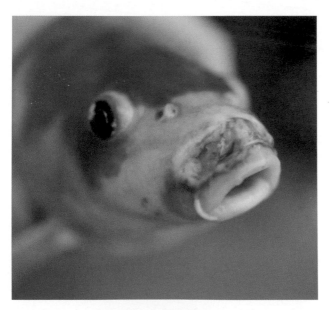

Fig. 11.4. Mouth ulceration due to *Flavobacteria*.

- Lymphocystis (iridovirus). Large, cauliflower like masses on fins and skin. Does not usually infect cyprinids, but may be seen in other pond or coldwater fish, e.g. sunfish (*Lepomis spp*)
- Epitheliocystis. Looks like lymphocystis but can infect cyprinids including carp
- Myxosporidae. Obvious nodules. Often fish displays dark or accentuating colouring, weight loss, whirling and fin rot
- *Henneguya koi*. Small, smooth rounded cyst-like nodules in the skin. Can also affect the gills and internal organs
- Wasting, darkening of skin colour and obvious boil-like swellings in the skin; in extreme cases it may have a sandpaper effect, due to the large number of granulomas present. Also exophthalmia, abnormal behaviour and swimming patterns (if the central nervous system is invaded). *(Ichthyophonus hoferi)*. See also *Neurological and Swimming Disorders, Ophthalmic Disorders* and *Systemic Disorders*
- Gas filled bubbles in the skin especially on the fins. Also occasionally behind the eye (gas bubble disease – usually secondary to oxygen supersaturation)
- Hypersensitivity reactions at attachment sites of parasites such as *Argulus* and *Lernea*.

Changes in pigmentation or colour

- Reddened fin and skin. Bacterial infection (see 'Erosions and ulceration' above), golden shiner virus (*Notemigonus crysoleucas* only), spring viraemia of carp (SVC; see *Systemic Disorders*), grass carp rheovirus (*Ctenopharygodon idella* only)
- Greying skin (secondary to excessive mucous production) (ectoparasites esp. *Chilonodella, Trichodina*) (Fig. 11.5)
- White tufts on surface, may look like cotton wool (*Epistylis, Saprolegnia*, Cytophaga-like bacteria). In pond fish, fungal infections that have been present for

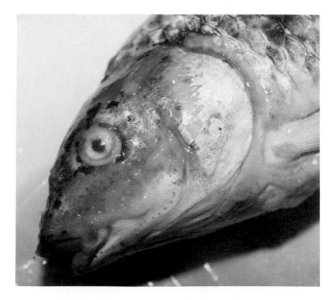

Fig. 11.5. Excess mucous on a koi with a *Chilonodella* infestation.

some time may be green or brown due to secondary colonization by algae. *Note* that mucous strands hanging from the skin can strongly resemble *Saprolegnia*
- 'Staff's disease' – *Saprolegnia* fungal growths present only in the nostrils. Seen in common carp in Poland during the winter months in 1–2 year old carp
- Obvious discrete white spots (*Ichthyophirius*). In koi, there is often a 'salt and pepper' dusting appearance rather than distinct white spots
- Dark or accentuating colouring (*Myxosporidae*)
- Dusty effect over body surface (*Oodinium*, velvet disease)
- Grey spots on gills and fins (*Glocchidia* – larval freshwater mussels)
- Whitish mucous tufts on hood (or wen) of fancy goldfish (see also *Ophthalmic Disorders*)
- Colour fading. In goldfish and koi it is likely to be a nutritional lack of appropriate carotenoids. Some goldfish on good diets do spontaneously turn white - this is likely to be genetic.
- Occasionally areas of dark pigment develop on the red areas of koi, particularly seen in kohakus. Known to koi-keepers as shimmies, these are merely changes in pigmentation and do not warrant removal except for aesthetic purposes.

Ectoparasites
- Protozoa
  - *Chilonodella* (see also *Respiratory Tract Disorders*)
  - *Trichodina*, *Trichodonella* and *Triparciella* (see also *Respiratory Tract Disorders*)
  - *Ichthyodo necator* (*Costia necatrix*) (see also *Respiratory Tract Disorders*)
  - *Epistylis* (*Heteropolaria*)
  - *Ichthyophthirius multifilis* (white spot) (see also *Respiratory Tract Disorders*)
  - *Oodinium* (velvet disease)
  - *Myxosporidea*
    - *Henneguya koi*
    - *Thelohanellus nikolskii*
    - *Thelohanellus hovorkai* (myxosporean) (Yokohama et al 1999)
- Helminths
  - *Gyrodactylus* (skin flukes)
  - *Dactylogyrus* (gill flukes) (see also *Respiratory Tract Disorders*)
  - Leeches, e.g. *Piscicola geometra*
- Molluscs
  - *Glocchidia* (larval freshwater mussels) (see also *Respiratory Tract Disorders*)
- Crustacean
  - *Argulus spp* (fish louse) (large, mobile disc-shaped parasite)
  - *Learnea spp* (anchor worm) (obvious Y-shaped parasites)
- Neoplasia
  - Carp pox (CHV-1, see above)
  - Squamous cell carcinoma (possibly triggered by CHV-1) (Fig. 11.6)
  - Erythrophoroma (esp. koi)
  - Fibromas (esp. goldfish) (Fig. 11.7)
  - Papillomas. *Note* that the lesions induced by CHV-1 histologically resemble papillomas.

Disorders of the fins
- Disorders of the fins largely follow those of the skin and are usually symptomatic of a more widespread dermal problem.

Fig. 11.6. Squamous cell carcinoma in a carp.

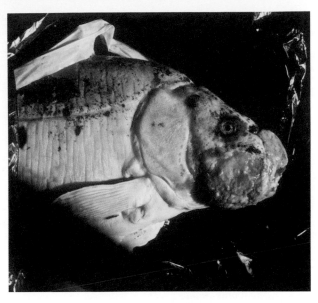

Fig. 11.7. Fibroma on a lionhead goldfish.

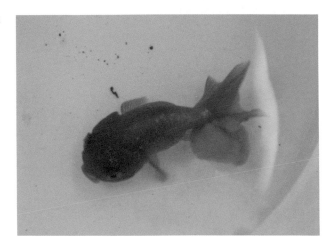

- Occasionally fins suffer traumatic injury and will split between the rays, or even fracture the rays. Often these heal uneventfully. Occasionally suturing may be undertaken to improve the aesthetic result.
- Damaged or diseased distal sections of the fins can be resected and usually the fin will regenerate over time.

Other findings on clinical examination

- Clamped fins, depression, sudden death (*Chilonodella*) (golden shiner virus)
- Skin ulceration, respiratory breathing problems
- Fish usually appear depressed, fins clamped shut, may 'wobble' as they swim or even 'shimmy', skin appears dull and grayish; ulceration may be seen, respiratory signs (*Ichthyobodo*)
- Breathing difficulties, irritation. Fins clamped (*Ichthyophthirius, Oodinium*)
- Dark or accentuating colouring, weight loss, whirling and fin rot (*Myxosporidea*)
- Open skin sores, wasting and protruding eyes. Possible spinal curvature (*Mycobacteriosis*)
- Exophthalmia, haemorrhages in grass carp (grass carp rheovirus)
- Gas bubbles behind eye (gas bubble disease)
- Darkened body colour, ascites, skin haemorrhages, anal prolapse (SVC).

Investigations

1. Skin scrape and microscopy (Fig. 11.8)
   a. Protozoa
      i. *Trichodina, Trichodonella* and *Triparciella:* circular, rotating parasites around 40 μm
      ii. *Ichthyophthirius;* large ciliate, horse-shoe shaped nucleus
      iii. *Chilonodella;* large protozoan (30–70 μm) that has an almost oval, flattened appearance. Obvious cilia; moves with gliding, slow circular movement
      iv. *Oodinium:* can be quite large, up to 1.0 mm diameter, oval shaped with a very dark appearance because of chloroplasts. Not usually mobile

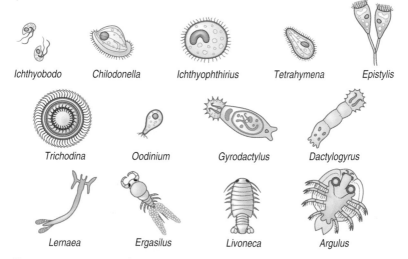

Ichthyobodo   *Chilodonella*   *Ichthyophthirius*   *Tetrahymena*   *Epistylis*

Trichodina   *Oodinium*   *Gyrodactylus*   *Dactylogyrus*

Lernaea   *Ergasilus*   *Livoneca*   *Argulus*

Fig. 11.8. Common fish ectoparasites (freshwater). (Not drawn to scale.)

    b. Flukes
      i. *Gyrodactylus*: live-bearing; can usually see large H-shaped hooks of both adult and unborn young
      ii. *Dactylogyrus*: egg-layer. Usually four black spots at caudal end. Can be quite large flukes
2. Radiography
3. Routine haematology and biochemistry
4. Culture and sensitivity
5. Endoscopy
6. Biopsy
    a. Intranuclear inclusions present with CHV-1 infections
    b. PCR for SVC
7. Ultrasonography
8. Postmortem examination
9. Viral isolation for SVC
10. Water-quality parameters – check temperature, ammonia, nitrite, nitrate and pH values.

Management

1. See under *Nursing Care*
2. Skin lesions and ulcers
    a. Maintain good water quality
    b. Clean once with topical iodine
    c. If large/deep then cover with barrier substance such as Orabase (Squibb) to reduce further secondary contamination and form a partial osmotic barrier
3. Antibiotic cover:
    a. Enrofloxacin at 5 mg/kg i.m. e.o.d. or as a bath at 2.5 mg/L for 5 h s.i.d.
    b. Marbofloxacin at 5 mg/kg every 3 days.
4. Alter management to reduce risk of recurrence.

Treatment/specific therapy

- Gas bubble disease
  - Oxygen supersaturation usually secondary to pressurized oxygenation (waterfalls, malfunctioning venturi pumps etc.), excess photosynthesis (high plant levels, suspended algae)
  - Correct source of problem
  - Rarely fatal – fish usually recover uneventfully
- Bacterial septicaemia and ulceration
  - See 'Management', above
  - Debridement of ulcers followed by packing with protective layer, e.g. Orabase (Squibb) – see *Nursing Care*
  - Some may benefit from long-term salt bath (see *Nursing Care*) to reduce osmotic gradient
- Sunburn
  - Treat as for bacterial ulceration above
- *Oodinium*:
  - Try a proprietary velvet treatment

- Metronidazole at 50 mg/L for up to 24 h daily for 10 days
- Quinine hydrochloride at 10–20 mg/L indefinitely. Some fish are sensitive to this
- The encysted stage is relatively resistant to chemical attack
- Can colonize the intestines of fish, where again it can be protected from medications
- Antibiotic cover should be considered as secondary infections are common at the areas where the skin is damaged
- Eliminate the parasite from a show aquarium by removing all fish, reducing or cutting out the light levels and raising the temperature to 30–32°C for 3 weeks
- *Ichthyophthirius multifillis* – white spot
  - Proprietary white spot remedy
  - Raising water temperature 1 or 2°C speeds up life cycle, promoting the exposure of the chemical-sensitive motile theront stage.
- *Epistylis* (*Heteropolaria*)
  - Commercial ectoparasitic preparations
- *Chilonodella*
  - Proprietary ectoparasitic medications
  - Glacial acetic acid dips at 8 mL/gallon for 30–45 s. May kill weak fish
  - *Chilonodella* prefers temperatures of 18–22°C, but for *Chilonodella cyprini*, temperatures of 5–10°C seem to be close to its optimum
- *Trichodina, Trichodonella* and *Triparciella*
  - Proprietary ectoparasitic medication
- *Ichthyobodo*
  - Standard proprietary anti-protozoan treatments
  - Remove all of the fish from the infected aquarium or pond for 24–48 h as the parasite can only survive without a host for a few hours
  - *Ichthyobodo* is able to survive temperatures down to 2°C and can cause mortalities in overwintering carp
- *Henneguya koi* and *Thelohanellus spp*
  - No effective treatment
  - Common carp are more susceptible to *Thelohanellus nikolsii* than koi or goldfish (Molnar 2002)
  - *Thelohanellus hovorkai* requires an intermediate oligochaete host
  - Feeding a diet of 0.1% fumagillin diet prevented mortalities in *Thelohanellus* infected koi (Yokohama et al 1999).
- Flukes (skin, gill)
  - Proprietary ectoparasitic preparations
  - *Praziquantel* at 10 mg/kg body weight by mouth; as a 1–2 h bath at 15–20 mg/L. With larger fish, in-feed medication at a rate of 400 mg/100 g food daily for 7 days
  - Dactylogyrids are egg-layers; the egg stage is resistant to treatment and so infestations require multiple treatments up to 4 weeks apart depending upon water temperature
- Glocchidia (larval freshwater mussels). Usually self-limiting. Larvae only transiently parasitic
  - Whitish tufts on hood. This is normal and may be linked to normal hood growth. No treatment needed
- Grass carp rheovirus
  - No treatment. Symptomatic treatment only
- Golden shiner virus
  - No treatment. Symptomatic treatment only

- Spring viraemia of carp
  - No treatment. Symptomatic treatment only
- Leeches
  - Remove individual parasites
  - Organophosphates (where legal to do so)
- *Learnea* (anchor worm)
  - Individual removal of parasites
  - Treat with lufenuron (Program, Novartis) at 0.088 mg/L as a once only treatment
  - Treat with organophosphates (where legal to do so)
- *Argulus* (fish louse)
  - Individual removal of parasites
  - Treat with lufenuron (Program, Novartis) at 0.088 mg/L as a once only treatment
  - Treat with organophosphates (where legal to do so)
  - A potassium permanganate bath at 10 p.p.m. (mg/L) for 5–60 min can be used to rid both individual fish and plants of this parasite
- *Dermocystidium koi*
  - Surgical removal
  - Consider itraconazole at 1.0–5.0 mg/kg p.o. every 1–7 days, either in feed or gavage
- Saprolegnia (fungal disease)
  - Proprietary medications containing malachite green
  - Remove visible hyphae and swab the affected area with a 10% povidone-iodine solution once daily
  - Maintain the fish in a salt solution as this will not only help to control the fungal infection, but will also help with the osmotic imbalance resulting from the infection. Even salt solutions as low as 10 parts per thousand (mg/100 mL) will inhibit Saprolegnia infections. Ideally aim for 1 to 3 g/L as a permanent solution until the problem has resolved
- Carp pox
  - No treatment. Will usually clear up in warmer water, but recrudescence common
- Lymphocystis
  - No direct cure. Usually self-limiting
  - Ozone or ultraviolet sterilization may reduce spread
  - Attempted surgical removal is usually followed by recurrence
- Epitheliocystis
  - *Chlamydophila*-like organism
  - Some antibiotics, e.g. chloramphenicol, recorded as effective
- Spring viraemia of carp – see *Systemic Disorders*
- Neoplasia
  - Chemotherapy in fish is in its infancy
  - Surgical removal followed by treatment of surgical wound as described under 'Management', above
  - Surgical debulking followed by injection of cisplatin directly into the tissue mass on a weekly basis.

Respiratory tract disorders

Viral

- Koi herpes virus (KHV, cyprinid herpes virus 3; CHV-3) (herpes virus)
- Gill necrosis virus.

Bacterial

* Bacterial (environmental) gill disease.

Fungal

* Branchiomycosis.

Protozoal

* White spot (*Ichtyophthirius*)
* *Chilonodella* (see also *Skin Disorders*)
* Ichthyobodo (Costia) necatrix
* Oodinium (velvet disease) (see also *Skin Disorders*)
* *Trichodina, Trichodonella* and *Triparciella* (see also *Skin Disorders*)
* *Henneguya koi* (see also *Skin Disorders*)
* *Myxosoma dujardini.*

Parasitic

* *Dactylogyrus spp* (gill flukes)
* Glocchidia (larval freshwater mussels)
* *Ergasilus* (gill maggot – large crustacean parasite).

Neoplasia

* Gill neoplasia.

Other non-infectious problems

* Hypoxia (high stocking levels, high temperatures, low atmospheric pressure)
* Poor water quality; can cause gill damage that predisposes to bacterial gill disease
* Ammonia toxicity (see also *Neurological and Swimming Disorders*)
* Nitrite toxicity
* Malachite green toxicity
* Stress.

Findings on clinical examination

* Moderate to extreme respiratory effort
* Rapid gill ventilation
* Apparent gasping at water surface
* Haemorrhage from the gills in koi following handling (stress)
* Grey spots on gills and fins (*Glocchidia*, larval freshwater mussels)
* Mottled coloured gills, necrotic gills or patches of gills, weak, lethargic (branchiomycosis; severe bacterial gill disease; in carp, koi – KHV, gill necrosis virus) (Fig. 11.9)
* Mass deaths in koi only. Goldfish, rudd, orfe, etc., unaffected (KHV)
* Extensive gill damage and haemorrhage (*Sanguinicola inermis*)
* Damaged gills, obvious large parasites (*Ergasilus*)
* Excess mucous production, clamped fins, depression, sudden death (*Chilonodella, Ichthyobodo*)
* Clamped fins, scratching and flashing; inactivity (gill flukes)
* Thickened gills, mucous trailing from gills (bacterial gill disease)

Fig. 11.9. Gill lesions of koi herpes virus (KHV).

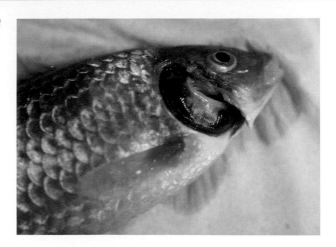

- Dusty effect over body surface (*Oodinium* – velvet disease)
- Cystic nodules on the gills (*Myxosoma dujardini, Henneguya koi*)
- Permissive temperature range for KHV (18–25°C)
- Brown discolouration of gills (nitrite toxicity – methaemoglobin formation).

Investigations

1. Water-quality tests especially ammonia, nitrite, nitrate, pH, temperature
2. Check dissolved oxygen levels
3. Gill scrape ('wet' prep under light microscope)
4. Radiography
5. Routine haematology and biochemistry
6. Culture and sensitivity
7. PCR for KHV
8. Endoscopy
9. Biopsy
   a. Gill and other organs: typical intranuclear inclusions for KHV. *Note* also seen with carp pox (CHV)
10. Ultrasonography
11. Water-quality parameters – check temperature, ammonia, nitrite, nitrate and pH values.

Management

1. See *Nursing Care*
2. Improve water quality
3. Vigorous aeration.

Treatment/specific therapy

- Ammonia toxicity
  - Partial water changes to dilute the ammonia levels
  - Adding zeolite will absorb large quantities of ammonia
  - Longer-term control may include addition of commercially available *Nitrosomonas* bacterial cultures or equivalent
- Nitrite toxicity
  - Add salt to the water to a concentration of 0.3%, the equivalent of 3.0 kg/1000 L, can be beneficial (chloride ions compete with the absorption of nitrite ions)
  - Partial water changes
  - Addition of extra bacterial (*Nitrobacter*) cultures in the form of commercially available freeze-dried or suspended cultures may be of some benefit
  - Dietary vitamin C may have a protective function, although its effect is less than that of salt
- Malachite green toxicity
  - Improved management only
  - Malachite green binds irreversibly to respiratory enzymes so increased aeration may not be beneficial
- Hypoxia
  - Increase water turnover by use of pumps and airstones to maximize gaseous exchange at the surface
  - Reduce stocking density
  - Pump liquid oxygen into water
- Gill necrosis virus: no treatment
- Koi herpes virus
  - No treatment
  - Reducing temperatures to below the permissive range may halt mortalities
  - Koi can be 'vaccinated' by exposing them to the virus at 23°C for 3–5 days and then transferring these fish to water held at the non-permissive temperature of 30°C. Such koi usually have high levels of KHV virus-specific antibodies
- Bacterial gill disease
  - Correct any underlying environmental problem
  - Chloramine-T at 10 mg/L – use less in soft water, down to 2 mg/L
  - Appropriate antibiosis
- Branchiomycosis
  - No known effective antifungals
  - Consider itraconazole at 1.0–5.0 mg/kg p.o. every 1–7 days, either in feed or gavage
- *Chilonodella*
  - Proprietary ectoparasitic medications
  - Glacial acetic acid dips at 8 mL per gallon for 30–45 s. May kill weak fish
  - *Chilonodella* prefers temperatures of 18–22°C, but for *Chilonodella cyprini* temperatures of 5–10°C seem to be close to its optimum
- *Ichthyobodo necator (Costia necatrix)*
  - Usual ectoparasitic treatments
  - Remove all of the fish from the infected aquarium for 24–48 h, as the parasite can only survive of the host for a few hours
  - *Ichthyobodo* is able to survive temperatures down to 2°C and can cause mortalities in overwintering carp

- *Oodinium* (velvet disease)
  - Proprietary velvet treatment
  - Metronidazole at 50 mg/L for up to 24 h daily for 10 days
  - Quinine hydrochloride at 10–20 mg/L indefinitely. Some fish sensitive to this
  - The encysted stage is relatively resistant to chemical attack
  - Can colonize the intestines of fish, where again it can be protected from medications
  - Antibiotic cover should be considered as secondary infections are common at the areas where the skin is damaged
  - Eliminate the parasite from a show aquarium by removing all fish, reducing or cutting out the light levels and raising the temperature to 30–32°C for 3 weeks
- *Ichthyophthirius multifilis* – white spot
  - Proprietary white spot remedy
  - Raising water temperature 1 or 2°C speeds up life cycle, promoting the exposure of the chemical-sensitive motile theront stage
- *Trichodina, Trichodonella* and *Triparciella*
  - Proprietary ectoparasitic medication
- *Myxosoma dujardini* and *Henneguya koi*
  - No effective treatment
- *Glocchidia* (larval freshwater mussels). Usually self-limiting. Larvae only transiently parasitic
- Flukes (skin, gill)
  - Proprietary ectoparasitic preparations
  - *Praziquantel* at 10 mg/kg by mouth or at 10 mg/L for a 3 h bath
  - *Dactylogyrus spp* are egg layers; the egg stage is resistant to treatment so praziquantel should be repeated every 2–4 weeks depending upon temperature, for at least 3 doses
- *Sanguinicola*
  - *Praziquantel* at 10 mg/kg in food
  - Control of snail intermediate hosts were possible
- Ergasilus
  - Individual removal of parasites
  - Organophosphates (where legal to do so)
  - Ivermectin at 0.1–0.2 mg/kg i.m. May be toxic to goldfish; may be persistent in environment
  - Treat with lufenuron (Program, Novartis) at 0.088 mg/L as a once only treatment.

Gastrointestinal tract disorders

Protozoal

- *Eimeria spp*, esp. *E. carpelli* and *E. subepithelialis* (young carp and koi).

Parasitic

- Nematodes
  - *Camallanus spp*
  - *Raphidascaris acus* (Dezfuli et al 2000)
- Helminths
  - *Bothriocephalus spp*
  - *Khawia spp.*

Nutritional

- Constipation/ diarrhoea (esp. fancy goldfish) (see also *Nutritional Disorders*)

Neoplasia

- Bucco-pharyngeal neoplasia
- Gill neoplasia
- Intestinal adenocarcinoma.

Other non-infectious disorders

- Foreign body, e.g. piece of gravel (especially goldfish).

Findings on clinical examination

- Emaciation, sunken eyes
- Diarrhoea
- Anorexia
- Long trails of faeces; may contain gas bubbles. Loss of balance (constipation/ diarrhoea)
- Weight loss; 'big-head' in carp. Swollen abdomen. May cause mass mortalities in young koi (tapeworms)
- Obvious red worms protruding from anus, especially with livebearers. Ulceration around anus may be apparent. Weight loss (*Camallanus*)
- Dysphagia (bucco-pharyngeal neoplasia, pharyngeal foreign body)
- Swimming with mouth permanently open (pharyngeal foreign body).

Investigations

1. Light microscopy
2. Faecal sample
   a. Floatation
3. Radiography
4. Routine haematology and biochemistry
5. Culture and sensitivity
6. Endoscopy
7. Biopsy/necropsy
   a. Larvae of *Raphidascaris acus* (European minnow *Phoxinus phoxinus*)
8. Ultrasonography
9. Water-quality parameters – check temperature, ammonia, nitrite, nitrate and pH values.

Treatment/specific therapy

- *Eimeria spp*
  - May respond to anticoccidial drugs such as amprolium as a continuous bath at 10 mg/L for 7–10 days or to sulphonamide antibiotics
- Constipation/diarrhoea
  - Feed higher fibre foods, e.g. shelled peas, live or frozen invertebrates, e.g. Daphnia or bloodworm (*Chironomus* larvae)

- Nematodes
  - Levamisol at 2 mg/L for up to 24 h
  - Fenbendazole at 20 mg/kg body weight given 7 days apart
  - Mebendazole at 20 mg/kg for 3 treatments given at weekly intervals
  - *Camallanus* has both a direct and indirect life cycle (small crustaceans, e.g. cyclops act as intermediate hosts)
- Tapeworms
  - *Praziquantel* at 10 mg/kg in food
  - Control of intermediates
    - *Bothriocephalus*: intermediate stages in copepods
    - *Khawia*: intermediate stages in Tubulicid worms
- Neoplasia
  - Usually inoperable by the time is identified
  - Accessible tumours may be managed by injecting cisplatin directly into the tissue mass on a weekly basis as a debulking exercise.

Nutritional disorders

- Hypovitaminosis E (Sekoke disease) (carp/koi)
  - Wasting when fed on vitamin E deficient diet – classically a diet of silkworm larvae only
  - Supplement with vitamin E or feed a commercially complete diet
- Hypovitaminosis C
  - Poor immune function; spinal deformities, possibly secondary to effects of collagen and cartilage integrity
- Hepatic lipidosis
  - Too high a protein and carbohydrate diet; often fed to achieve maximum growth rates in koi
  - Switch to lower energy foods and supplement with vitamin E
- Constipation/diarrhoea
  - Difficult in practice to distinguish between the two
  - Typically a problem with fancy goldfish characterized by long trails of faeces
  - Gas bubbles may be present in the faeces; in the gut these may cause a loss of balance, mimicking swimbladder disease
  - Feed higher fibre foods, e.g. shelled peas, live or frozen invertebrates, e.g. Daphnia or bloodworm (*Chironomus* larvae).

Hepatic disorders

Protozoal

- *Chloromyxum cyprini* and *C. koi*.

Nutritional

- Hepatic lipidosis (see *Nutritional Disorders*).

Neoplasia

- Hepatocellular tumours.

Findings on clinical examination

- Vague signs of ill-health
- Unexpected mortalities in 'healthy' fish
- Large females particularly susceptible (hepatic lipidosis)
- Incidental finding of protozoa in gall bladder (*Chloromyxum spp*).

Investigations

1. Radiography
2. Routine haematology and biochemistry
3. Culture and sensitivity
4. Endoscopy
5. Biopsy
6. Ultrasonography
7. Water-quality parameters – check temperature, ammonia, nitrite, nitrate and pH values.

Treatment/specific therapy

- Hepatic neoplasia
  - Usually no viable treatment – often sizable by the time of diagnosis
- *Chloromyxum spp*
  - Usually incidental finding. No effective treatment.

Pancreatic disorders

Parasitic

- Nematodes.

Neoplasia

Findings on clinical examination

- Vague signs of ill-health
- May be incidental finding.

Investigations

1. Radiography
2. Routine haematology and biochemistry
3. Culture and sensitivity
4. Endoscopy
5. Biopsy
6. Ultrasonography
7. Water-quality parameters – check temperature, ammonia, nitrite, nitrate and pH values.

- Nematodes (see *Gastrointestinal Tract Disorders*).

Cardiovascular and haematological disorders

Bacterial

- Endocarditis.

Protozoal

- Haemoparasites (see *Systemic Disorders*)
- *Trypanoplasma borreli* (see also *Urinary Disorders*)
- *Trypanosoma carassii*
- *Trypanosoma danilewskyi*.

Parasitic

- *Sanguinicola inermis* (see *Respiratory Tract Disorders*).

Neoplasia

Other non-infectious problems

- Cardiomyopathy.

Findings on clinical examination

- Apparent respiratory disease secondary to anaemia (see also *Respiratory Tract Disorders*)
- Ascites, bloated abdomen
- Exophthalmus (see also *Ophthalmic Disorders*).

Investigations

1. Radiography
2. Routine haematology and biochemistry
   a. Cytology – stained blood smears for haemoparasites
3. Culture and sensitivity
4. Endoscopy
5. Biopsy/necropsy
6. Ultrasonography
7. Water quality parameters – check temperature, ammonia, nitrite, nitrate and pH values.

Management

- See *Nursing Care*
- Keeping fish in a permanent 5 g/L solution of salt (not table or rock salt) will reduce the osmotic load on a sick koi or goldfish.

- Vegetative endocarditis
  - Antibiotics
  - Guarded prognosis
- Haemoparasites
  - Methylene blue by mouth at 60 mg/kg per day for 4 days
  - Metronidazole at 50 mg/kg per day
  - Note that the leech *Piscicola geometra* acts as a vector for *Trypanosoma danilewskyi.*

Systemic disorders

Viral

- Spring viraemia of carp virus (SVC) (*Rhabdovirus*)
- Lymphocystis (*Iridovirus*). Usually forms masses on skin, but rarely occurs in coelom (see *Skin Disorders*)
- Cyprinid herpes virus 1 (in carp fry <8 weeks old) (see also *Skin Disorders*)
- Infectious haematopoetic necrosis virus (IHN) (herpes virus) in goldfish.

Bacterial

- Mycobacteriosis (see *Musculoskeletal Disorders*)
- Septicaemia
- Typically *Aeromonas spp, Pseudomonas spp Flavibacterium spp.* Rarely *Vibrio cholerae.*

Fungal

- *Ichthyophonus hoferi* (see also *Neurological and Swimming Disorders, Ophthalmic Disorders* and *Skin Disorders*).

Protozoal

- Haemoparasites
- *Trypanosoma spp*
- *Trypanoplasma borreli* (Bunnajirakul et al 2000)
- *Hoferrellus carassii* (goldfish only – see *Urinary Disorders*).

Nutritional

- Vitamin E deficiency (Sekoke disease).

Neoplasia

- Gonadal neoplasia (see *Reproductive Disorders*)
- Liver neoplasia
- Renal neoplasia, polycystic kidney disease (see *Urinary Disorders*)
- Oral/pharyngeal neoplasia (fish unable to feed).

Other non-infectious problems

- Polycystic renal disease (goldfish – see *Urinary Disorders*)
- Metabolic acidosis/delayed capture mortality.

Findings on clinical examination

- Lethargy
- Wasting (mycobacteriosis, haemoparasites, neoplasia (especially oral), hypovitaminosis E). See also *Gastrointestinal Tract Disorders*.
- Wasting, darkening of skin colour and obvious boil-like swellings in the skin. Also exophthalmia, abnormal behaviour and swimming patterns *(Ichthyophonus hoferi)*.
- Swollen abdomen:
  - Haemorrhages, mucoid faecal casts from rectum. Lethargy. Seen in carp, koi, goldfish, grass carp and tench. Occasionally pike *(Esox)* and Wels catfish *(Siluris glanis* (SVC). Differentiate from non-SVC ascites
  - Scales protruding, haemorrhages. *(Ascites* – known to aquarists as *dropsy)* Usually secondary to multi-organ failure especially heart, gill and kidney disease
  - Goldfish only. Scales not protruding. *(Hoferellus carassii*, polycystic renal disease)
  - Non-symmetrical swelling, ulceration, loss of balance (internal neoplasia)
  - Exophthalmus, swimming disorders ('sleeping sickness') in carp *(T. borreli)*
- Mass mortalities in young (<8 weeks old) carp fry. Typically show swimming abnormalities, haemorrhages, swollen abdomen (CHV-1) (Sano et al 1991)
- Listlessness, followed by mortalities (IHN)
- Following a difficult capture, fish may exhibit incoordination, weakness, poor vision and mortalities (often several days later) (metabolic acidosis) (see Jepson 2001)
- Tumours.

Investigations

1. Radiography
2. Routine haematology and biochemistry
   a. Cytology/blood smears (haemoparasites)
   b. Anaemia (haemoparasites)
3. Culture and sensitivity
4. PCR test for SVC (notifiable in UK)
5. Virus isolation for SVC
6. Endoscopy
7. Biopsy
8. Ultrasonography
9. Water-quality parameters – check temperature, ammonia, nitrite, nitrate and pH values.

Treatment/specific therapy

- Bacterial disease
  - Appropriate antibiosis
- Haemoparasites
  - Methylene blue by mouth at 60 mg/kg per day for 4 days
  - Metronidazole at 50 mg/kg per day

- Spring viraemia of carp. No effective treatment
- IHN. No effective treatment. Usually a post-mortem diagnosis
- Neoplasia
  - Surgery or euthanasia
- Ascites
  - Poor prognosis
  - Often involves multi-organ failure
  - Attempt to correct osmotic imbalance by keeping in either salt solution (0.55%) or magnesium sulphate solution
  - Often bacterial in origin so consider antibiotics
- Lymphocystis
  - No treatment – usually self-limiting but may cause significant problems internally
- *Ichthyophonus hoferi*
  - No efficacious treatment available
- Cyprinid herpes virus 1
  - No efficacious treatment available
- Metabolic acidosis
  - Difficult to treat; best avoided by patient, low stress capture techniques involving two nets (use one net to guide the fish towards the other).

Musculoskeletal disorders

Bacterial

- Mycobacteriosis (fish tuberculosis). Primarily *Mycobacterium marinum, M. fortuitum, M. cheloni,* occ. other *Mycobacterium spp* implicated.

Fungal

- *Dermocystidium koi.*

Nutritional

- Hypovitaminosis C (see *Nutritional Disorders*)
- Tryptophan deficiency
- Sekoke disease (see *Nutritional Disorders*).

Neoplasia

Other non-infectious problems

- Electrocution (see *Neurological Disorders*)
- Organophosphate exposure
- Trauma.

Findings on clinical examination

- Spinal curvature/scoliosis (*Mycobacteriosis*, electrocution, trauma, hypovitaminosis C, tryptophan deficiency, organophosphates)
- Open skin sores, wasting and protruding eyes with or without spinal curvature (*Mycobacteriosis*)
- Cysts in skin and muscles (*Dermocystidium*).

Investigations

1. Radiography
2. Routine haematology and biochemistry
3. Culture and sensitivity
4. Endoscopy
5. Biopsy
6. Ultrasonography
7. Water-quality parameters – check temperature, ammonia, nitrite, nitrate and pH values.

Treatment/specific therapy

- Mycobacteriosis
  - Antibiotic treatment often not very effective
  - Kanamycin at 50 mg/L every 48 h for 4 treatments was successful in guppies (Conroy & Conroy 1999)
  - Consider euthanasia, especially due to zoonotic risk.
- *Dermocystidium koi*
  - See *Skin Disorders*
- Spinal curvature/scoliosis
  - Treatment difficult. Surgical internal fixation to stabilize condition has been attempted (Govett et al 2004)
- Tryptophan deficiency
  - Supplement with tryptophan.

Neurological and swimming disorders

Viral

- Spring viraemia of carp (swimbladder inflammation) (see *Systemic Disorders*).

Bacterial

- Central nervous system infection/granuloma.

Fungal

- *Ichthyophonus hoferi*
- Central nervous system infection/granuloma.

Protozoal

- Myxosporidea (see also *Skin Disorders*)
- *Myxosoma encephalina*
- *Sphaerospora renicol.*

Neoplasia

- Internal neoplasia compressing swimbladder.

Other non-infectious problems

- Electrocution/lightning strike (sudden onset spinal deformities, sudden death, especially in pond fish) (Pasnik et al 2003)

- Whirling and erratic swimming. Dark or accentuating colouring, weight loss, and fin rot. There may be obvious nodules (Myxosporidea)
- Poor water quality especially high ammonia and/or nitrite levels. New tank/pond syndrome
- Sudden onset poisoning, e.g. zinc (galvanized buckets, etc.), pesticides
- Swimbladder dysfunction. A particular problem with fancy goldfish. Often due to anatomical malformation of swimbladder in fancy breeds of goldfish, but can be due to infection (bacterial, fungal) or compression from surrounding organs, e.g. gonadal neoplasia
- Abnormal swimbladder functioning secondary to compression from internal space-occupying lesions, e.g. neoplasia
- Swimbladder torsion.

Findings on clinical examination

- Sudden darting movements, loss of balance, rapid respiration (water-quality, poisoning)
- Loss of balance. Unable to swim down from surface or up from bottom (swimbladder dysfunction, enteritis, SVC)
- Swimbladder signs but in carp fry (*Sphaerospora*)
- Wasting, darkening of skin colour and obvious boil-like swellings in the skin. Also exophthalmia, abnormal behaviour and swimming patterns (*Ichthyophonus*)
- Abnormal swimming posture, whirling (*Myxosporidea, Myxosoma encephalina*).

Investigations

1. Water quality tests
2. Radiography
   a. Swimbladder disease (Figs 11.10–11.12)
3. Routine haematology and biochemistry
4. Culture and sensitivity
5. PCR test for SVC (notifiable in UK)
6. Virus isolation for SVC
7. Endoscopy
8. Biopsy
9. Ultrasonography
10. Water-quality parameters – check temperature, ammonia, nitrite, nitrate and pH values.

Management

- Maintain optimum water conditions.

Treatment/specific therapy

- Poor water quality
  - Address which parameter(s) are abnormal. Multiple partial water changes often beneficial in short-term. Many need to review stocking, filtration system or husbandry management

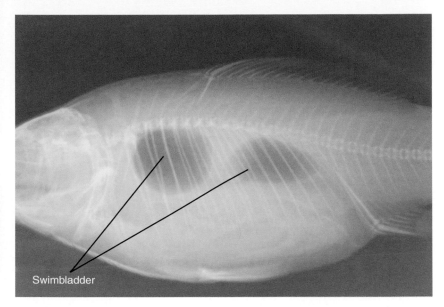

Swimbladder

Fig. 11.10. Comparative radiograph of a normal goldfish showing relative size and position of the cranial and caudal sections of the swimbladder (labelled).

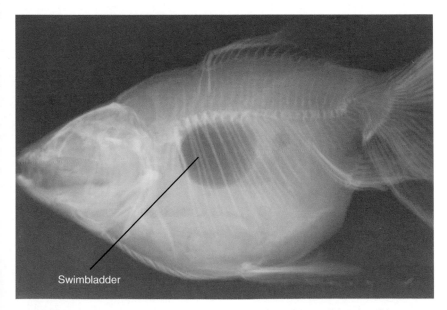

Swimbladder

Fig. 11.11. Same view of a fantail goldfish showing poor inflation of the caudal portion of the swimbladder.

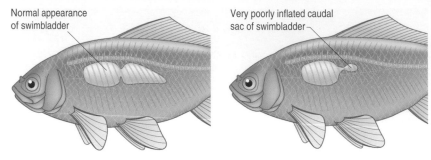

Fig. 11.12. Diagrammatic explanation of Figures 11.10 and 11.11.

- Ammonia toxicity
- Partial water changes to dilute the ammonia levels
  - Adding zeolite will absorb large quantities of ammonia
  - Longer-term control may include addition of commercially available *Nitrosomonas* bacterial cultures or equivalent
- Swimbladder disease
  - Usually no effective treatment for fancy goldfish. May develop ulceration on areas persistently floating above water level
  - Pneumocystocentesis can provide temporary relief but the problem is likely to recur
  - Try antibiotics if suspect bacterial infection
  - If goldfish is floating can implant small sterile counterweight into ventral coelomic cavity, but is difficult to judge correct weight
  - Pneumocystoplasty has been attempted (Britt et al 2002) and with refinement could prove useful
  - Enteritis may trigger gas formation in the gut mimicking swimbladder dysfunction. Offer high-fibre feeds such as live or frozen bloodworm or daphnia
  - Surgical removal of internal neoplasia.
- SVC (see *Systemic Disorders*)
- Swimbladder torsion
  - Surgical correction
- *Sphaeropsora renicola*
  - Fumigillin at 1 g/kg food for 10–14 days for prevention
- Myxosporidea/*Myxosoma encephalina*
  - No effective treatment. Try fumigilin as above
- *Ichthyophonus hoferi*
  - No efficacious treatment available
- Central nervous system infection/granuloma
  - Attempt antibiotic or antimycotic treatment. Poor prognosis
- Electric shock
  - Supportive treatment.

Ophthalmic disorders

Viral

- Grass carp rheovirus (grass carp *Ctenopharyngodon idella*) (see *Skin Disorders*).

Bacterial

- Mycobacteriosis (see also *Musculoskeletal Disorders* and *Skin Disorders*)
- Retrobulbar granuloma
- Bacterial keratitis (often cytophaga-like bacteria).

Fungal

- *Fusarium spp* (see also *Skin Disorders*)
- *Ichthyophonus hoferi.* See also *Neurological and Swimming Disorders, Skin Disorders* and *Systemic Disorders*
- Retrobulbar granuloma.

Protozoal

- *Ichthyophthirius.*

Parasitic

- *Diplostomum* (intermediate stage of avian tapeworm).

Nutritional

- Riboflavin deficiency
- Ascorbic acid deficiency
- Hypovitaminosis A.

Neoplasia

- Retrobulbar neoplasm.

Other non-infectious problems

- Overgrowth of the eye by the hood in certain breeds of fancy goldfish such as lionheads and orandas (Fig. 11.13)

Fig. 11.13. Overgrowth of the eye by the hood of an oranda goldfish.

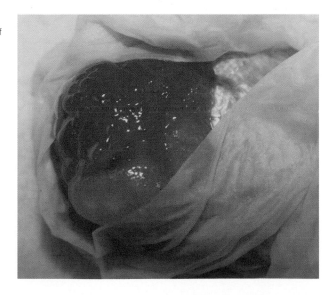

- Gas bubble disease (see *Skin Disorders*)
- Cataracts
- Erythrophoroma
- Cardiomyopathy.

Findings on clinical examination

- Exophthalmia (grass carp rheovirus, SVC, retrobulbar mass, cardiomyopathy)
- Opacity of the cornea – keratitis
- Opacity of lens in eye
- Corneal ulceration
- Blindness. Fish may be able to compensate to some extent by use of lateral line
- Exophthalmia accompanied by wasting, darkening of skin colour and obvious boil-like swellings in the skin, abnormal behaviour and swimming patterns (*Ichthyophonus hoferi*)
- Gas bubbles around and behind eye (gas bubble disease)
- Glaucoma (usually secondary to intraocular disease)
- Overgrowth of both eyes by exuberant growth of the hood in fancy goldfish.

Investigations

1. Ophthalmic examination
2. Radiography
3. Routine haematology and biochemistry
4. Culture and sensitivity
5. PCR test for SVC (notifiable in UK)
6. Virus isolation for SVC
7. Endoscopy
8. Biopsy
9. Ocular ultrasonography
10. Water-quality parameters – check temperature, ammonia, nitrite, nitrate and pH values.

Treatment/specific therapy

- *Ichthyophonus hoferi*
  - No efficacious treatment available
- *Diplostomum*
  - No effective treatment
  - Consider praziquantel at 10 mg/kg body weight by mouth; as a 1–2 h bath at 15–20 mg/L. With larger fish, in-feed medication at a rate of 400 mg/100 g food daily for 7 days. This should eliminate the cestode but there is unlikely to be any resolution of ocular damage
  - Attempt to break life cycle by:
    - Control of aquatic snails as source of disease
    - Prevent predation by birds (primary hosts)
- Glaucoma
  - Enucleation

- Cataracts
  - Ageing change; occasionally can be due to nutritional deficiencies, e.g. riboflavin or parasitism, but these are rare
  - In globe-eyed goldfish is very common
- Corneal ulceration
  - Systemic antibiosis
  - Scarification and application of tissue glue can protect the cornea and aid re-epithelialization
- Erythrophoroma
  - If partially or completely covering the cornea then a superficial keratectomy may be necessary. Treat subsequently as for corneal ulceration
- Overgrowth of hood
  - Resect part of hood covering eye under GA.

Urinary disorders

Bacterial

- Nephritis.

Protozoal

- *Hoferrellus carassii* (goldfish)
- *Hoferellus cyprini* (carp)
- *Trypanoplasma borreli* (Meyer et al 2002) (see *Cardiovascular and Haematological Disorders*).

Neoplasia

Other non-infectious problems

- Polycystic renal disease (goldfish).

Findings on clinical examination

- Lethargy
- Ascites
- Swollen abdomen in goldfish. Loss of balance. Scales not protruding (*Hoferellus carassii*, polycystic renal disease) (differentiate from Ascites – see *Systemic Disorders*)
- Carp cease feeding, are 'off colour', deaths after 7–14 days (*H. cyprini*)
- Abdominal distension, exophthalmus, swimming disorders ('sleeping sickness') (*T. borreli*).

Investigations

1. Radiography
2. Routine haematology and biochemistry
3. Culture and sensitivity
4. Endoscopy
5. Biopsy/necropsy

a. Progressive nephritis (*T. borreli*)
b. Dilated renal tubules and collecting ducts. Trophozoites or spores visible (*H. carassii*)
c. Trophozoites or spores visible (*H. cyprini*)
6. Ultrasonography
7. Water-quality parameters – check temperature, ammonia, nitrite, nitrate and pH values.

Treatment/specific therapy

- Polycystic renal disease
  - Genetic disorder – autosomal recessive. No treatment
- *Hoferellus spp*
  - No reliable treatment
  - Try toltrazuril at 30 mg/L as a 60-min bath e.o.d. for 3 treatments
  - Intermediate stages found in Tubulicid worms
- Trypanoplasma – see *Cardiovascular and Haematological Disorders*.

Reproductive disorders

Neoplasia

- Ovarian neoplasia
- Testicular neoplasia.

Other non-infectious problems

- Egg retention.

Findings on clinical examination

- Pronounced swelling of the coelomic cavity; may be asymmetrical (gonadal neoplasia) or symmetrical (egg retention)
- Other differentials for a symmetrical swollen coelom
  - Scales not prominent (in goldfish consider also *Hoferellus*, polycystic kidney disease – see *Urinary Disorders*)
  - Scales prominent – ascites (see *Systemic Disorders*).

Investigations

1. Radiography
2. Routine haematology and biochemistry
3. Culture and sensitivity
4. Endoscopy
5. Biopsy
6. Ultrasonography
7. Water-quality parameters – check temperature, ammonia, nitrite, nitrate and pH values.

Treatment/specific therapy

- Gonadal neoplasia
  - Surgical resection
- Egg retention.

Treatment of egg retention

Goldfish

1. Buserelin at a 1:10 dilution applied to the gills.
2. Human chorionic gonadotrophin (hCG) at 700–1000 IU/kg i.m.
3. In both cases, followed by manual stripping 6–12 h later.

Koi

1. In general koi will only respond to injections of carp pituitary extract.
2. Maintain temperature around 25°C.
3. Priming dose of 0.3 mg/kg of reconstituted carp pituitary extract.
4. Second dose of 3.0 mg/kg 12–18 h later.
5. Attempt manual stripping 6–12 h later.
6. Cool temperatures (<20°C) and/or lack of sufficient or large enough sexually active males contribute to the aetiology of this condition.
7. Koi may, however respond to GnRH analogues in combination with dopamine antagonists, e.g. domperidone or metoclopramide (Patino 1997).

References

Britt T, Weisse C, Weber S et al 2002 Use of pneumocystoplasty for overinflation of the swim bladder in a goldfish. J Am Vet Med Assoc 221(5):690–693

Bunnajirakul S, Steinhagen D, Hetzel U et al 2000 A study of histopathology of Trypanoplasma borreli (Protozoa: Kinetoplastida) in susceptible common carp Cyprinus carpio. Dis Aquat Organ 39(3):221–229

Conroy G, Conroy D A 1999 Acid-fast bacterial infection and its control in guppies (Lebistes reticulatus) reared on an ornamental fish farm in Venezuela. Vet Rec 144:177–178

Dezfuli B S, Simoni E, Rossi R et al 2000 Rodlet cells and other inflammatory cells of Phoxinus phoxinus infected with Raphidascaris acus (Nematoda). Dis Aquat Organ 43 (1):61–69

Govett P D, Olby N J, Marcellin-Little D J et al 2004 Stabilisation of scoliosis in two koi (Cyprinus carpio) Vet Rec 155:115–119

Jepson L 2001 Koi medicine. Kingdom Books, Havant

Meyer C, Ganter M, Korting W et al 2002 Effects of a parasite-induced nephritis on osmoregulation in the common carp Cyprinus carpio. Dis Aquat Organ 8:50(2):127–135

Molnar K 2002 Differences between the European carp (Cyprinus carpio carpio) and the coloured carp (Cyprinus carpio haematopterus) in susceptibility to Thelohanellus nikolskii (Myxosporea) infection. Acta Vet Hung 50(1):51–57

Pasnik DJ, Smith S A, Wolf J C 2003 Accidental electroshock of fish in a recirculation facility. Veterinary Record 153:562–564

Patino R 1997 Manipulations of the Reproductive system of fishes by means of exogenous chemicals. Prog Fish Cult 59(1):18–128

Sano T, Morita N, Shima N et al 1991 Herpesvirus cyprini: lethality and oncogenicity. J Fish Dis 14:533–543

Yokohama H, Liyanage Y S, Sugai A et al 1999 Efficacy of fumagillin against haemorrhagic thelohanellosis caused by Thelohanellus hovorkai (Myxosporea:Myyxozoa) in coloured carp, Cyprinus carpio L. J Fish Dis 22:243–245

Tropical freshwater fish

CHAPTER 12

Around 80–90% of tropical freshwater fish are captive bred, with typical hot spots of production being Singapore (e.g. Fig. 12.1), Malaysia, Israel, Florida and the Czech and Slovak Republics. Some important fish to the industry are still wild-caught however, such as the cardinal tetra (*Paracheirodon axelrodi*) from the Amazon basin.

For general information on fish consultations, examination, nursing care and anaesthesia, see Chapter 11, *Goldfish and Koi*.

Recommended water quality parameters for different aquariums are listed in Table 12.1. Water hardness is measured in a variety of different ways with mg $CaCO_3$ as international standard. Conversion factors from other units are given in Table 12.2. Common species of tropical freshwater fish presented to the veterinarian are listed in Table 12.3.

Skin disorders

Structure and function of skin (see Ch. 11, *Goldfish and Koi*).

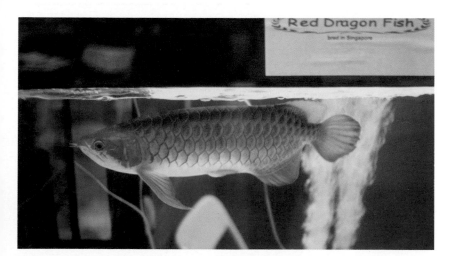

Fig. 12.1. The Asian Dragonfish (*Scleropages formosus*).

Table 12.1 Recommended parameters for: typical community aquarium; rift lake aquarium; discus aquarium

Parameter	Typical community aquarium	Rift lake aquarium (Lake Malawi/Tanganyika)	Discus aquarium
Temperature (°C)	22–26	22–26	26–30°C (higher for spawning)
pH	6.8–7.5	8.0–8.3	5.0–7.5 (lower range for wild caught discus)
General hardness (GH) (mg CaCO₃)	60–200	200+	50–100
Carbonate hardness (KH) (mg CaCO₃)	50–100	>80	20–80
Conductivity (µs/cm)	500–800	800+	180–480
Ammonia (total) (mg/L)	<0.02	<0.02 mg/L but the high pH requires ammonia should be 0.0 mg/L	<0.02
Nitrite (mg/L)	<0.02	<0.02	<0.02
Nitrate (mg/L)	<40 mg above ambient tapwater levels	<40 mg above ambient tapwater levels	<40 mg above ambient tapwater levels
Oxygen (mg/L)	5.0–8.0	5.0–8.0	5.0–8.0
Chlorine (mg/L)	<0.002	<0.002	<0.002

Table 12.2 Water hardness conversion factors

Unit	Conversion factor to (mg CaCO₃)
dH	17.85
Clark	0.07
f (French)	0.1
Hardness	1
Milliequivalent (mEq)	0.02

Differential diagnoses for skin disorders

Pruritus

- Ectoparasites
- Poor water quality.

Table 12.3 Common species of tropical freshwater fish: Key facts

Species	Temperature (°C)	pH	Hardness	Common disorders
Discus (*Symphysodon spp*)	26–30	5.0–7.5	Soft	*Capillaria, Hexamita* and *Spironucleus* are common diseases encountered with discus. 'Discus Plague' may be another up and coming disease
Angelfish (*Pterophyllum spp*)	23–28	6.5–7.6	Soft to medium hard (aquarium stocks)	*Capillaria*, gill flukes, *Hexamita* and *Spironucleus* can be troublesome. Also *Pleistophora* and bacterial infections occasionally. Deep angelfish herpes virus should be considered for unexplained deaths in this species
Oscar (*Astronotus occellatus*)	23–30	6.5–7.8	Moderately soft to moderately hard	Veil-tail varieties have their fins easily damaged and should be kept individually or in mated pairs. Very good at begging, this can lead to overfeeding and degeneration of water quality. *Hexamita* and *Spironucleus* can be a problem. Trauma from damage, with a consequent risk of bacterial or fungal infection. Many oscars die from poor water quality due to overfeeding and inadequate filtration
Rift Lake cichlids (originating from Lakes Malawi, Tanganyika and Victoria)	22–26	8.0–8.3	Hard to very hard	Many species such as the Mbuna group require a higher vegetable intake than cichlids from other continents and failure to provide this may predispose to gut-related problems. Also overfeeding leads to some individuals attaining a larger size than they would in the wild. Such 'giants' can dominate an aquarium leading to stress and trauma-related damage. Best kept in crowded communities where no one individual can dominate and where aggression is dissipated amongst a group. Bacterial diseases are common, as are external parasites such as white spot. *Cryptobia* is considered by many to the main cause of Malawi Bloat. Outbreaks of this may be related to an improper diet

Continued

Table 12.3 Common species of tropical freshwater fish: Key facts—cont'd

Species	Temperature (°C)	pH	Hardness	Common disorders
Arowanas; Dragonfish (*Osteoglossum* and *Scleropages spp*) (Fig.12.1)	24–30	6.5–7.5	Moderately soft to moderately hard	Many arowanas die either from poor water quality (high ammonia levels) or injuries sustained from leaping – either hitting the lid or lighting apparatus, or from periods spent drying outside of water. Common parasites include fish lice, anchor worm and white spot. Two common but poorly understood conditions in captive arowanas are overturned gill covers and 'drop eye'
Freshwater stingrays (*Potomotrygon spp*)	24–27	6.0–7.0	Soft to medium hard	The sting is often damaged during transit and can become infected – it may need removal under sedation. Stingrays will bite each other, especially during courtship and such bites can become secondarily infected. Fungal infections are common – usually *Saprolegnia*. Bacterial infections, especially of the fins around the disc, are also regularly seen. Protozoan parasites appear to be a rare problem, although fish lice such as *Argulus* and *Livoneca* may be seen on recently caught specimens. Very sick stingrays will often show obvious upward curling of the disc. Heater burns may be seen. These are live-bearers so dystocia is occasionally encountered

Erosions and ulceration including fin rot

- Bacterial disease, typically *Aeromonas spp*, cytophagic-like bacteria, *Flavobacterium spp*. Also mycobacteriosis (see *Musculoskeletal Disorders*)
- Ulceration, haemorrhage, darkening of colour and exophthalmus in cichlids (*Streptococcal* infections)
- Often secondary to trauma or ectoparasites (esp. *Tetrahymena, Ichthyobodo*)
- *Flexibacter columnaris*. Whitish erosive areas especially along back of fish, mouth fungus and shimmying (mollies) and tail rot (guppies). Sometimes known as false neon tetra disease when it occurs on small tetras
- In snakehead, striped snakehead skin ulcerative disease (*Rhabdovirus*)
- *Fusarium* Mycosis. May also cause blindness
- *Aphanomyces invadens* mycosis (epizootic ulcerative syndrome, EUS). Susceptible species include striped snakehead (*Channa striata*), giant gourami (*Osphronemus gouramy*) and silver barb (*Barbodes gonionotus*) (see Miles et al 2001)
- Channel catfish virus disease is a herpes virus that affects fry and fingerling catfish. Infected fish swim erratically, are pale with multiple skin haemorrhages, severe exophthalmia and swollen abdomens
- Lymphosarcoma (see *Neoplasia*).

Nodules and non-healing wounds

- Large, cauliflower-like masses on fins and skin (*Lymphocystis* – an iridovirus) (Fig. 12.2)
- Uneven skin surface in angelfish (*Pterophyllum spp*) (*Pleistophora*)
- Lip fibroma in angelfish (*Pterophyllum spp* suspected retrovirus; Francis-Floyd et al 1993)
- Obvious skin nodules (*Myxosporidea*, see below)
- Hole-in-the-head disease (head and lateral line disease) (*Spironucleus*). Especially in discus, angelfish, oscars and other cichlids. Ulceration on the head and along lateral line (see also *Gastrointestinal Tract Disorders*)
- Wasting, darkening of skin colour and obvious boil-like swellings in the skin; in extreme cases it may have a sandpaper effect, due to the large number of

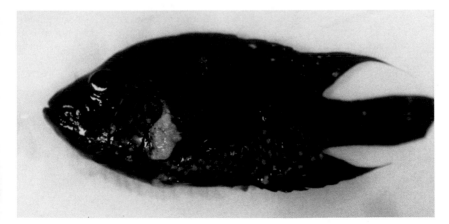

Fig. 12.2. Lymphocystis on a Texas cichlid (*Herichthys cyanoguttatum*).

granulomas present. Also exophthalmia, abnormal behaviour and swimming patterns (if the central nervous system is invaded) (*Ichthyophonus hoferi*). See also *Neurological and Swimming Disorders, Ophthalmic Disorders* and *Systemic Disorders*
- Pentastomids
- Gas-filled bubbles in the skin especially on the fins. Also occasionally behind the eye (gas bubble disease – usually secondary to oxygen supersaturation)
- Yellowish cystic lesions up to 5 mm diameter *Clinostomum spp*, a digenetic trematode (Wildgoose 1998).

Changes in pigmentation and colour
- Lethargy and reddened areas of skin. Fish stop feeding (bacterial septicaemia, *Edwardsiella ictaruli* in catfish)
- Obvious discrete white spots visible on skin and fins. *Ichthyophthirius multifilis* (white spot disease)
- Whitened areas of muscle, often accompanied by loss of colour, especially with neon tetras, other small tetras, killifish. Also may see emaciation and spinal curvature (*Pleistophora* – neon tetra disease). In white angelfish may cause localized accumulations of melanophores producing 'black holes'
- Dark or accentuating colouring, obvious nodules. weight loss, whirling and fin rot (*Myxosporidea*)
- Darkened colours, emaciation, abnormal swimming behaviour and mortalities in tilapia (Piscirickettsiosis-like organisms, PLOs). Some respiratory signs (gill hyperplasia)
- Enhanced colouration, especially Malawi cichlids (haemoparasites). May see wasting
- White tufts on surface that may resemble cotton wool (*Epistylis, Saprolegnia, Flexibacter columnaris*). *Note* that mucus strands hanging from the skin can strongly resemble *Saprolegnia*
- 'Mouth fungus' (along with fin-rot) is often described as a fungal infection, especially live-bearers such as mollies and guppies. This is usually due to cytophagiclike bacteria such as *Flexibacter columnaris*
- Greying skin (due to excessive mucus production). Ectoparasites – typically *Trichodina, Chilonodella, Ichthyobodo, Gyrodactylus, Dactylogyrus*
- Multiple small black spots in the skin and deeper in the muscles – so-called black spot disease. Digenetic trematodes, e.g. *Neascus*. The blackened cysts appear particularly obvious in light coloured fish such as silver dollars (*Metynnus argentius*)
- Darkening of body colouration, lethargy, loss of appetite, abdominal distension and mortalities in varieties of the three spot gourami (*Trichogaster trichopterus*). Also mortalities in the dwarf gourami (*Colisia lalia*) – an unspecified iridovirus
- Black spots – melanin concentrations – described in *Mycobacterium marinum* skin granulomas in *Oreochromis mossambassicus* (Noga et al 1990)
- Darkened colour, weight loss, excessive mucus production, rapid respiration, lethargy ('discus plague'). Discus, occasionally angelfish (*Pterophyllum* species) (see *Systemic Disorders*)
- Algal dermatitis in farmed *Metriaclima zebra* has been described associated with deep invasion and persistent skin infections with *Chlorochytrium* and *Scenedesmus spp* of algae
- Colour fading. Likely to be nutritional lack of appropriate carotenoids
- Planaria (flatworms) visible in aquaria. Rarely cause problems. Usually due to overfeeding. Consider praziquantel (toxic to corydoras catfish).

Ectoparasites

- Protozoa
  - *Ichthyophthirius multifilis* (white spot disease)
  - *Oodinium* (velvet disease). Dusty effect over body surface
  - *Tetrahymena*. Whitish areas or 'spots' often with ulceration. Commoner on live-bearers, cichlids (particularly dwarf cichlids) and tetras. Often associated with bacterial infections and white spot
  - *Icthyobodo necator (Costia necatrix)*. Common on catfish, killifish, anabantids, swordtails (*Xiphophorus spp*) and cichlids. See also *Respiratory Tract Disorders*
  - *Epistylis (Heteropolaria)*
  - *Chilonodella*
  - *Spironucleus*
  - *Trichodina, Trichodonella* and *Triparciella*
  - Myxosporidea including *Henneguya, Myxidium and Mitaspora*
- Helminths
  - *Gyrodactylus, Enterogyrus* and *Cichlidogyrus spp* (skin flukes)
  - Digenetic trematodes (black spot disease)
  - *Clinostomum spp*
  - Leeches
  - *Batracobdelloides tricarinata* (Negm-Eldin & Davies 1999) (see also *Cardiovascular and Haematological Disorders*)
  - Flatworms on glass and substrate (*Planaria*). Not parasitic, but may indicate over feeding
- Molluscs
  - *Anodonites trapesialis* (Silva-Souza & Eiras 2002)
- Crustaceans
  - *Argulus* (fish louse)
  - *Livoneca* (usually on wild caught South American fish) See also *Respiratory Tract Disorders*
- Pentastomes.

Neoplasia

- Lymphosarcoma. Start as nodules in the skin; eventually the overlying skin becomes devitalized and sloughs, leaving an ulcer. Internal lesions may also occur. Lymphosarcoma has been identified in pike (*Esox spp*) and Malawi cichlids (*Metriaclima spp*)
- *Xiphophorus* (swordtails and platies) hybrids are very prone to developing melanomas and neuroblastomas. *Note* that at least three viruses, a papovavirus and two retroviruses, have been implicated as predisposing factors
- Papillomas
- Odontomas appear as swellings around the mouth on freshwater angelfish (*Pterophyllum spp*)
- Lip fibroma in angelfish (*Pterophyllum spp* (suspected retrovirus – Francis-Floyd et al 1993).

Other findings on clinical examination

- Loss of fins and/or eyes
- Irritation, ulceration (ectoparasites)

- Breathing difficulties, irritation. Fins clamped. (*Ichthyophthirius, Oodinium, Trichodina* (see also *Respiratory Tract Disorders*)
- Clamped fins, depression, sudden death (*Chilonodella*)
- Slimey droppings, weight loss, no appetite, secondary infections (*Spironucleus*).

Investigations

1. Skin scrape under light microscopy (see 'Fig. 11.8', in *Goldfish and Koi*)
   a. Protozoa
      i. *Chilonodella* is a large protozoan (30–70 µm) that has an almost oval, flattened appearance. Obvious cilia; moves with gliding, slow circular movement
      ii. *Icthyobodo*: even on high power, a small coma-shaped, very mobile parasite seen gyrating through the water
      iii. *Oodinium:* can be quite large, up to 1.0 mm diameter, oval shaped with a very dark appearance because of chloroplasts. Not usually mobile
      iv. *Trichodina, Trichodonella* and *Tripartiella*: circular, rotating parasites around 40 µm
      v. *Ichthyophthirius*: large ciliate, horse-shoe shaped nucleus
      vi. *Epistylis*: stalked, cup-shaped ciliates in colonies
   b. Flukes
      i. Gyrodactylus: live-bearing; can usually see large H-shaped hooks of both adult and unborn young
      ii. Dactylogyrids: egg-layer. Usually four black spots at caudal end. Can be quite large flukes
   c. Fungi
      i. *Saprolegnia*: a meshwork of mycelium and fruiting bodies should be easily identifiable
      ii. *Ichthyophonus*: squash preparation of nodule. The spores can be readily seen as spherical bodies, varying from 10 to 100 µm in diameter. There is much variation in the appearance of these multinucleate spores
2. Radiography
3. Routine haematology and biochemistry
4. Culture and sensitivity
5. Endoscopy
6. Biopsy
7. Ultrasonography
8. Water-quality parameters – check temperature, ammonia, nitrite, nitrate and pH values.

Management

- See *Nursing Care.*

Treatment/specific therapy

- Gas bubble disease
  - Oxygen supersaturation usually secondary to pressurized oxygenation (waterfalls, malfunctioning venturi pumps, etc.), excess photosynthesis (high plant levels, suspended algae)

- Correct source of problem
- Rarely fatal – fish usually recover uneventfully
- Algal dermatitis
  - No treatment. Usually of no consequence to the fish
- *Lymphocystis*
  - No direct cure. Usually self-limiting
  - Ozone or ultraviolet sterilization may reduce spread
  - Attempted surgical removal is usually followed by recurrence
- Striped snakehead skin ulcerative disease (viral infection)
  - No treatment
- Channel catfish virus disease
  - No treatment
  - Covering antibiotics as it may be secondary infections that cause mortalities
- Bacterial infections
  - Antibiotics
  - Debridement of ulcers followed by packing with protective layer, e.g. Orabase (Squibb)
  - Change management system, e.g. separation of aggressive individuals, removal of damaging aquarium furniture, improved water quality
- *Flexibacter columnaris*
  - Antibiotics
  - Copper-based medications can work
  - Surfactants such as benzalkonium chloride are useful as a bath. *Note* that toxicity of benzalkonium chloride is increased in soft water so doses should be reduced if used in soft water (or if hardness not known) and the fish monitored closely for signs of distress
  - Recommended dose rate for benzalkonium chloride (Table 12.4)
  - Improved management
- Piscirickettsiosis-like organisms (PLOs)
  - Antibiotics
- Mycobacteriosis
  - Difficult to treat and potential zoonosis
  - Kanamycin at 50 mg/L every 48 h for 4 treatments was successful in guppies (Conroy & Conroy 1999)
- *Ichthyophonus hoferi*
  - No efficacious treatment available
- *Ichthyophthirius multifillis* white spot
  - Proprietary white spot remedy

Table 12.4 Recommended dose rate for benzalkonium chloride

Benzalkonium chloride concentration (mg/L)	Duration of bath (min)
10	5–10
5	30
2	60
1	Several hours

- Raising water temperature 1 or 2°C speeds up life cycle, promoting the exposure of the chemical-sensitive motile theront stage
- *Oodinium*
  - Proprietary velvet treatment
  - Metronidazole at 50 mg/L for up to 24 h daily for 10 days
  - Quinine hydrochloride at 10–20 mg/L indefinitely. *Some fish are sensitive*
  - The encysted stage is relatively resistant to chemical attack
  - Can colonize the intestines of fish, where again it can be protected from medications
  - Antibiotic cover should be considered as secondary infections are common at the areas where the skin is damaged
  - Eliminate the parasite from a show aquarium by removing all fish, reducing or cutting out the light levels and raising the temperature to 30–32°C for 3 weeks
- *Tetrahymena*
  - Predisposes to secondary infections
  - Often found associated with *Ichthyophthirius*
  - Poor environmental conditions (high ammonia, high organic load, low water temperatures) predispose (Pimenta Leibowitz et al 2005)
  - Try proprietary ectoparasitic medication. Can spread internally through the body musculature so treatment may not work
  - Chloramine-T at an average dose rate of 10 mg/L – use less in soft water, down to 2 mg/L
  - Recommended chloramine-T concentrations for different pH and water hardness combinations (Table 12.5)
- *Epistylis* (*Heteropolaria*)
  - Commercial ectoparasitic preparations
- Chilonodella
  - Proprietary ectoparasitic medications.
  - Glacial acetic acid dips at 8 mL/gallon for 30–45 s. May kill weak fish
- *Trichodina*
  - Proprietary ectoparasitic medication
  - Flukes (skin, gill)
  - Proprietary ectoparasitic preparations
  - *Praziquantel* at 10 mg/kg body weight by mouth; as a 1–2 hour bath at 15–20 mg/L. With larger fish, in-feed medication at a rate of 400 mg/100 g food daily for 7 days. *Toxic to corydoras catfish*

Table 12.5 Recommended chloramine-T concentrations for different pH and water hardness combinations

pH	Concentration in soft water (mg/L)	Concentration in hard water (mg/L)
6.0	2.5	7.0
6.5	5.0	10.0
7.0	10.0	15.0
7.5	18.0	18.0
8.0	20.0	20.0

- Dactylogyrids are egg-layers; the egg stage is resistant to treatment and so infestations require multiple treatments up to 4 weeks apart depending upon water temperature
- Digenetic trematodes
  - Complex life cycle involving a primary host such as a piscivorous bird, reptile or fish, and secondary snail hosts, so they rarely become a problem in aquaria
  - Treat with praziquantel as described above for skin flukes
  - Alternatively treat in a bath for 1 h with a combination of salt, acriflavine and formalin or in the aquarium with acriflavine and salt only for 36 h. *Care with corydoras catfish*
- Haemoparasites, e.g. *Trypanosoma spp*
  - Methylene blue by mouth at 60 mg/kg per day for 4 days, or metronidazole at 50 mg/kg per day
- Myxosporidea. No treatment available. Try fumagillin at 1 g/kg food for 10–14 days for prevention
- Neon tetra disease (*Pleistophora*)
  - No good treatment. Options would include:
    - Feeding a diet of 0.1% fumagillin
    - Toltrazuril at 30 mg/L as a 60-min bath e.o.d. for 3 treatments
    - Transmitted via consumption of infected cadavers or food crustaceans (cyclops)
- Spironucleus
  - Treat with metronidazole
  - Dimetridazole appears to be linked with sterility in fish
- Fusarium mycosis
  - No effective treatment
- *Aphanomyces invadens* (EUS)
  - No effective treatment
  - Temperature – dependant pathology; EUS not seen at 32°C but does occur at lower temperatures (20°C)
- Saprolegnia (fungal disease)
  - Proprietary medications containing malachite green
  - Remove visible hyphae and swab the affected area with a 10% povidone–iodine solution once daily
  - Maintain the fish in a salt solution, as this will not only help to control the fungal infection, but will also help with the osmotic imbalance resulting from the infection. Salt solutions as low as 10 parts per thousand (ppt) (mg/100 mL) will inhibit Saprolegnial infections. Ideally aim for 1–3 g/L as a permanent solution until the problem has resolved. *Care with corydoras catfish*
  - Usually secondary invader so may need to treat underlying ulceration and secondary bacterial infections
- *Anodonites trapesialis*
  - Larval stages described as parasitizing the epidermis of the cichlid *Tilapia rendalli* and the suckermouth catfish *Hypostomus regani* (Silva-Souza & Eiras 2002)
  - Little inflammatory response but multiple microscopic skin lesions may predispose secondary skin infections
  - Usually self-limiting. Larvae only transiently parasitic
- Fish louse (*Argulus*) or *Livoneca*
  - Individual removal of parasites
  - Treat with lufenuron (Program, Novartis) at 0.088 mg/L as a once only treatment

- Treat with organophosphates where legal
- Placing fish in a potassium permanganate bath at 10 p.p.m. (mg/L) for 5–60 min can be used to rid both individual fish and plants of this parasite. Care with sensitive species
- Pentastomids
  - No treatment
  - Prevent by removal of other hosts from life cycle especially reptile predators, e.g. turtles, snakes
- Discus plague
  - Unknown cause. No effective treatment. May be linked, or initiated by, stress
- Lip fibromas, odontomes, neoplasia
  - Debulking/surgical removal
  - Surgical debulking followed by injection of cisplatin directly into the tissue mass on a weekly basis.

Respiratory tract disorders

Note that many freshwater fish can utilize atmospheric air. Lungfish (*Protopterus spp*) anabantids (including the popular gouramies (*Trichogaster spp*), fighting fish (*Betta spp*) and paradisefish (*Macropodus spp*)) and some South American catfish such as *Hypostomus punctatus* and *corydoras* are common examples. Gulping for air in these species may not necessarily indicate a respiratory problem.

Bacterial

- Bacterial gill disease
- Piscirickettsiosis-like organisms (PLOs) in tilapia. See also *Skin Disorders*.

Fungal

- Fungal gill diseases.

Protozoal

- *Oodinium* (velvet disease) (see *Skin Disorders*)
- *Trichodina* (see *Skin Disorders*)
- *Ichthyophthirius* (white spot) (esp. catfish) (see *Skin Disorders*)
- *Icthyobodo necator* (*Costia necatrix*) (see also *Skin Disorders*)
- *Cryptobia iubilans* (indirect – respiratory signs secondary to anaemia – see *Systemic Disorders*)
- Myxosporidea including *Henneguya* (esp. corydoras catfish), *Myxidium* and *Myxobolus*.

Parasitic

- Helminths – Dactylogyrus (gill flukes)
- Crustaceans – *Livoneca*.

Neoplasia

- Gill tumours are common in *Poecilia* hybrids (molly-guppy).

Other non-infectious problems

- Hypoxia
- Ammonia toxicity (see also *Neurological Disorders*)

- Nitrite toxicity
- Malachite green toxicity
- Overturned operculae in dragonfish (*Sclerohages spp*) and arowanas (*Osteoglossum spp*)
- Complete or partial absence of operculae (unilateral or bilateral).

Findings on clinical examination

- Moderate to extreme respiratory effort
- Rapid gill ventilation
- Apparent gasping at water surface or at areas of high turbulence, e.g. water inlets (Fig. 12.3)
- Anaemia (chronic disease, *Cryptobia*)
- Breathing difficulties, dusty effect over body surface (*Oodinium*)
- White spots on skin/fins (*Ichthyophthirius*). White spots not always obvious

Fig. 12.3. A group of discus with high respiratory rates aggregate at the surface in one corner. Contrast this with the behaviour of fish in the other aquaria.

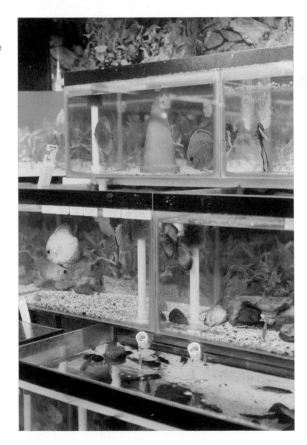

- Visible gill flukes
- Respiratory distress, clamped fins, flashing. One-sided breathing in discus (*Dactylogyrus*)
- Fish usually appear depressed, fins clamped shut, may 'wobble' as they swim or even 'shimmy', skin appears dull and greyish; ulceration may be seen, respiratory signs (*Ichthyobodo*)
- Brown colour to gills (nitrite toxicity)
- Respiratory signs, darkened colours, emaciation, abnormal swimming behaviour and mortalities in tilapia (piscirickettsiosis-like organisms, PLOs)
- Large woodlouse-resembling parasite (*Livoneca*). Up to 2.5 cm long; the adult parasites burrow into the gills and mouth cavity but they may also attach and burrow into the flank. *Livoneca* are protoandrous hermaphrodites. The larger female is often found in the mouth, while the smaller male is attached to the gills
- The soft edging to the operculum gradually curls outward and can become permanently deformed (overturned operculae).

Investigations

1. Gill scrape under light microscopy
   a. Thickening of the secondary lamellae (gill hyperplasia)
   b. Large ciliate, horse-shoe shaped nucleus (*Ichthyophthirius*)
   c. *Chilonodella* is a large protozoan (30–70 μm) that has an almost oval, flattened appearance. Obvious cilia; moves with gliding, slow circular movement
   d. *Oodinium*: can be quite large, up to 1.0 mm diameter, oval shaped with a very dark appearance because of chloroplasts. Not usually mobile
   e. Circular, rotating parasites around 40 μm (*Trichodina*, *Trichodonella* and *Triparciella*)
2. Radiography
3. Routine haematology and biochemistry
4. Culture and sensitivity
5. Endoscopy
6. Biopsy
7. Ultrasonography
8. Water-quality parameters
   a. Check temperature, ammonia, nitrite, nitrate and pH values
   b. Recommended levels of oxygen are above 6.0 mg/L at 25°C for tropical freshwater fish.

Management

- Improve circulation and/or aeration.

Treatment/specific therapy

- Ammonia toxicity
  - Partial water changes to dilute the ammonia levels
  - Adding zeolite will absorb large quantities of ammonia
  - Longer-term control may include addition of commercially available *Nitrosomonas* bacterial cultures or equivalent

- Nitrite toxicity
  - Partial water changes
  - Salt (chloride ions compete with nitrite binding sites at the gills). Ideally aim for 1–3 g/L as a permanent solution until the problem has resolved. *Care with corydoras catfish*
  - Commercially available *Nitrobacter* cultures (long term)
- Malachite green toxicity
  - Improved management only
  - Malachite green binds irreversibly to respiratory enzymes so increased aeration may not be beneficial
- Bacterial gill disease
  - Correct any underlying environmental problem
  - Consider surfactants such as:
    - Chloramine-T (see 'Tetrahymena', in *Skin Disorders*)
    - Benzalkonium chloride (see 'Flexibacter', in *Skin Disorders*)
- Fungal gill disease
  - As for bacterial gill disease
  - Salt at 1–3 g/L as a permanent solution until the problem has resolved if *Saprolegnia* involved. *Care with corydoras catfish*
- Piscirickettsiosis-like organisms
  - Antibiotics
- *Oodinium* (velvet disease) (see *Skin Disorders*)
- *Chilonodella*
  - Proprietary ectoparasitic medications
  - Glacial acetic acid dips at 8 mL/gallon for 30–45 s. May kill weak fish
  - *Chilonodella* prefers temperatures of 18–22°C
- *Ichthyobodo*
  - Standard proprietary anti-protozoan treatments
  - With species of fish able to cope with high temperatures (like discus and fighting fish *Betta spp*), raise the temperature to over 30°C
  - Remove all of the fish from the infected aquarium for 24–48 h as the parasite can only survive away from the host for a few hours
- *Dactylogyrus spp*
  - Proprietary ectoparasitic preparations
  - *Praziquantel* at 10 mg/kg by mouth or at 10 mg/L for a 3 h bath. *Toxic to corydoras catfish*
  - *Dactylogyrus spp* are egg-layers; the egg stage is resistant to treatment so praziquantel should be repeated every 2–4 weeks depending upon temperature, for at least 3 doses. *Toxic to corydoras catfish*
- *Livoneca*
  - See *Skin Disorders*
- Overturned gill covers
  - Linked to poor water quality, especially high ammonia and nitrite levels
  - If caught in the early stages transferring the arrowana to highly oxygenated, good-quality water may reverse the condition
  - For advanced cases, surgical removal of the affected part is undertaken
  - This operation is regularly described for the highly prized Asian Dragonfish (see Fig. 12.1), but it may be more for aesthetic reasons than of benefit to the fish
- Partial or complete absence of operculum
  - Congenital problem. No treatment.

Gastrointestinal tract disorders

Bacterial

- Enteritis.

Protozoal

- *Protopalina* (very large ciliate) (esp. discus, kissing gouramis)
- *Spironucleus*. Especially in discus, angelfish, oscars and other cichlids (see *Skin Disorders*)
- *Hexamita*. Especially in cichlids and anabantids
- *Cryptosporidium*. Especially angelfish (*Pterophylllum* species)
- *Coccidia*
- *Piscicryptospordium cichlidaris*. Uncertain pathogenicity; encysts deep in the lining of the stomach so has the potential to cause much damage
- *Crytobia iubilans*.

Parasitic

- Nematodes
  - *Camallanus spp*
  - *Spirocamallanus rebecae* (Vidal-Martinez & Kennedy 2000)
  - *Raillietnema kritscheri* (Vidal-Martinez & Kennedy 2000)
  - *Capillaria spp* (esp. discus)
  - *Atractis vidali* (in wild *Vieja intermedia* and *Cichlasoma pearsei*) (Gonzalez-Solis & Moravec 2002)
  - *Contracaecum spp* (in *Oreochromis leucostictus*)
- Cestodes
  - Tapeworms
    - *Crassicutis cichlasomae* (Vidal-Martinez & Kennedy 2000).
    - *Amirthalingamia spp* (Aloo 2002)
    - *Cyclustera spp* (Aloo 2002)
    - *Enterogyrus cichlidarum* (tilapine cichlids)
  - Thorny-headed worms
    - *Acanthocephalus spp* (esp. wild caught Malawi cichlids)
    - *Neoechinorhynchus golvani* (Vidal-Martinez & Kennedy 2000)
    - *Polyacanthorhynchus kenyensis* (Aloo 2002).

Nutritional disorders

- Lack of dietary fibre, especially Lake Malawi cichlids. In highly adapted vegetarian cichlids such as many of the Rift Lake species a diet low in dietary fibre appears to predispose to *Cryptobia iubilans*
- Lack of bogwood. Some loricarid catfish (South American sucking catfish) – particularly some of the panaques – have specialist dietary requirements including bogwood on which to feed. Failure to provide this causing a progressive fading and loss of condition
- Hypovitaminosis C. Classic sign is spinal curvature, typically in livebearers. Supplement with vitamin C and increase greens/algae in diet. See *Musculoskeletal Disorders*

- Vitamin E deficiency. Muscle wastage. Especially large, fast-growing predatory fish fed on dead fish. Supplement with vitamin E, and alter diet appropriately
- Hepatic lipidosis. Seen often in rapidly growing large fish such as red-tailed catfish (*Phractocephalus*), which are fed excessively to maximize growth rate. Reduce feeding and supplement with vitamin E.

Neoplasia

- Bucco-pharyngeal neoplasia
- Gill neoplasia.

Other non-infectious problems

- Incisor teeth overgrowth in pufferfish
- Foreign body.

Findings on clinical examination

- Weight loss
- Stunting/poor growth (intestinal parasites)
- Listlessness and weight loss especially in wild caught Malawi cichlids (*Acanthocephalus*)
- Emaciation (*Coccidiosis*)
- Stringy, white faeces (*Protopalina, Spironucleus, Capillaria, Cryptobia*)
- Diarrhoea, darkened colouration in discus (*Capillaria*)
- Anorexia, regurgitation of food, diarrhoea, death in angelfish (*Pterophyllum spp*) (*Cryptosporidium*)
- Weight loss, poor growth (tapeworms, *Enterogyrus cichlidarum*)
- Slimey droppings, head and lateral line lesions, weight loss, no appetite, secondary infections (*Spironucleus*)
- Anorexia, lethargy and weight loss. Some fish may develop ascites (*Hexamita*)
  - In Siamese fighting fish (*Betta splendens*) *hexamita* can cause dropsy-like signs due to multi-organ damage. The liver and kidneys are especially affected
  - In kissing gouramis (*Helostoma temmincki*) it has been linked to swimming abnormalities, emaciation, white stringy faeces and secondary bacterial infections of the skin
  - Severely affected angelfish will show a distended abdomen and may lie flat at the water surface
  - Less severely affected adult cichlids may have reduced fertility, egg hatchability and increased loss of fry
- Obvious red worms protruding from anus, especially with livebearers. Ulceration around anus may be apparent. Weight loss (*Camallanus*)
- Weight loss in spite of good appetite in pufferfish (incisor teeth overgrowth)
- Dysphagia (bucco-pharyngeal or gill neoplasia, overgrown incisors).

Investigations

1. Anaesthetize and examine teeth/oral cavity (esp. pufferfish)
2. Light microscopy of faeces
   a. Large, capsule-shaped ciliated protozoan (*Protopalina*)
   b. Typical capillarid eggs (*Capillaria*)

3. Radiography
4. Routine haematology and biochemistry
5. Culture and sensitivity
6. Endoscopy
7. Biopsy/necropsy with histopathology
   a. Granulomatous gastritis; other organs affected (*Cryptobia, mycobacteriosis*). Use MZN stain to differentiate (positive for *mycobacteriosis*)
8. Ultrasonography
9. Water-quality parameters – check temperature, ammonia, nitrite, nitrate and pH values.

Management

• Routine removal of dead fish to prevent scavenging (and hence cross-infection) by other aquarium inhabitants.

Treatment/specific therapy

• *Protopalina* (protozoal parasite)
  • Proprietary ectoparasitic medication
• *Hexamita*
  • Metronidazole at 50 mg/L as a bath for up to 24 h daily for 10 days or as a bath at 5 mg/L every other day for a total of 3 treatments
• *Coccidia*
  • May respond to amprolium as a continuous bath at 10 mg/L for 7–10 days
  • Potentiated sulphonamide antibiotics:
    • 30 mg/kg s.i.d. i.m. for 7–10 days
    • 30 mg/kg body weight in feed every 24 h for 10–14 days
  • Toltrazuril at 30 mg/L as a 60-min bath e.o.d. for 3 treatments
• *Cryptosporidium*
  • Treatment is difficult. Consider sulphonamide antibiotics, but success unlikely
• *Cryptobia iubilans* – see *Systemic Disorders*
• Tapeworms (including *Enterogyrus cichlidarum*)
  • Worming with praziquantel at 10 mg/kg body weight by mouth; as a 1–2 h bath at 15–20 mg/L. With larger fish, in-feed medication at a rate of 400 mg/100 g food daily for 7 days. *Toxic to corydoras catfish*
  • Avoid feeding live foods to complete life cycle
• *Enterogyrus cichlidarum* may escape from the stomach and anterior intestine to invade other organs, e.g. liver, coelomic cavity, swimbladder and braincase (Noga & Flowers 1995). See *Systemic Disorders*
• *Camallanus, Capillaria* and *Acanthocephalous*
  • Levamisol at 2 mg/L for up to 24 h
  • Fenbendazole at 20 mg/kg body weight given 7 days apart
  • Mebendazole at 20 mg/kg for 3 treatments given at weekly intervals
  • *Camallanus* has both a direct and indirect life cycle (small crustaceans, e.g. cyclops act as intermediate hosts)
• Incisor teeth overgrowth
  • Burr back under anaesthetic
  • Offer foods that increase normal wear, e.g. cockles still in shell

- Foreign body
  - Retrieval from stomach, possibly with aid of endoscopy
  - Coeliotomy and surgical retrieval.

Hepatic disorders

Bacterial
- Hepatitis
- Mycobacteriosis (see *Systemic Disorders*).

Nutritional
Hepatic lipidosis (see *Nutritional Disorders*).

Neoplasia

Other non-infectious problems
- Hypoxia/anoxia, e.g. gill disease (areas of liver necrosis)
- Heavy metal toxicity.

Findings on clinical examination

- Non-specific signs of ill-health
- Anorexia
- Loss of balance (displacement of swimbladder)
- Swollen coelom
- Ascites (see *Systemic Disorders*).

Investigations

1. Radiography
   a. Abnormal position of swimbladder secondary to hepatomegaly
2. Routine haematology and biochemistry
   a. Raised liver enzymes
3. Culture and sensitivity
4. Endoscopy
5. Biopsy
6. Ultrasonography
7. Water-quality parameters – check temperature, ammonia, nitrite, nitrate and pH values, ammonia, nitrite, nitrate and pH values.

Management

- Try milk thistle mixed in feed or via gavage.

Treatment/specific therapy

- Neoplasia
  - No treatment
- Heavy metal poisoning
  - Remove suspected source
  - Remove to unaffected water
  - Oxygenate or aerate water well.

Cardiovascular and haematological disorders

Bacterial

- Endocarditis.

Protozoal

- *Cryptobia iubilans* (see *Systemic Disorders*)
- *Trypanosoma mukasai* (Negm-Eldin & Davies 1999)
- *Babesiosoma mariae* (Negm-Eldin & Davies 1999)
- *Cyrilia nili* (Negm-Eldin & Davies 1999).

Neoplasia

Other non-infectious problems

- Cardiomyopathy.

Findings on clinical examination

- High respiratory rate. Anaemia (haemoparasites)
- Death occurring within 24 h of respiratory disease (*Cryptobia*)
- Ascites (see *Systemic Disorders*).

Investigations

1. Radiography
2. Routine haematology and biochemistry
3. Cytology (haemoparasites)
4. Culture and sensitivity
5. Endoscopy
6. Biopsy
7. Ultrasonography
8. Water-quality parameters – check temperature, ammonia, nitrite, nitrate and pH values.

Treatment/specific therapy

- Bacterial endocarditis
  - Antibiosis

- *Cryptobia* – see *Systemic Disorders*
- Haemoparasites (*Trypanosoma, Babesiosoma and Cyrilia*)
  - Methylene blue by mouth at 60 mg/kg per day for 4 days
  - Metronidazole at 50 mg/kg per day
- Cardiomyopathy
  - No treatments described, possibly due to difficulty in diagnosis. May be worth adapting reptile protocols.

Systemic disorders

Viral

- Lymphocystis (iridovirus) (see *Skin Disorders*). Lymphocystis-induced masses can occur internally, acting as space occupying lesions
- Rio Grande perch rhabdovirus; Texas cichlid (*Herichthys cyanoguttatum*), convict cichlid (*Archocentrus nigrofasciatum*) and *Tilapia zilli*
- Ramirez dwarf cichlid virus (in Ramirez dwarf cichlid, *Microgeophagus ramirezi*)
- Channel catfish virus disease (herpes virus)
- Piscirickettsiosis-like organisms (PLOs), in blue-eyed panaque (*Panaque suttonorum*).

Bacterial

- Multi-organ systemic infections
- *Mycobacteriosis*
- *Lactococcus garvieae* (syn *Enterococcus seriolicida*)
- *Clostridium difficile*. Possible link with 'Malawi Bloat'.

Fungal

- (*Ichthyophonus hoferi*). See also *Neurological and Swimming Disorders, Ophthalmic Disorders, Reproductive Disorders* and *Skin Disorders*.

Protozoal

- *Hexamita* (see *Gastrointestinal Tract Disorders*)
- *Cryptobia* (see *Musculoskeletal Disorders*)
- *Cryptosporidiosis* (angelfish *Pterophyllum spp*) (see *Gastrointestinal Tract Disorders*).

Parasitic

- *Enterogyrus cichlidarum* (visceral invasion from gut; see *Gastrointestinal Tract Disorders*)
- Infectious conditions of unknown aetiology
- 'Discus plague'.

Nutritional

- See *Nutritional Disorders*.

Neoplasia

Other non-infectious problems

- Nitrite toxicity.

Findings on clinical examination

- Fish may separate themselves from the main group
- Weight loss. Obvious loss of muscle mass of epaxial muscles
- Ascites. Known to aquarists as dropsy this is often considered a disease in its own right. Typical signs include a swollen abdomen, raised scales and protruding eyes. Commonly due to multi-organ failure from systemic bacterial infection.
- In Siamese fighting fish (*Betta splendens*) *Hexamita* can cause dropsy-like signs due to multi-organ damage, in particular the liver and kidneys
- Haemorrhages and mortalities (systemic bacterial infections, *Lactococcus garvieae*)
- Spinal curvature, open skin sores, protruding eyes, especially anabantids (mycobacteriosis)
- Erratic swimming, palor, multiple skin haemorrhages, severe exophthalmia and swollen abdomens in fry and fingerling Channel catfish (*Ictarulus puntatus*) (Channel catfish virus disease)
- Progressive loss of appetite and wasting (*Cryptobia*). Can affect all cichlid species, but it is a particular cause of mortalities in the Rift Lake cichlids. Some of these fish will develop ascites known as 'Malawi bloat'. *Note* that C. *difficile* has also been implicated with 'Malawi bloat'
- Weight loss, darkened colour, excessive mucus production, rapid respiration, lethargy ('discus plague'). Seen in discus (*Symphysodon spp*), occasionally angelfish (*Pterophyllum* species). See *Skin Disorders*
- Lethargy and mortalities in Texas, convict and *Tilapia zilli* (Rio Grande perch rhabdovirus)
- Lethargy, loss of appetite, incoordination, emaciation and death in Ramirez dwarf cichlids (Ramirez dwarf cichlid virus)
- Head standing (tiger barbs); respiratory signs (nitrite toxicity)
- Wasting, darkening of skin colour and obvious boil-like swellings in the skin. Also exophthalmia, abnormal behaviour and swimming patterns (if the central nervous system is invaded). Sex reversal in guppies (female to male) (*Ichthyophonus*)
- Mortalities in blue-eyed panaque (*Panaque suttonorum*) (piscirickettsiosis-like organisms).

Investigations

1. Radiography
2. Routine haematology and biochemistry
3. Culture and sensitivity
4. Endoscopy
5. Biopsy
6. Postmortem
   a. Multiple granulomas in internal organs (mycobacteriosis, cryptobia). Differentiate with MZN (positive for mycobacteria)
7. Ultrasonography
8. Water-quality parameters – check temperature, ammonia, nitrite, nitrate and pH values.

Management

- See *Nursing Care*.

Treatment/specific therapy

- Rio Grande perch rhabdovirus – no treatment
- Ramirez dwarf cichlid virus – no treatment
- Channel catfish virus – no effective treatment
  - Antibiotics, as secondary infection often cause of mortalities
- Ascites (dropsy)
  - Without definite diagnosis prognosis is poor. Attempt use of antibiotic
- Bacterial infections (including *Lactococcus garvieae*)
  - Antibiotics
- Mycobacteriosis
  - Difficult. Potential zoonosis so euthanasia. See *Musculoskeletal Disorders*
- Piscirickettsiosis-like organisms
  - PLOs can be treated with a variety of antibiotics
- Cryptobia
  - Metronidazole helps but does not appear to eradicate the organism (see *Gastrointestinal Tract Disorders – Hexamita*, for suggested dose rates). Yanong et al (2004) found metronidazole ineffective in discus (*Symphysodon aequifasciatus*) but dimetridazole (80 mg/L for 24 h repeated daily for 3 days) or 2-amino-5-nitrothiazol (10 mg/L for 24 h repeated daily for 3 days) reduced infection
  - In some collections virtually all the cichlids can be infected and the disease will show itself as a low-grade loss of fish over a period of time
- *Ichthyophonus hoferi*
  - No efficacious treatment available
- Discus plague
  - Unquantified disease; may actually outbreaks of other undiagnosed diseases such as *Hexamita* or *Capillaria*. However, there is some suggestion that an as yet unidentified infectious agent may be responsible
  - Concentrate on maintaining optimum water quality and minimize stress, e.g. provide hiding places
  - Quarantine all new stock.

Musculoskeletal disorders

Viral

- *Chromide Iridovirus* (Chromide cichlids, *Etroplus maculates*, *E. canariensis* and *E. suratensis*)

Bacterial

- Mycobacteriosis. Typically *M. marinum*, *M. cheloni* and *M. fortuitum*

Fungal

Protozoal

- *Pleistophora* (neon tetra disease)
- *Cryptobia iubilans* (see *Systemic Disorders*).

Nutritional

* Hypovitaminosis C (esp. live-bearers) (see *Nutritional Disorders*)
* Starvation; inappetence, through failure to provide correct environment or diet. See comments on stingrays, below.

Neoplasia

Other non-infectious problems

* Electroshock (Pasnik et al 2003).

Findings on clinical examination

* Weight loss, muscle wastage (see also *Systemic Disorders* and *Gastrointestinal Tract Disorders*)
* In freshwater stingrays (*Potamotrygon spp*) weight loss over the pelvic bones can be prominent
* Spinal curvature (hypovitaminosis C, mycobacteriosis, *Pleistophora*)
* White patches, loss of colour and emaciation (*Pleistophora*) (see *Skin Disorders*)
* Open skin sores, wasting and protruding eyes (mycobacteriosis)
* Poor growth (hypovitaminosis C)
* Weight loss and weakness in chromide cichlids *Etroplus spp* (*Chromide Iridovirus*).

Investigations

1. Radiography
2. Routine haematology and biochemistry
3. Culture and sensitivity
4. Endoscopy
5. Biopsy
6. Postmortem
   a. Multiple granulomas in internal organs (mycobacteriosis, *Cryptobia*, *Flavobacteria*). Differentiate with MZN (positive for mycobacteria)
7. Ultrasonography
8. Water-quality parameters – check temperature, ammonia, nitrite, nitrate and pH values.

Treatment/specific therapy

* *Chromide Iridovirus* – no treatment
* *Pleistophora*, see *Skin Disorders*
* Mycobacteriosis
  * Potential zoonosis so consider euthanasia
  * Treatment problematical. Kanamycin at 50 mg/L every 48 h for 4 treatments was successful in guppies (Conroy & Conroy 1999)
* Hypovitaminosis C, see *Nutritional Disorders*.

Neurological and swimming disorders

Viral

- Ramirez dwarf cichlid virus in Ramirez dwarf cichlid (*Microgeophagus ramirezi*)
- Deep angelfish disease (herpesvirus), altum (deep) angelfish (*Pterophyllum altum*) only. Other *Pterophyllum* species unaffected.

Bacterial

- *Flavobacterium spp* (esp. live-bearers)
- *Streptococcal* infections esp. *S. iniae*
- Bacterial meningitis
- Central nervous system infection/granuloma.

Fungal

- (*Ichthyophonus hoferi*). See also *Systemic Disorders, Ophthalmic Disorders, Reproductive Disorders* and *Skin Disorders*
- Central nervous system infection/granuloma.

Protozoal

- Myxosporidea (see *Skin Disorders*)
- Hexamita (see *Gastrointestinal Tract Disorders*).

Neoplasia

Other non-infectious problems

- Ammonia toxicity (see also *Respiratory Tract Disorders*)
- Abnormal swimbladder functioning secondary to compression from internal space-occupying lesions, e.g. neoplasia
- Swimbladder disease
- Swimbladder torsion
- Nicotine toxicity.

Findings on clinical examination

- Whirling swimming pattern, dark or accentuating colouring, sudden death (meningitis, Myxosporidea – especially if obvious nodules visible). There may be weight loss and fin rot
- Swimming abnormalities, emaciation, white stringy faeces and secondary bacterial infections of the skin in kissing gouramis (*Helostoma temmincki*) (*Hexamita* – see *Gastrointestinal Tract Disorders*)
- Incoordination, muscle spasms, lethargy, loss of appetite, emaciation and death in Ramirez dwarf cichlids
- Aimless swimming (shimmying), loss of balance, death (*Flavobacterium*)
- Loss of balance, spinning, pale gills, ulcers, death in altum angelfish (deep angelfish disease)
- Abnormal behaviour and swimming patterns accompanied by wasting, darkening of skin colour and obvious boil-like swellings in the skin; in extreme cases it may have a sandpaper effect, due to the large number of granulomas present, exophthalmia, and sex reversal in guppies (female to male) (*Ichthyophonus*)

- All or most fish affected – consider environmental disease, e.g. water quality
- Upward curling of the disc in freshwater stingrays (*Potamotrygon spp*) is often a sign of ill-health and is usually either poor water quality or bacterial infection
- Stiffened pectoral fins, muscular spasms (nicotine toxicity).

Investigations

1. Radiography
2. Routine haematology and biochemistry
3. Culture and sensitivity
4. Endoscopy
5. Biopsy or postmortem
   a. Multiple granulomas (*Flavobacterium*, mycobacteriosis, see *Systemic Disorders*)
6. Ultrasonography
7. Water quality parameters – check temperature, ammonia, nitrite, nitrate and pH values
8. Assessment of environment (nicotine toxicity).

Treatment/specific therapy

- Ammonia toxicity
  - Partial water changes to dilute the ammonia levels
  - Adding zeolite will absorb large quantities of ammonia
  - Longer-term control may include addition of commercially available *Nitrosomonas* bacterial cultures or equivalent
- Deep angelfish disease
  - No treatment – supportive only
- Flavobacteria and bacterial meningitis
  - Antibiotics
- *Ichthyophonus hoferi*
  - No efficacious treatment available
- Swimbladder disease
  - Usually no effective treatment. May develop ulceration on areas persistently floating above water level
  - Pneumocystocentesis can provide temporary relief but the problem is likely to recur
  - Try antibiotics if suspect bacterial infection
  - If the fish is floating, may implant small sterile counterweight into ventral coelomic cavity, but is difficult to judge correct weight
  - Pneumocystoplasty (Britt et al 2002) and pneumocystectomy (Lewbart et al 1995) have been attempted, and with refinement could prove useful
- Swimbladder torsion
  - Surgical correction
- Central nervous system infection/granuloma
  - Attempt antibiotic or antimycotic treatment. Poor prognosis
- Nicotine toxicity
  - 10 ppmm can kill guppies within 5 min
  - Lower doses can cause low-grade mortalities, infertility and other reproductive problems
  - No direct treatment. Situate air pumps away from smoky atmospheres.

Ophthalmic disorders

Viral

- Channel catfish virus (herpesvirus). See also *Skin Disorders* and *Systemic Disorders*.

Bacterial

- Systemic bacterial infection/multi-organ failure
- Retrobulbar granuloma
- *Streptococcal* infections especially *S. iniae*
- *Edwardsiella ictaruli* (catfish). See also *Skin Disorders*.

Fungal

- *Fusarium mycosis*
- *Ichthyophonus hoferi*. See also *Systemic Disorders, Neurological and Swimming Disorders, Reproductive Disorders* and *Skin Disorders*
- Retrobulbar granuloma.

Protozoal

- *Ichthyophthirius*
- *Tetrahymena*.

Nutritional

- Riboflavin deficiency
- Ascorbic acid deficiency
- Hypovitaminosis A.

Neoplasia

- Retrobulbar neoplasia.

Other non-infectious problems

- Traumatic damage or loss of eye. Often due to inter-specific or con-specific aggression, especially cichlids
- Gas bubble disease (see *Skin Disorders*)
- Cardiomyopathy
- 'Drop eye' in dragonfish (*Sclerohages spp*) and arowanas (*Osteoglossum spp*) (Fig. 12.4).

Findings on clinical examination

- Blindness (*Fusarium*)
- Exophthalmus. Often accompanied by ascites
- Exophthalmus, lethargy, pale skin, sex reversal in guppies (female to male) (*Ichthyophonus*)
- Exophthalmus, panophthalmitis, darkening of colour, haemorrhage, ulceration in cichlids (*Streptococcal* infections)
- Exophthalmus in Channel catfish fry and fingerlings, accompanied by skin haemorrhages, severe abnormal swimming swollen abdomens (Channel catfish virus)
- Glaucoma (usually secondary to intraocular disease)
- One or both eyes is turned permanently downward in arowanas (drop eye).

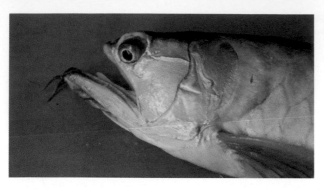

Fig. 12.4. 'Drop-eye' in a large silver arowana (*Osteoglossum birchirrosum*).

Investigations

1. Ophthalmic examination
2. Radiography
3. Routine haematology and biochemistry
4. Culture and sensitivity
5. Endoscopy
6. Biopsy
7. Ultrasonography
8. Water-quality parameters – check temperature, ammonia, nitrite, nitrate and pH values.

Management

- Maintain optimum water quality
- See *Nursing Care.*

Treatment/specific therapy

- Traumatic damage/loss of eye
  - Consider antibiotic therapy
  - Removal of aggressive individuals, sharp aquarium furniture, etc.
- Bacterial infections
  - Antibiotics
- Fusarium mycosis – no effective treatment
- *Ichthyophonus*
  - No effective treatment
  - Enucleation
- Glaucoma
  - Enucleation
- 'Drop eye'
  - Aetiology unknown

- Likely to be a neurological problem leading to loss of function of the muscles that control the eye, possibly as a result of head trauma while jumping
- Neoplasia
  - Enucleation
  - Euthanasia
- Cardiomyopathy, see *Cardiovascular and Haematological Disorders*
- Nutritional disorders
  - Feed analysis
  - Correction with dietary supplements.

Endocrine disorders

Goitre in freshwater stingrays, see *Endocrine Disorders* in *Tropical Marine Fish.*

Renal disorders

In many fish, the kidney is divided into two sections. The caudal pole excretes urine and, along with the gills, is important in osmoregulation. The other section is involved with hematopoiesis and immune function, including white blood cell production and antibody formation. The osmoregulatory function means that freshwater fish excrete prodigious amounts of dilute urine to eliminate excess water entering across the skin and gills. Severe renal disease may result in severe osmoregulatory upset, with extreme cases developing into ascites.

Bacterial

- Nephritis.

Fungal

Protozoal

- Myozoans.

Neoplasia

- Renal cyst adenomas (possibly genetic in red oscars, *Astronotus occellatus*).

Other non-infectious problems

- Prolonged exposure to free CO_2 levels >10–20 mg/L has been associated with nephrocalcinosis, mineral deposits forming in the renal tubules, collecting ducts and ureters.

Findings on clinical examination

- Wasting and general malaise
- Anaemia
- Ascites due to osmoregulatory disruption
- Mortalities
- Swollen abdomen.

Investigations

1. Radiography
   a. Swimbladder displacement (renal and other coelomic neoplasia)
2. Routine haematology and biochemistry
3. Culture and sensitivity
4. Endoscopy
5. Biopsy
6. Ultrasonography
7. Postmortem examination
8. Water-quality parameters
   a. Check temperature, ammonia, nitrite, nitrate and pH values
   b. High CO_2 levels may be linked with low pH levels, high stocking densities, poor water circulation, excess CO_2 infusion in planted aquaria.

Treatment/specific therapy

- CO_2 excess
  - Assess possible underlying causes and correct (see above)
- Neoplasia
  - Surgical resection
  - Euthanasia.

Reproductive disorders

Fungal

- *Ichthyophonus hoferi* (see also *Skin Disorders, Neurological and Swimming Disorders, Ophthalmic Disorders* and *Systemic Disorders*).

Protozoal

- *Hexamita*.

Other non-infectious problems

- Functional sterility in fancy strains of live-bearers (guppies, swordtails) where there is increased length or branching of the gonopodium – the modified anal fin used for sperm transfer in these fish. In these strains it is usually only young males without full gonopodial development that are used for breeding. In the guppy this is a dominant autosomal mutation in which increased branching of the fins produces a veil-tail appearance
- Lethal gene in certain strains of black Siamese fighting fish (*Betta splendens*). Such strains must be outcrossed to be propagated
- Nicotine toxicity (see also *Neurological and Swimming Disorders*)
- Egg retention (see *Reproductive Disorders* in Ch. 11, *Goldfish and Koi*)
- Dystocia in live-bearing species, e.g. freshwater stingrays.

Findings on clinical examination

- Poor reproductive performance in cichlids (*Hexamita*)
- Sex reversal in guppies (female to male). Also lethargy, pale skin, protruding eyes (*Ichthyophonus*)
- Swollen body cavity (dystocia in stingrays).

Investigations

1. Radiography
2. Routine haematology and biochemistry
3. Culture and sensitivity
4. Endoscopy
5. Biopsy
6. Ultrasonography
   a. Check for foetal heartbeats in dystocic stingrays
7. Water-quality parameters – check temperature, ammonia, nitrite, nitrate and pH values.

Treatment/specific therapy

- *Ichthyophonus* – no treatment. Consider euthanasia
- *Hexamita*
  - See *Gastrointestinal Tract Disorders*
- Nicotine toxicity (see also *Neurological and Swimming Disorders*)
- Dystocia
  - If possible calculate if over due date (in stingrays gestation is around 2.5–3 months; young females will have one to two young, older, full-sized females can have eight or more)
  - Under GA, assess if young are alive either by observation/palpation of young or ultrasonography
  - Young may be delivered per cloaca or via surgical salpingotomy.

References

Aloo P A 2002 A comparative study of helminth parasites from the fish Tilapia zillii and Oreochromis leucostictus in Lake Naivasha and Oloidien Bay, Kenya. J Helminthol 76 (2):95–104

Britt T, Weisse C, Weber S et al 2002 Use of pneumocystoplasty for overinflation of the swim bladder in a goldfish. J Am Vet Med Assoc 221(5):690–693

Conroy G, Conroy D A 1999 Acid-fast bacterial infection and its control in guppies (Lebistes reticulatus) reared on an ornamental fish farm in Venezuela. Vet Rec 144:177–178

Francis-Floyd R, Bolon B, Frase W et al 1993 Lip fibromas associated with retrovirus-like particles in angelfish. J Am Vet Med Assoc 202(10):1547–1548

Gonzalez-Solis D, Moravec F 2002 A new atractid nematode, Atractis vidali sp. n. (Nematoda: Atractidae), from cichlid fishes in southern Mexico. Folia Parasitol (Praha) 49 (3):227–230

Lewbart G A, Stone E A, Love N E 1995 Pneumocystectomy in a Midas cichlid. J Am Vet Med Assoc 207:319–321

Miles D J, Kanchanakhan S, Lilley J H et al 2001 Effect of macrophages and serum of fish susceptible or resistant to epizootic ulcerative syndrome (EUS) on the EUS pathogen, Aphanomyces invadans. Fish Shellfish Immunol 11(7):569–584

Negm-Eldin M M, Davies R W 1999 Simultaneous transmission of Trypanosoma mukasai, Babesiosoma mariae and Cyrilia nili to fish by the leech Batracobdelloides tricarinata. Dtsch Tierarztl Wochenschr 106(12):526–527

Noga E J, Flowers J R 1995 Invasion of Tilapia mossambica (cichlidae) viscera by the monogenean Enterogyrus cichlidarum. J Parasitol 81(5):815–817

Noga E J, Wright J F, Pasarell L 1990 Some unusual features of mycobacteriosis in the cichlid fish Oreochromis mossambicus. J Comp Pathol 102(3):335–344

Pasnik D J, Smith S A, Wolf J C 2003 Accidental electroshock of fish in a recirculation facility. Vet Rec 153:562–564

Pimenta Leibowitz M, Ariav R, Zilberg D 2005 Environmental and physiological conditions affecting Tetrahymena sp infection in guppies, Poecilia reticulata Peters. J Fish Dis 28:539–547

Silva-Souza A T, Eiras J C 2002 The histopathology of the infection of Tilapia rendalli and Hypostomus regani (Osteichthyes) by lasidium larvae of Anodontites trapesialis (Mollusca, Bivalvia). Mem Inst Oswaldo Cruz 97(3):431–433

Vidal-Martinez V M, Kennedy C R 2000 Potential interactions between the intestinal helminths of the cichlid fish Cichlasoma synspilum from southeastern Mexico. J Parasitol 86(4):691–695

Wildgoose W 1998 Skin disease in ornamental fish: identifying common problems. In Practice 20:226–243

Yanong R P, Curtis E, Russo R et al 2004 Cryptobia iubilans infection in juvenile discus. J Am Vet Med Assoc 224(10):1644–1650

Tropical marine fish

Over 90% of tropical marine fish are wild-caught. This means that, although they are robust as individuals (they are the Darwinian survivors of the rigours of planktonic survival), the stress of capture, transportation plus the mingling of species from different continents and biotopes at the wholesaler and retailer, mean that disease outbreaks are not uncommon. Some captive breeding does occur, principally with those species with either short or no planktonic larval stage, e.g. clownfish (*Amphiprion spp*), seahorses (*Hippocampus spp*) and Banggai cardinals (*Pterapogon kauderni*).

Most marine fish are net-caught, but in some countries there is still an unacceptable willingness to use cyanide to catch fish hidden in coral crevices; an action that causes both immediate and later mortalities when the fish have entered the ornamental fish trade.

Recommended water-quality parameters are listed in Table 13.1.

Table 13.1 Recommended water quality parameters: Fish-only community aquarium; reef aquarium

Parameter	Fish-only community aquarium	Reef aquarium (with photosynthetic invertebrates)
Temperature (°C)	22–26	24–28
pH	8.0–8.3	8.0–8.4
Salinity (measured as specific gravity)	1.020–1.027	1.022–1.027
Carbonate hardness (KH) (mg $CaCO_3$)	116	116–267
Ammonia (total) (mg/L)	<0.02	<0.02 mg/L but the high pH requires ammonia should be 0.0 mg/L
Nitrite (mg/L)	<0.02	<0.02
Nitrate (mg/L)	<40 mg above ambient tapwater levels	<5–10
Calcium (mg/L)	300–500	300–500
Oxygen (mg/L)	5.0–8.0	5.0–8.0
Phosphate (mg/L)	<0.2	<0.036
Water volume turnover	Dependant upon fish housed in aquarium	15–20 times per hour
Lighting	Dependant upon fish housed in aquarium	10–14 h daylight; 0.6–5.5 Watts/L

Consultation and handling

See *Goldfish and Koi.*

Nursing care

The same principles apply as for goldfish and koi but differ significantly in some areas. Salt water holds less oxygen than fresh water at an equivalent temperature, so stocking densities are more critical. The high pH of marine aquaria means that excreted ammonia is more toxic. Lowering the salinity to a specific gravity of 1.020 is often beneficial – it reduces osmotic stress on the fish and is less well tolerated by many ectoparasites. Protein skimming is an important method of removing proteinaceous and other dissolved and suspended materials from salt water. However, zeolite is ineffective in salt water.

Proprietary products containing copper are commonly available medications for marine fish. Copper is toxic to certain groups of fish including the elasmobranchs (sharks and rays) and many invertebrate species. It may also interfere with the normal gut flora of herbivorous fish such as tangs and surgeonfish. Signs of toxicity include stress colouration, loss of appetite, excessive mucous production and respiratory distress. Copper levels, therefore, require daily monitoring with a copper test kit (Table 13.2). Never use copper-based treatments in aquaria containing invertebrates, and ideally always use a separate dedicated treatment aquarium.

Analgesia and anaesthesia

See Chapter 11, *Goldfish and Koi.*

Species commonly presented to the veterinarian include those listed in Table 13.3.

Skin disorders

Structure and function of skin (see Ch. 11, *Goldfish and Koi*).

Pruritus

* *Note* that for wrasses, apparent scratching against the substrate can be normal behaviour thought to be linked to foraging for hidden invertebrates
* Scratching and irritation (flukes, protozoa)

Table 13.2 Therapeutic use of copper

Free copper ion concentration	Result
0.2 p.p.m.	Therapeutic
<0.15 p.p.m.	Non-therapeutic
>0.25 p.p.m.	Toxic

Table 13.3 Species of tropical marine fish commonly encountered: Key facts

Species	Notes	Common disorders
Clownfish (*Amphiprion spp*)	Most species available are captive bred. Host anemone not often required in captivity	Ectoparasites especially *Crytocaryon, Brooklynella, Uronema* and *amyloodinium*
Angelfish (*Pomacanthus, Holacanthus* and *Centropyge spp*)	Natural diet high in algae and sponges	*Cryptocaryon*, skin flukes, head and lateral line disease. Variably susceptible to poor water quality
Lionfish (*Pterois spp* and *Dendrochirus spp*)	Venomous dorsal spines	Hepatic lipidosis
Hippocampus spp	Live-bearers; commercially bred for both the ornamental fish-trade and traditional Chinese medicine	Ectoparasites, brood pouch emphysema

- Sudden darting movements, loss of balance, rapid respiration (sudden-onset water poisoning; new tank syndrome) See *Systemic Disorders* and *Neurological and Swimming Disorders*
- Seahorses with *Glugea* (see below) appear pruritic and induce serious excoriation by rubbing affected areas.

Erosions and ulceration including fin rot

- Respiratory distress, irritation, ulceration (*Brooklynella, Uronema, Miamiensis marinum*, esp. seahorses) See *Respiratory Tract Disorders*.
- Damage to skin and/or loss of eyes and fins (bacterial infections – typically *Vibrio spp* (for *Vibrio parahaemolyticus*, see also *Gastrointestinal Tract Disorders*), but *Pasteurella, Myxobacteria, Streptococci* are also recorded; mycobacteriosis, *Nocardia kampachi*, trauma
- Weight loss, thickened areas of inflammation, ulceration, fin rot (*Nocardia*)
- Ulcers on snout and mouth of puffer fish (*Tetraodon spp*). Increased aggression (tiger puffer virus)
- Erosions at cephalic sensory pits and along lateral line, often involving surrounding muscles, in marine angelfish, surgeonfish and tangs. Slimy faeces (head and lateral line disease, HLLD)
  - Linked to an aquareovirus in marine angelfish (*Pomacanthus spp*) (Varner & Lewis 1991)
  - Possible hypovitaminosis A
  - Suggested protozoal aetiology (see Ch. 12, *Tropical Freshwater Fish*) but unconfirmed in marine fish
- Foreign body reaction to fibreglass in moray eels
- Neoplasia
- Excessively low pH.

Nodules and non-healing wounds

- Wasting, darkening of skin colour and obvious boil-like swellings in the skin; in extreme cases it may have a sandpaper effect, due to the large number of granulomas present. Also exophthalmia, abnormal behaviour and swimming patterns (if the central nervous system is invaded) *(Ichthyophonus hoferi)*. See also *Neurological and Swimming Disorders, Ophthalmic Disorders* and *Systemic Disorders*
- Non-ulcerative skin masses in seahorses *(Hippocampus spp)*. Also lethargy and disorientation (Exophthalia)
- Whitish skin nodules in seahorses especially *H. erectus* *(Glugea heraldi)* (Vincent & Clifton-Hadley 1989)
- Nodules, darkened colouring, emaciation, abnormal swimming (Myxosporidea)
- Cauliflower-like growths on fins and skin *(Lymphocystis)* (Fig. 13.1)
- Epitheliocystis. Looks like lymphocystis *(Chlamydophila*-like organism)
- Goitre in marine elasmobranchs, see *Endocrine Disorders*
- Gas filled bubbles in the skin especially on the fins. Also occasionally behind the eye (gas bubble disease – usually secondary to oxygen supersaturation). See also 'seahorse gas bubble disease', in *Systemic Disorders*
- Neoplasia.

Changes in pigmentation

- Large discrete white spots. Laboured breathing, flashing. *Cryptocaryon irritans* (marine white spot)
- Fine white 'dusting' on skin. Laboured breathing, flashing, *Amyloodinium* (coral fish disease), *Crepidoodinium*

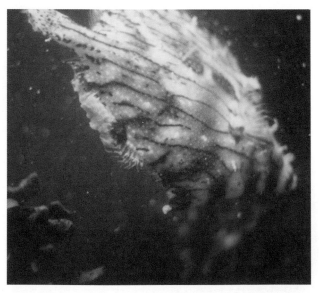

Fig. 13.1. A tesselated file fish (*Chaetoderma pencilligerus*) with yellow lymphocystic lesions on the ventral fin.

- Grey skin due to excessive mucous production, reddened skin, ulceration (skin flukes, ectoparasites)
- Haemorrhages, ulceration, abnormal swimming, shimmying (bacterial disease)
- Small black spots over body, cloudy skin, respiratory distress, especially in laterally compressed fish such as yellow tangs (*Zebrasoma flavescens, Turbellaria*)
- Fingerprint-like marks on skin of tangs and surgeonfish (tang fingerprint disease virus)
- Colour fading. Likely to be nutritional lack of appropriate carotenoids
- Light grey patches that are multi-focal, well defined and ovoid in blacktip sharks (*Carcharinus limbatus*) (Dermopthirus) (Bullard et al 2000).

Ectoparasites

- Protozoa
  - *Cryptocaryon irritans* (see also *Respiratory Tract Disorders*)
  - *Amyloodinium* and *Crepidoodinium* (see also *Respiratory Tract Disorders*)
  - *Brooklynella hostilis* (see also *Respiratory Tract Disorders*)
  - *Uronema marinum* (see also *Respiratory Tract Disorders*)
  - *Miamiensis marinum,* esp. seahorses
  - Turbellaria (see also *Respiratory Tract Disorders*)
  - Microsporideans, e.g. *Glugea, Pleistophora, Sprauga spp*
- Helminths
  - Skin flukes (*Gyrodactylus*)
  - Gill flukes (*Dactylogyrids*). See also *Respiratory Tract Disorders*
  - *Dermopthirius penneri*
- Crustacea
  - *Livoneca*
  - Lerneascus spp
- Neoplasia
  - Non-symmetrical swelling, ulceration, loss of balance
  - Epithelioma
  - Papillomas.

Investigations

1. Skin scrape and light microscopy
   a. Protozoa
      i. *Brooklynella*: large (55–85 μm) and mobile ciliates, with the basket-shaped 'mouth' and cilia very apparent
      ii. *Cryptocaryon*: large (48 × 27 to 450 × 350 μm) oval-shaped ciliated protozoa with a characteristic four-lobed nucleus
      iii. *Amyloodinium*: can be quite large, up to 1.0 mm diameter, oval shaped with a very dark appearance because of chloroplasts. Not usually mobile
      iv. *Uronema*: motile, oval shaped protozoan parasites.
   b. Flukes
      i. *Gyrodactylus*: live-bearing; can usually see large H-shaped hooks of both adult and unborn young
      ii. *Dactylogyrids*: egg-layer. Usually four black spots at caudal end. Can be quite large flukes

c. Fungi
   i. *Ichthyophonus*: squash preparation of nodule. The spores can be readily seen as spherical bodies, varying from 10 to 100 µm in diameter. There is much variation in the appearance of these multinucleate spores
2. Radiography
3. Routine haematology and biochemistry
4. Culture and sensitivity
5. Endoscopy
6. Biopsy
7. Ultrasonography
8. Water-quality parameters – check as a minimum: temperature, ammonia, nitrite, nitrate and pH values.

Treatment/specific therapy

- Gas bubble disease (see also 'seahorse gas bubble disease', in *Systemic Disorders*)
  - Oxygen supersaturation usually secondary to pressurized oxygenation (e.g. malfunctioning venturi pumps), excess photosynthesis (high algae levels)
  - Correct source of problem
  - Rarely fatal – fish usually recover uneventfully
- Head and lateral line disease
  - No treatment for aquareovirus
  - Vitamin A supplementation, either in commercial supplement or as 'greens', e.g. suchi seaweed wraps
  - Metronidazole at 50 mg/kg per day if suspect protozoal involvement
- Tiger puffer virus
  - No treatment available. Supportive care only
- Tang fingerprint disease virus
  - No treatment available. Supportive care only
- Lymphocystis
  - No direct cure. Usually self-limiting
  - Ozone or ultraviolet sterilization may reduce spread
  - Attempted surgical removal is usually followed by recurrence
- Epitheliocystis
  - Some antibiotics, e.g. chloramphenicol, recorded as effective
- Bacterial infections
  - Antibiotics
  - Debridement of ulcers followed by packing with protective layer, e.g. Orabase (Squibb)
- *Nocardia* and mycobacteriosis
  - Antibiotic treatment not very effective
  - Consider euthanasia, especially because of zoonotic risk
- *Exophthaliosis*
  - Ketoconazole at 5.0 mg/kg. p.o. s.i.d.
  - Itraconazole at 1–10 mg/kg s.i.d. p.o. (in feed) for 1–7 days
- *Ichthyophonus hoferi*
  - No efficacious treatment available. Try treatment as for *Exophthaliosis*, above.
- *Glugea*
  - No effective treatment. Consider:
    - Toltrazuril at 30 mg/L bath for 60 min repeated every other day for 3 treatments
    - Feeding a diet of 0.1% fumagillin

- Myxosporidea
  - No effective treatment – try as for *Glugea* above
- *Cryptocaryon irritans* (marine white spot)
  - Sensitive to copper-based ectoparasitic treatments (see *Nursing Care*, above)
  - Formalin baths
  - Freshwater dips
  - *Cryptocaryon tomonts* cannot survive at salinities with a specific gravity below around 1.015 (a salinity of around 16 ppt). Maintaining *Cryptocaryon*-infested fish at 1.015 or below for a minimum of 6 days can effect a cure at standard tropical temperatures. Examples of fish groups able to adapt to such low levels of salt include the blennies (*Blenniidae*), groupers (*Serranidae*), target fish (*Theraponidae*), jacks (*Carangidae*), snappers (*Lutja*), rabbitfishes (*Siganidae*), damselfish and clowns (*Pomacentridae*), left-eye flounders (*Bothidae*) and even some marine angelfish (*Pomacanthids*). Estuarine and rock pool fish will also have little difficulty osmoregulating at such low salinities. Some invertebrates such as cleaner shrimps (*Lysmata* spp) may well not survive such treatment.
- *Amyloodinium* and *Crepidoodinium*
  - Sensitive to copper-based ectoparasitic treatments
  - The encysted stage is relatively resistant to chemical attack
  - Can colonize the intestines of fish, where again it can be protected from medications
  - In such cases, treat with metronidazole at 50 mg/L daily for 10 days, changing the water daily
  - Antibiotic cover should be considered as secondary infections are common at the areas where the skin is damaged
  - Eliminate the parasite from a show aquarium by removing all fish, reducing or cutting out the light levels and raising the temperature to 30–32°C for 3 weeks
- *Brooklynella*, *Uronema* and *Miamiensis*
  - Sensitive to proprietary formalin/malachite green and/or copper-based ectoparasitic treatments
  - Freshwater baths for larger/tougher fish
  - Covering antibiosis
- Skin flukes
  - Proprietary ectoparasitic preparations
  - *Praziquantel* at 10 mg/L for a 3 h bath , or in feed at a rate of 400 mg/100 g food daily for 7 days (but see *Neurological and Swimming Disorders*)
  - Freshwater dips 5 min once daily for 5 days
- *Dermophthirius penneri*
  - Consider praziquantel as above
- Turbellariae
  - Formalin bath at 2 mL formalin per litre for up to 1 h
  - 5 min freshwater bath daily for 5 days
- Crustacean ectoparasites
  - Individual removal of parasites
  - Treat with lufenuron (Program, Novartis) at 0.088 mg/L as a once only treatment
  - Treat with organophosphates if legal to do so
- Neoplasia
  - Surgery or euthanasia
  - Surgical debulking followed by injection of cisplatin directly into the tissue mass on a weekly basis.

Respiratory tract disorders

Bacterial

- Bacterial gill disease.

Fungal

- Fungal gill disease.

Protozoal

- *Cryptocaryon irritans* (see also *Skin Disorders*)
- *Amyloodinium* and *Crepidoodinium* (see also *Skin Disorders*)
- *Brooklynella hostilis* (see also *Skin Disorders*)
- *Uronema marinum* (see also *Skin Disorders*)
- *Miamiensis marinum* esp. seahorses
- *Turbellaria* (see also *Skin Disorders*)
- *Coccomyxa hoffmani* (Myxosporidean).

Parasitic

- Gill flukes (*Dactylogyrus, Microcotyle, Haliotrema, Ancyrocephalus, Pseudoancyrocephalus, Cleithrarticus, Neohaliotrema* and *Pseudempleurosoma*).

Neoplasia

Other non-infectious problems

- Hypoxia
- Ammonia toxicity (see also *Neurological Disorders*)
- Copper toxicity.

Findings on clinical examination

- Moderate-to-extreme respiratory effort
- Rapid gill ventilation
- Apparent gasping at water surface
- Abnormal colour of gills, necrosis, exposure of underlying cartilage
- Respiratory distress, irritation, ulceration (*Brooklynella, Uronema*)
- Respiratory distress, small black spots over body with cloudy skin (*Turbellaria*)
- Respiratory distress, clamped fins, scratching and flashing. Inactivity (gill flukes)
- Gill or intra-oral mass.

Investigations

1. Gill scrape and light microscopy
   a. Protozoa
      i. *Brooklynella*: large (55–85 μm) and mobile ciliates, with the basket-shaped 'mouth' and cilia very apparent
      ii. *Cryptocaryon*: large (48 × 27 to 450 × 350 μm) oval-shaped ciliated protozoa with a characteristic four-lobed nucleus
      iii. *Amyloodinium*: can be quite large, up to 1.0 mm diameter, oval-shaped with a very dark appearance because of chloroplasts. Not usually mobile

    iv. *Uronema* and *Miamiensis*: motile, oval shaped protozoan parasites

    v. *Coccomyxa hoffmani* cartilage of the gill filaments of coral catfish (*Plotosus anguillaris*)

  b. Flukes

    i. *Gyrodactylus*: live-bearing; can usually see large H-shaped hooks of both adult and unborn young

    ii. *Dactylogyrus*: egg-layer. Usually four black spots at caudal end. Can be quite large flukes

2. Radiography
3. Routine haematology and biochemistry
4. Culture and sensitivity
5. Endoscopy
6. Biopsy
7. Ultrasonography
8. Water-quality parameters – check as a minimum: temperature, ammonia, nitrite, nitrate and pH values.

Management

- Good oxygenation of water; recommended level of oxygen is above 5.5 mg/L at 25°C, for tropical marine fish.

Treatment/specific therapy

- Ammonia toxicity
  - Partial water changes to dilute the ammonia levels
  - Longer-term control may include addition of commercially available Nitrosomonas bacterial cultures or equivalent
- Bacterial gill disease
  - Correct any underlying environmental problem
  - Chloramine-T at 5–10 mg/L
  - Appropriate antibiosis
- Fungal gill disease
  - Consider itraconazole at 1.0–5.0 mg/kg p.o. every 1–7 days, either in feed or gavage
- *Brooklynella*, *Uronema* and *Miamiensis*
  - Sensitive to proprietary formalin/malachite green and/or copper-based ectoparasitic treatments
  - Freshwater baths for larger/tougher fish
  - Covering antibiosis
- *Cryptocaryon irritans* (marine white spot)
  - Sensitive to copper-based ectoparasitic treatments (see *Nursing Care* above)
  - Formalin baths
  - Freshwater dips
- *Amyloodinium* and *Crepidoodinium*
  - Sensitive to copper-based ectoparasitic treatments (see *Nursing Care* above)
  - The encysted stage is relatively resistant to chemical attack
  - Can colonize the intestines of fish, where again it can be protected from medications

- In such cases, treat with metronidazole at 50 mg/L daily for 10 days, changing the water daily
- Antibiotic cover should be considered as secondary infections are common at the areas where the skin is damaged
- Eliminate the parasite from a show aquarium by removing all fish, reducing or cutting out the light levels and raising the temperature to 30–32°C for 3 weeks
- *Turbellaria*
  - Formalin bath at 2 mL formalin per litre for up to 1 h
  - 5 min freshwater bath daily for 5 days
- Gill flukes
  - Proprietary ectoparasitic preparations
  - *Praziquantel* at 10 mg/L for a 3 h bath, or in feed at a rate of 400 mg/100 g food daily for 7 days (but see *Neurological and Swimming Disorders*)
  - Freshwater dips 5 min daily for 5 days
  - *Dactylogyrus spp* are egg-layers; the egg stage is resistant to treatment so treatment should be repeated every 2–4 weeks depending upon temperature, for at least 3 doses
- *Coccomyxa hoffmani*
  - No treatment
- Copper toxicity
  - Multiple partial water changes
  - See also (see *Nursing Care* above)
- Neoplasia
  - Surgical debulking followed by injection of cisplatin directly into the tissue mass on a weekly basis
  - Euthanasia if inoperable.

Gastrointestinal tract disorders

Bacterial

- *Vibrio parahaemolyticus* (Oestmann 1985).

Protozoal

- *Cryptosporidium nasoris* (in tangs).

Parasitic

- Tapeworms
  - *Tetraphyllidea*
  - *Spathbothriidea*
  - *Trypanorhyncha*
  - *Pseudophyllidea*
- Nematodes
  - *Spirocamallanus*
  - *Cucullanus*
  - *Camallanus.*

Nutritional

- Inappropriate feeding.

Neoplasia

Other non-infectious problems
- Overgrowth of incisor teeth in pufferfish, parrotfish and trigger fish
- Foreign body
- Air ingestion by neonatal seahorses.

Findings on clinical examination

- Weight loss, poor growth, swollen abdomen (tapeworms)
- A cluster of worms protruding from the anus of an infested fish often accompanied by extensive damage and erosion around this area (*Spirocamallanus*). Also weight loss, failure to thrive, stringy or slimy faeces and a susceptibility to secondary infections including tail and fin rot
- Weight loss, regurgitation, undigested food in faeces and anorexia in tangs (*Cryptosporidium*)
- Chronic weight loss in pufferfish, triggerfish or parrotfish; appetite still good, difficulty feeding (incisor overgrowth)
- Haemorrhagic faeces, reddening around cloaca. Also erythematous skin lesions and boil-like lesions following septicaemia (*Vibrio parahaemolyticus*)
- Swollen coelom, lethargy (foreign body, inappropriate nutrition, neoplasia, egg retention, see *Reproductive Disorders*)
- Neonatal seahorses with gas bubbles visible in their guts; trapped floating at surface.

Investigations

1. Faecal examination
2. Anaesthetize and examine teeth/buccal cavity
3. Radiography
4. Routine haematology and biochemistry
5. Culture and sensitivity
6. Endoscopy
7. Biopsy
8. Ultrasonography
9. Water-quality parameters – check as a minimum: temperature, ammonia, nitrite, nitrate and pH values.

Treatment/specific therapy

- *Vibrio parahaemolyticus*
  - Antibiotics
  - Quarantining/removal of infected fish.
- *Cryptosporidium nasoris* – no effective treatment
- Tapeworms
  - *Praziquantel* at 10 mg/L for a 3 h bath (but see *Neurological and Swimming Disorders*)
- *Cucullanus*, *Camallanus* and *Spirocamallanus*

- Levamisole at 10 mg/L as a single dose added to the water. This is particularly good for killing larval worms. Suspend carbon filtration
- Piperazine at 2.5 mg/g of feed, added to the food. This may only kill adult worms
- Fenbendazole at 50 mg/kg body weight added to feed, or by stomach tube if the fish is large enough. Fish are quick to refuse medicated food, so it is best to starve for 24–48 h prior to offering such feed
- Camallanus has both a direct and indirect life cycle (small crustaceans, e.g. cyclops act as intermediate hosts)
- Incisor teeth overgrowth
  - Burr back under anaesthetic
  - Offer foods that increase normal wear, e.g. cockles still in shell
- Inappropriate nutrition
  - Some marine fish fed on foods designed for other fish, e.g. koi foods can develop a gastric or intestinal bloat and ileus as a result of excessive carbohydrate intake
  - Starve for 24–48 h
  - Gavage activated charcoal
  - Covering antibiosis
- Neoplasia
  - Surgical resection
- Air ingestion in neonatal seahorses
  - Neonatal seahorses are often fed on *artemia nauplii* (brine shrimp); these larvae are positively phototactic and accumulate at the surface where the light intensity is strongest. Neonatal seahorses accidentally ingest air at the surface while feeding
  - Cover the surface so as too darken it and light from below and to the side to attract the *Artemia* (and so the neonates) away from the surface
- Foreign body
  - Retrieval from stomach, possibly with aid of endoscopy
  - Coeliotomy and surgical retrieval.

Nutritional disorders

- Hypovitaminosis A
  - Suggested as a cause of head and lateral line disease in marine angelfish and tangs (see *Skin Disorders*). Provide either with a commercial vitamin A supplement or offering more vegetable foods, e.g. suchi mori seaweed wraps or lightly boiled greens
- Highly unsaturated fatty acid (HUFAs) deficiency
  - Commonly seen in captive bred marine fry, e.g. clownfish (*Amphiprion spp*) fed wholly or largely on unsupplemented brine shrimp *nauplii*. Jerky spasmic swimming and mass deaths are often triggered by external stimuli such as a loud noise or water change. Supplement with commercially available HUFA products
- Hepatic lipidosis
  - Frequently seen in large predatory species such as groupers (*Serranidae*) and lionfish (*Pterois spp*) that are overfed; often exacerbated by the feeding of freshwater fish such as goldfish which are deficient in HUFAs
  - Failure to provide appropriate foods

Note that many marine fish are specialist feeders. Those that prey primarily on coral polyps such as the exquisite butterflyfish (*Chaetodon austriacus*) or sponges (such as the rock beauty *Holocanthus tricolour*) may receive inadequate diets and fail to thrive

- Underfeeding
  - Some aquarists may deliberately underfeed to reduce the levels of metabolites in reef systems
- Overfeeding
  - In addition to hepatic lipidosis and other obesity-related problems, overfeeding can cause rapid and dangerous changes in the water quality, particularly triggering falls in the pH and KH.

Findings on clinical examination

- Weight loss
- Inappetence
- Lethargy
- Mass mortality of larvae or fry (HUFA insufficiency)
- Ulcerative lesions on the head and lateral line of marine angelfish, surgeonfish and tangs.

Investigations

1. Review species identification and husbandry
2. Radiography
3. Routine haematology and biochemistry
4. Culture and sensitivity
5. Endoscopy
6. Biopsy
7. Ultrasonography
8. Water-quality parameters – check as a minimum: temperature, ammonia, nitrite, nitrate and pH values
9. Postmortem
   a. Lack of food in stomach/intestines
   b. Loss of body fat.

Treatment/specific therapy

- Address obvious deficiencies
- Otherwise as described above.

Hepatic disorders

Bacterial
- Hepatitis.

Fungal
- Hepatitis.

Protozoal

- Myxosporideans, e.g. *Ceratomyxa, Myxidium, Leptotheca* and *Sphaeromyxa spp.*

Nutritional

- Hepatic lipidosis (see *Nutritional Disorders*).

Neoplasia

- Liver neoplasia.

Findings on clinical examination

- Weight loss
- Inappetence
- Lethargy.

Investigations

1. Radiography
2. Routine haematology and biochemistry
3. Culture and sensitivity
4. Endoscopy
5. Biopsy
   a. Histopathology
      i. *Myxosporideans* in the gall bladder. Large numbers may affect function of gall bladder
      ii. *Sphaeromyxa* spores in the gall bladder of seahorses (*Hippocampus spp*) (Vincent & Clifton-Hadley 1989)
6. Ultrasonography
7. Water-quality parameters – check as a minimum: temperature, ammonia, nitrite, nitrate and pH values.

Treatment/specific therapy

- *Myxosporideans*
  - No treatment. Usually an incidental finding
- Bacterial and fungal hepatitis
  - Treat as for similar infections in *Systemic Disorders*.

Pancreatic disorders

Viral

- Infectious pancreatic necrosis virus (see *Systemic Disorders*).

Cardiovascular and haematological disorders

Bacterial

- Endocarditis.

Protozoal

- Haemoparasites, e.g. *Trypanosoma, Trypanoplasma, Haemogrergarina spp* (see *Systemic Disorders*).

Neoplasia

- Mesothelioma (Shields & Popp 1979).

Other non-infectious problems

- Cardiomyopathy.

Findings on clinical examination

- Anaemia, abnormal swellings (*Trypanoplasma spp*)
- Lethargy
- Anorexia
- Non-specific signs of ill-health.

Investigations

1. Radiography
2. Routine haematology and biochemistry
3. Culture and sensitivity
4. Endoscopy
5. Biopsy
6. Ultrasonography
7. Water-quality parameters – check as a minimum: temperature, ammonia, nitrite, nitrate and pH values.

Treatment/specific therapy

- Haemoparasites
  - Try methylene blue by mouth at 60 mg/kg per day for 4 days
  - Metronidazole at 50 mg/kg per day
- Bacterial endocarditis
  - Likely to be diagnosed on postmortem
  - Appropriate antibiosis
- Cardiomyopathy
  - Likely to be diagnosed on postmortem.

Systemic disorders

Viral

- Infectious pancreatic necrosis virus
- Angelfish encephalitis virus (*Pomacanthus, Holocanthus* and *Centropyge spp*). See also *Neurological Disorders*.

Bacterial

- Abnormal swimming, shimmying. May also see haemorrhages, ulceration (bacteriaemia, septicaemia)
- *Mycobacteria*, esp. *M marinum*, *M. fortuitum* and *M. cheloni* (fish tuberculosis), esp. seahorses (*Hippocampus spp*). See also *Skin Disorders* and *Musculoskeletal Disorders*
- *Nocardia asteroides*
- *Renibacterium (Corynebacterium) spp.*

Fungal

- *Ichthyophonus hoferi*. See also *Skin Disorders, Neurological and Swimming Disorders* and *Ophthalmic Disorders*.

Protozoal

- Haemoparasites (see *Cardiovascular and Haematological Disorders*).

Neoplasia

Other non-infectious problems

- Sudden-onset water quality toxicity; new tank syndrome
- Pouch and systemic emphysema of male seahorses (seahorse gas bubble disease)
- Cyanide toxicity (in recently caught wild marine fish).

Findings on clinical examination

- Sudden darting movements, loss of balance, rapid respiration (poor water quality)
- Anorexia, lethargy, abdominal fluid accumulation, sudden death (infectious pancreatic necrosis virus)
- Weight loss, thickened areas of inflammation, ulceration, fin rot (*Nocardiosis, mycobacteriosis*)
- Loss of balance in male sea horses (*Hippocampus spp*) accompanied by obviously swollen brood pouch. May float at surface. Emboli may also be found subcutaneously, especially at the tail (Fig. 13.2) (seahorse gas bubble disease)
- Weakness, wasting and anaemia (haemoparasites)
- Lethargy, weight loss, excessive mucous production, loss of balance and death in marine angelfish (angelfish encephalitis virus)
- Wasting, darkening of skin colour and obvious boil-like swellings in the skin. Exophthalmia, abnormal behaviour and swimming patterns (*Ichthyophonus hoferi*)
- Swollen abdomen, ascites (*Renibacterium spp*)
- Anorexia, excessive bright colours, deaths in recently caught fish (cyanide toxicity).

Investigations

1. Radiography
2. Routine haematology and biochemistry
3. Culture and sensitivity
4. Endoscopy
5. Biopsy
6. Ultrasonography

Fig. 13.2. Seahorse with systemic emphysema affecting the tail. *Note* how the tail floats at the surface.

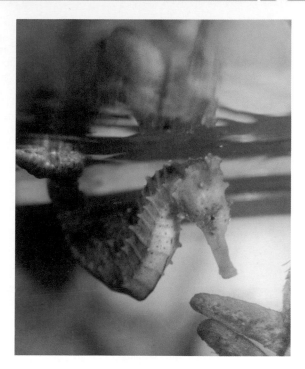

7. Assay for cyanide on postmortem
8. Water-quality parameters – check as a minimum: temperature, ammonia, nitrite, nitrate and pH values.

Treatment/specific therapy

- Water-quality problem
  - Identify and address problem
- Infectious pancreatic necrosis virus – no treatment. Supportive only
- Angelfish encephalitis virus – no treatment. Supportive only
- Bacterial disease (bacteriaemia, septicaemia)
  - Antibiotics
- Nocardiosis – see *Skin Disorders*
- *Mycobacteriosis* – see *Musculoskeletal Disorders*
- *Ichthyophonus hoferi* – no efficacious treatment available
- Haemoparasites
  - Methylene blue by mouth at 60 mg/kg per day for 4 days
  - Metronidazole at 50 mg/kg per day

- Seahorse gas bubble disease (pouch and systemic emphysema of (male) seahorses)
  - Unknown aetiology – often linked to subclinical mycobacteriosis, metabolic disturbances, and occasionally brood pouch infections
  - Gently release trapped air from brood pouch. For systemic emphysema aspirate gas from obvious gas pockets
  - Acetazolamide. Three treatment options:
    - 2–3 mg/kg i.m. every 5–7 days for up to 3 treatments
    - Flush the brood pouch with an acetazolamide solution daily for 3 days
    - 2–4 mg/L as a 24 treatment over 3 consecutive days. Perform a 100% water change between treatments
      Note that acetazolamide may temporarily affect both vision (Fairbanks et al 1974) and balance (Beier et al 2002), potentially giving rise to apparent inappetence
    - High-pressure treatment (exposing affected seahorses to great depth) has been successful in curing this condition
    - Antibiotics if appropriate
- Cyanide toxicity
  - No effective treatment – supportive therapy only.

Musculoskeletal disorders

Bacterial

- *Mycobacteria* esp. *M marinum*, *M. fortuitum* and *M. cheloni* (fish tuberculosis). See also *Skin Disorders* and *Systemic Disorders*.

Parasitic

- Tapeworms (see *Gastrointestinal Tract Disorders*).

Neoplasia

Other non-infectious problems

- Electrocution (Pasnik et al 2003).

Findings on clinical examination

- Spinal curvature, ulceration, weight loss (mycobacteriosis, electrocution)
- Chronic weight loss, skin ulceration (mycobacteriosis)
- Weight loss (mycobacteriosis, tapeworms)
- Sudden multiple mortalities (electrocution).

Investigations

1. Check electrical equipment for faults
2. Radiography
   a. Vertebral fractures (electric shock)
3. Routine haematology and biochemistry
4. Culture and sensitivity

5. Endoscopy
6. Biopsy
7. Ultrasonography
8. Water-quality parameters – check as a minimum: temperature, ammonia, nitrite, nitrate and pH values.

Treatment/specific therapy

- Mycobacteriosis
  - Antibiotic treatment not very effective
  - Kanamycin at 50 mg/L every 48 h for 4 treatments was successful in guppies (Conroy & Conroy 1999)
  - Consider euthanasia, especially because of zoonotic risk
- Electrocution
  - No specific treatment.

Neurological and swimming disorders

Viral

- Angelfish encephalitis rhabdovirus (*Pomacanthus, Holocanthus* and *Centropyge spp*) See also *Systemic Disorders*.

Bacterial

- Central nervous system infection/granuloma
- *Eubacterium tarantellus.*

Fungal

- *Ichthyophonus hoferi.* See also *Skin Disorders, Ophthalmic Disorders* and *Systemic Disorders*
- Central nervous system infection/granuloma.

Protozoal

- *Septemcapsula plotosi* (*Myxosporidea*) in coral catfish (*Plotosus anguillaris*).

Nutritional

- HUFAs deficiency. See *Nutritional Disorders*.

Neoplasia

Other non-infectious problems

- Sudden onset water quality problem; new tank syndrome
  - Ammonia toxicity (see also *Respiratory Tract Disorders*)
- Abnormal swimbladder functioning secondary to compression from internal space-occupying lesions, e.g. neoplasia
- Swimbladder torsion
- Praziquantel toxicity
- Nicotine toxicity
- Heavy metal poisoning.

Findings on clinical examination

- Sudden darting movements, loss of balance, rapid respiration (water-quality problem)
- Lethargy, weight loss, excessive mucous production, loss of balance and death in marine angelfish (angelfish encephalitis virus)
- Abnormal behaviour and swimming patterns (*Ichthyophonus*). Also wasting, darkening of skin colour and obvious boil-like swellings in the skin. Exophthalmia (*Ichthyophonus hoferi*)
- Spasmic, jerky swimming movements accompanied by sudden mass deaths in captive-bred marine fish, e.g. clownfish fed wholely or largely on brine shrimp *nauplii* (ω-3-fatty acid deficiency)
- Whirling behaviour, death in coral catfish (*Septemcapsula*)
- Stiffened pectoral fins, muscular spasms (nicotine toxicity).

Investigations

1. Radiography
2. Routine haematology and biochemistry
3. Culture and sensitivity
4. Endoscopy
5. Biopsy
6. Ultrasonography
7. Water-quality parameters – check as a minimum: temperature, ammonia, nitrite, nitrate and pH values.

Treatment/specific therapy

- Water-quality problem
  - Identify and address problem
  - Ammonia toxicity
    - Partial water changes to dilute the ammonia levels
    - Longer-term control may include addition of commercially available *Nitrosomonas* bacterial cultures or equivalent
- Angelfish encephalitis rhabdovirus – no treatment. Supportive only
- *Ichthyophonus hoferi* – no efficacious treatment available
- Swimbladder torsion
  - Surgical correction
- Central nervous system infection/granuloma
  - Attempt antibiotic or antimycotic treatment. Poor prognosis
- *Eubacterium tarantellus*
  - Antibiotic therapy
- *Septemcapsula plotosi*
  - No effective treatment
- Praziquantel toxicity
  - Terminate treatment
- Nicotine toxicity
  - No direct treatment. Situate air pumps away from smoky atmospheres
- Heavy metal poisoning
  - Partial water changes
  - Remove possible sources, e.g. piping, equipment not designed for marine aquaria, e.g. central heating pumps.

Ophthalmic disorders

Bacterial

- Bacterial granuloma
- Uveitis.

Fungal

- Fungal granuloma
- *Ichthyophonus hoferi.* See also *Skin Disorders, Neurological and Swimming Disorders* and *Systemic Disorders*
- Uveitis.

Protozoal

- *Cryptocaryon*
- *Henneguya.*

Nutritional

- Lipid keratopathy (in green moray eels, see Greenwell & Vainisi 1994)
- Riboflavin deficiency
- Ascorbic acid deficiency
- Hypovitaminosis A.

Neoplasia

- Thyroid neoplasia
- Lymphoma.

Other non-infectious problems

- Blindness secondary to exposure to excessive bright light in nocturnal species, especially lionfish *(Pterois* and *Dendrochirus spp)*
- Gas bubble disease (see also *Skin Disorders, Reproductive Disorders* and *Systemic Disorders)*
- Trauma (Carrillo et al 1999)
- Cardiomyopathy.

Findings on clinical examination

- Blindness (may present as inability to locate food in predatory species)
- Cataracts
- Exophthalmus
- Exophthalmia accompanied by wasting, darkening of skin colour and obvious boil-like swellings in the skin. Abnormal behaviour and swimming patterns if the central nervous system is invaded *(Ichthyophonus)*
- Glaucoma (usually secondary to intraocular disease)
- Gas bubbles around and behind eye (gas bubble disease).

Investigations

1. Ophthalmic examination (under sedation/GA)
2. Radiography
3. Routine haematology and biochemistry

4. Culture and sensitivity
5. Endoscopy
6. Biopsy
7. Ultrasonography
8. Water-quality parameters – check as a minimum: temperature, ammonia, nitrite, nitrate and pH values.

Treatment/specific therapy

- Bacterial or fungal uveitis
  - Appropriate antibiosis
  - Enucleation
- Gas bubble disease
  - If only eyes affected (frequently in seahorses) consider acetazolamide:
    - 2–3 mg/kg i.m. every 5–7 days for up to 3 treatments.
    - 2–4 mg/L as a 24 treatment over 3 consecutive days. Perform a 100% water change between treatments
      Note that acetazolamide may temporarily affect vision, giving rise to apparent inappetence
  - Species other than seahorses – likely to be connected to supersaturation of water, see *Skin Disorders*
- Blindness secondary to excessive exposure to bright light
  - Reduce lighting levels
  - Supplement with vitamin A
- *Ichthyophonus hoferi*
  - No efficacious treatment available
- Glaucoma
  - Enucleation
- Lipid keratopathy
  - Keratoplasty (see Greenwell & Vainisi 1994).

Endocrine disorders

Neoplasia
- Thyroid adenoma
- Thyroid adenocarcinoma (Blasiola et al 1981).

Other non-infectious problems
- Goitre (hypothyroidism) in marine elasmobranchs.

Findings on clinical examination

- Swelling in the thyroid region (especially visible in sharks and rays).

Investigations

1. Radiography
2. Routine haematology and biochemistry
   a. Blood thyroid levels (Table 13.4)

Table 13.4 Blood thyroid levels

Species	Total T4 (µg/dL)
Dusky shark (*Carcharinus obscurus*)	4.5
Scalloped hammerhead shark (*Sphyrna lewini*)	2.9
Sharpnose shark (*Scoliodon terraenovae*)	2.9

Adapted from Stoskopf (1993).

3. Culture and sensitivity
4. Endoscopy
5. Biopsy
6. Ultrasonography
7. Water-quality parameters
   a. Check as a minimum: temperature, ammonia, nitrite, nitrate and pH values.
   b. High nitrate levels antagonize iodine uptake.

Treatment/specific therapy

- Goitre
  - Supplement with dietary iodine at 20 µg/kg p.o. or every 48 h i.m.
  - Reduce nitrate levels to below 40 mg/L, preferably below 10 mg/L
- Thyroid adenoma
  - May require surgery but likely to be technically very difficult.

Urinary disorders

Bacterial

- *Renibacterium spp* (*Corynebacterium*).

Fungal

Protozoal

- *Myxosporidea.*

Neoplasia

Other non-infectious problems

Findings on clinical examination

- Swollen body, ascites (*Renibacterium spp*)
- Non-specific signs of ill health including anorexia and lethargy.

Investigations

1. Radiography
2. Routine haematology and biochemistry

3. Culture and sensitivity
4. Endoscopy
5. Biopsy
6. Ultrasonography
7. Water-quality parameters – check as a minimum: temperature, ammonia, nitrite, nitrate and pH values.

Treatment/specific therapy

- *Renibacterium*
  - Appropriate antibiosis
  - Reduce salinity to 1.020 to reduce osmotic stress
- *Myxosporidea*
  - No effective treatment, but see *Skin Disorders*.

Reproductive disorders

See *Reproductive Disorders* in *Goldfish and Koi* and *Tropical Freshwater Fish*.

Non-infectious problems

- Pouch emphysema of seahorses – see *Systemic Disorders*.
- Egg retention – see *Reproductive Disorders* in *Goldfish and Koi* (Ch. 11) and *Tropical Freshwater Fish* (Ch. 12).

References

Beier M, Anken R H, Rahmann H 2002 Susceptibility to abnormal (kinetotic) swimming fish correlates with inner ear carbonic anhydrase-reactivity. Neurosci Lett 335(1):17–20

Blasiola G C, Turnier J C, Hurst E E 1981 Metastatic thyroid adenocarcinomas in a captive population of kelp bass, Paralabrax clanthatus. J Nat Cancer Inst 66:51–59

Bullard S A, Frasca S Jr, Benz G W 2000 Skin lesions caused by Dermophthirius penneri (Monogenea Microbothriidae) on wild-caught blacktip sharks (Carcharinus limbatus). J Parasitol 86(3):618–622

Carrillo J, Martinez J, Divanach P et al 1999 Unilateral eye abnormalities in reared Mediterranean gilthead sea bream. Vet Rec 145:494–487

Conroy G, Conroy D A 1999 Acid-fast bacterial infection and its control in guppies (Lebistes reticulatus) reared on an ornamental fish farm in Venezuela. Vet Rec 144:177–178

Fairbanks M B, Hoffert J R, Fromm P O 1974 Short circuiting of the ocular oxygen concentrating mechanism in the Teleost Salmo gairdneri using carbonic anhydrase inhibitors. J Gen Physiol 64:263–273

Greenwell M G, Vainisi S J 1994 Surgical management of lipid keratopathy in green moray eels (Gynothorax funebris). Proc Am Assoc Zoo Vet 179–181

Oestmann D J 1985 Environmental and disease problems in ornamental marine aquariums. Comp Cont Ed Pract Vet 7(8):656–667

Pasnik D J, Smith S A, Wolf J C 2003 Accidental electroshock of fish in a recirculation facility. Vet Rec 153:562–564

Shields R P, Popp J A 1979 Intracardial mesotheliomas and a gastric papilloma in a giant grouper, Epinephelus itajara. Vet Pathol 16:191–198

Stoskopf M K 1993 Clinical pathology of sharks, skates and rays. Fish medicine. Saunders, Philadelphia

Varner P W, Lewis D H 1991 Characterization of a virus associated with head and lateral line erosion syndrome in marine angelfish. J Aquat Health 3:198–205

Vincent A C J, Clifton-Hadley R S 1989 Parasitic infection of the seahorse (Hippocampus erectus). A case report. J Wildl Dis 25(3):404–406

Index

G

yellow fungus disease, bearded dragons 275, 277
yellow skin, bearded dragons 275
yellow urates
  lizards 289
  parrots and related species 202, 219
  tortoises and turtles 400
Yersinia 156, 214, 217
  Y. pestis 146
  Y. pseudotuberculosis 109, 121, 153, 213, 221,
      251, 252, 259, 262
yersiniosis
  hystricomorphs 122, 123
  songbirds and softbills 253, 263

Z

zidovudine, snakes 348
zinc toxicity

amphibians 426, 429
parrots and related species 194, *195*, 207, 211,
    232, 233, 238
songbirds and softbills 250, 255, 256
tortoises and turtles 389
zolazepam toxicity, rabbits 86
zoonosis
  amphibians 424, 427
  ferrets 11, 15, 26
  hystricomorphs 124
  lizards 287, 291, 297, 305
  parrots and related species 192, 204
  small rodents 147, 148, 161, 169
  snakes 334, 342, 347
  songbirds and softbills 253, 256, 260
  tortoises and turtles 390
  tropical freshwater fish 493, 494
Zygomycete 341